LIPOPROTEIN LIPASE

edited by

Jayme Borensztajn
Department of Pathology
Northwestern University Medical School
Chicago, Illinois

Evener Publishers, Inc.
Chicago

EVENER PUBLISHERS
227 East Ontario Street, P.O. Box 11379
Chicago, Illinois 60611

Library of Congress Catalog Card Number 86-82837

ISBN 0-940327-24-4

Printed in the United States of America

Dedicated to the memory of

Esko A. Nikkilä, M.D.

CONTRIBUTORS

GREGORY J. BAGBY
Department of Physiology
Louisiana State University Medical Center
New Orleans, LA 70112

GUNILLA BENGTSSON-OLIVECRONA
Department of Physiological Chemistry
University of Umea
Umea, Sweden

JAYME BORENSZTAJN
Department of Pathology
Northwestern University Medical School
Chicago, IL 60611

SIDNEY S. CHERNICK
Endocrinology Section
Laboratory of Cellular and Developmental Biology
National Institutes of Health
Bethesda, MD 20892

ANTHONY CRYER
Department of Biochemistry
University College
Cardiff, CF1, 1XL
Wales, United Kingdom

ROBERT H. ECKEL
Division of Endocrinology
University of Colorado Health Sciences Center
Denver, CO 80262

ESKO A. NIKKILÄ (Deceased)
Third Department of Medicine
University of Helsinki
Helsinki, Finland

PETER NILSSON-EHLE
Department of Clinical Chemistry
University of Lund
Lund, Sweden

THOMAS OLIVECRONA
Department of Physiological Chemistry
University of Umea
Umea, Sweden

PATRICIA A. O'LOONEY
The George Washington University
Department of Biochemistry
School of Medicine and Health Sciences
Washington, D.C. 20037

PHILLIP H. PEKALA
Department of Biochemistry
East Carolina University School of Medicine
Greenville, NC 27834

DONALD S. ROBINSON
Department of Biochemistry
University of Leeds
Leeds LS2 9JT
United Kingdom

ROBERT O. SCOW
Endocrinology Section
Laboratory of Cellular and Developmental Biology
National Institutes of Health
Bethesda, MD 20892

MARJA-RIITTA TASKINEN
Second Department of Medicine
University of Helsinki
Helsinki, Finland

GEORGE V. VAHOUNY (Deceased)
The George Washington University
Department of Biochemistry
School of Medicine and Health Sciences
Washington, D.C. 20037

CONTENTS

PREFACE

During the past three decades lipoprotein lipase has emerged as one of the most important enzymes involved in the metabolism of plasma lipoproteins. This importance is reflected in the increasingly greater number of publications aimed at elucidating the properties and structure of the enzyme, its physiological functions and its involvement in the pathogenesis of lipid-associated disorders. Several reviews—some authored by contributors to this book— have been published in the past several years in an effort to summarize the existing knowledge on lipoprotein lipase. However, because of the extensive literature available, most of these reviews have been limited to the detailed examination of only certain aspects of the enzyme. In this monograph, all aspects of work carried out to date on lipoprotein lipase are reviewed in detail by several investigators, each from different perspectives in his/her area of interest. The result of this collaborative effort constitutes the first comprehensive text on lipoprotein lipase intended to serve as a major source of reference to investigators interested in this enzyme and its functions in normal and pathological conditions.

I should like to acknowledge the invaluable contributions made by Jerold L. Kellman, Barbara Ferencz, Mary Ann Moore, and last, but not least, my wife Anne in the publication of this book.

J.B.

Chapter 1

LIPOPROTEIN LIPASE— PAST, PRESENT AND FUTURE

Donald S. Robinson

In 1943 *Science* published a brief note by Dr. Paul Hahn in which he reported as follows: 'During the course of determining red cell circulating mass in dogs by the donor-isotope red cell procedure, an occasional animal of irregular eating habits showed a marked lipaemia in the initial control blood sample. When injected with whole blood containing tagged cells, in the instances in which heparin was used as an anticoagulant, this lipaemia had completely disappeared in the blood sample taken three to five minutes later'.* Later in the same publication he noted: 'It was finally found that the same amount of heparin as used in the earlier experiments when dissolved in saline and given by vein would in itself abolish the lipaemia' and 'Addition of 5 mg of heparin to 5 ml of lipaemic plasma *in vitro* with mixing showed no reaction on standing'(1). This was the first description of the 'clearing reaction' (as it came to be called) whereby the alimentary lipemia, which is normally associated with the absorption of a fatty meal in most animal species, is rapidly cleared when heparin is injected intravenously.

Little notice was taken of Hahn's study until 1950, when Anderson and Fawcett (2) suggested that the injection of heparin caused the release of a 'clearing factor' into the blood from the tissues. Although Anderson and Fawcett thought that the factor was a surface-active agent and that clearing was a physical phenomenon, Anfinsen, Boyle and Brown in 1952 published convincing evidence that the reaction was in fact an enzymic one (3). My personal involvement began about this time** and, in 1953, a group of

---

**When Anfinsen, Boyle and Brown were carrying out the studies on which their 1952 paper was based in the National Heart Institute of the National Institutes of Health in Bethesda, Washington, D.C., I was working as a postdoctoral fellow on an entirely different project in the nearby National Cancer Institute with the late Jesse P. Greenstein. Oddly enough, I had just accepted a post back in England with the late Lord (then Sir Howard) Florey to work on the self-same 'clearing factor' in the Sir William Dunn School of Pathology in Oxford. Florey's work on penicillin was almost complete and he had decided

papers was published (one of them by the late John French and myself) that together established the factor as a lipase which produced its 'clearing reaction' through hydrolysis of the chylomicron triglycerides present in lipemic blood (4–7). The unesterified fatty acids that were produced formed water-soluble complexes with the plasma albumin so that the lipemia caused by the water-insoluble chylomicrons disappeared as lipolysis took place.

In 1955, Korn showed that a lipase, with many of the properties of the 'clearing factor lipase' present in the plasma after the intravenous injection of heparin, was also to be found in extracts of delipidated preparations of a number of extrahepatic tissues, including heart and adipose tissue (8–10). The finding clearly supported Anderson and Fawcett's earlier suggestion that the enzyme was released into the blood from a site in the tissues. However, although Korn's preparations rapidly broke down chylomicron triglycerides, they were found to have only a very limited ability to hydrolyse the triglycerides of artificial lipid emulsions, except in the presence of added plasma high density lipoproteins. This observation was eventually accounted for by the identification of the CII apoprotein, present in both plasma cylomicrons and high density lipoproteins, as an essential co-factor for the action of the lipase on its triglyceride substrate (11–13). More immediately, however, it led Korn to identify his tissue enzyme as a 'lipoprotein lipase'. The name is not ideal, since it does not indicate the origin of the enzyme or its particular lipoprotein substrates, and could equally well be applied to a second lipase that is now known to be released from the liver after heparin injection. Although this second lipase does not require an apoprotein co-factor, it also has lipoprotein lipid, either triglyceride or phospholipid, as its physiological substrate (14). Nevertheless, the term was rapidly accepted, particularly in the United States, and although 'clearing factor lipase' persisted as an alternative in Europe for several years thereafter, its use has now been virtually abandoned.

Probably no more than twenty people world-wide were directly involved in work on lipoprotcin lipase at the time of Korn's study. However, mainly through the pioneering investigations of Gofman and his colleagues (15,16), a substantially larger number were concerned with the positive link between

---

to establish a small research group to carry out basic work in the atherosclerosis field because, as he somewhat grandly wrote at the time, 'now that the infectious diseases are under control, it is time that the degenerative diseases were tackled'. He had been particularly impressed by the work of Gofman and his colleagues (15,16) suggesting a direct relationship between the concentrations of particular plasma lipoprotein classes and atherosclerosis and showing that heparin injection drastically altered the plasma lipoprotein distribution. He speculated that heparin's effect on the plasma lipoprotein pattern might be related to its release of the 'clearing factor', and decided therefore that some studies on this last would be of interest. Hence, when he learnt of my proximity to Anfinsen and his colleagues, he encouraged me to spend a few days with them. This I promptly did and, thereby, established links that extended over many years with colleagues such as Frederickson, Bragdon, Gordon, Havel and Korn, who all joined Anfinsen's group at the National Heart Institute at, or shortly after, that time.

the plasma concentrations of particular plasma lipids and lipoproteins and the incidence of ischaemic heart disease. Indeed, such was the interest in this topic that a conference entitled 'The Blood Lipids and the Clearing Factor' was organized in Brussels in 1956. In retrospect, this meeting can be seen as the occasion when lipoprotein lipase finally established itself. Thus, the view that the 'clearing reaction' was due to an enzyme which was able to hydrolyse chylomicron triglycerides in the bloodstream was by no means generally accepted at the time, the alternative notion being that it essentially represented a physical dispersion or dissolution of chemically-unaltered particulate lipid. From the report of the conference discussions (17), however, it is evident that, without any experimental evidence to support it, a physical explanation for the phenomenon was rejected at the meeting and, indeed, it was never seriously considered thereafter.

Nevertheless, because lipoprotein lipase was only present in the blood at a significant level under the special circumstances created by the injection of heparin intravenously, the physiological role of the enzyme and its normal site of action remained uncertain (18). Answers to these questions, in fact, required the coming together of several distinct lines of evidence. One was the discovery by Havel and Gordon of lipoprotein lipase-deficient states in man that were associated with dramatic increases in the plasma concentrations of chylomicron triglycerides (19). Another derived from work by Borgstrom and Jordan (20) and by Olivecrona (21) using chylomicrons in which the glycerol and the fatty acid moieties of the triglycerides were labelled with ^{14}C and with ^{3}H respectively. When these were injected intravenously in rats, the $^{14}C/^{3}H$ ratios of the radio-labelled triglycerides that appeared a short time thereafter in white adipose tissue and in heart were much lower than those of the injected double-labelled triglycerides, indicating that lipolysis and subsequent triglyceride resynthesis had occurred before the lipid was deposited. The third related to the very rapid appearance of the enzyme in the blood, not only after heparin injection (22), but also following the injection of dextran sulphates of high molecular weight which could not be expected to escape readily from the circulation in the extrahepatic tissues (23).

Taken together, these findings led, first, to the suggestion that lipoprotein lipase was normally located at the luminal surfaces of the capillary endothelial cells of the extrahepatic tissues where it acted on the triglycerides of the plasma chylomicrons and very low density lipoproteins and, second, to the further proposal that hydrolysis at this site was necessary for the rapid transport of the constituent fatty acids of the chylomicron and very low density lipoprotein triglycerides out of the blood and into the tissues (24–26). It was suggested that the enzyme was anchored at the endothelial cell surface by ionic linkage to heparin-like molecules associated with the cell plasma membrane, and that its release into the blood following heparin injection depended on competition for the enzyme between injected and endogenous glycosaminoglycans (27).

The essential role of lipoprotein lipase in facilitating triglyceride fatty acid removal from the bloodstream has, of course, now been amply confirmed by studies in experimental animals showing that the injection of antibodies to the enzyme causes a marked rise in the plasma triglyceride concentration and, at the same time, prevents the uptake of chylomicron triglyceride fatty acids by the tissues (28,29). It has also been found that elevations of plasma triglyceride levels occur, not only in association with a familial deficiency of lipoprotein lipase, but also in individuals with genetic deficiencies of the CII lipoprotein apoprotein that mediates the action of the enzyme on its physiological substrates (30,31). Electron microscope studies have, in their turn, supported the proposal that the enzyme normally acts at the capillary endothelial cell surface by showing that chylomicrons are sequestered at this site in tissues rich in lipoprotein lipase, presumably as a result of their association with the enzyme (32,33); while the view that the enzyme is itself anchored to the cell surface through its association with heparin-like molecules has been established on a sound experimental basis by extensive work on the interactions of lipoprotein lipase with sulphated glycosaminoglycans *in vitro,* particularly by Olivecrona and Bengtsson (34,35). Heparan sulphate is the likely endogenous species involved.

Recognition of the essential role of lipoprotein lipase in facilitating the removal of triglyceride fatty acids from the bloodstream was soon followed by evidence that the activity of the enzyme in a particular tissue could change with alterations in the physiological state. The first example to be reported was a fall in the lipoprotein lipase activity of white adipose tissue on starvation and its rise again on refeeding (36–38). Then came the observation of reciprocal activity changes in muscle and in adipose tissue—for example, on starvation, during exercise, and in the diabetic (39–42)—and, most dramatically, the discovery in 1963 of a massive rise in the activity of the enzyme in the mammary gland at parturition that coincided with the beginning of plasma triglyceride fatty acid uptake by the gland (43–45). The significance of such tissue-specific changes in lipoprotein lipase activity was rapidly appreciated, and the general proposition was advanced that the enzyme not only facilitates triglyceride removal from the circulation, but also directs it, so that the uptake of triglyceride fatty acids by particular tissues occurs according to their needs (27).

During the 1960's, a number of studies began into the mechanisms whereby such tissue-specific changes in lipoprotein lipase activity might be achieved, particular attention being focused on the possibilities for hormonal control of the enzyme's activity. Such work had, however, soon to take account of an important observation by Rodbell in 1964 who, in the course of work that is mainly remembered now for its introduction of the use of collagenase to disrupt intact adipose tissue, found that lipoprotein lipase was associated with the fat cell component of that tissue (46). The presence of the enzyme at a site other than the endothelial cell surface led to the conclusion that, in adipose tissue at least, the enzyme must first be synthesized within the fat cell and then secreted and transported to its functional site in the capillary bed (47,48). It was quickly recognized that control of the enzyme's activity could be exercised at a number of points in this sequence of events.

Work that has been carried out since 1970, including studies with a variety of isolated cell preparations, has amply supported the general concept of lipoprotein lipase synthesis within the parenchymal cells of a tissue, followed by release and transport within the tissue to the luminal surfaces of the capillary endothelial cells (49,50)* Hormonal control of the enzyme's activity has also been demonstrated in a variety of tissues (50) and direct effects of insulin and glucocorticoids on the synthesis, and of adrenaline on both the synthesis and the degradation, of the enzyme have recently been observed during incubations of adipose tissue *in vitro* (51—54). However, the precise mechanisms of action of individual hormones and their overall physiological significance, as well as the way in which the tissue-specific effects are achieved, remain in large part unknown (*see below*).

For many years, studies on the interactions of lipoprotein lipase at a molecular level lagged behind work on the control of the enzyme's activity because of the enzyme's instability, its tendency to form aggregates in solution, and, most particularly, through the lack of a straightforward procedure for its purification. However, during the 1970's glycerol and detergents were introduced, variously to stabilize the enzyme, to solubilize it, and to maintain it in an unaggregated state (55—58). Moreover, in 1971 an important fractionation procedure was introduced by Olivecrona and his colleagues, based on the ionic binding of the enzyme to heparin-agarose and elution of the bound enzyme at sodium chloride concentrations above 1M (59).

The method was first applied by Egelrud and Olivecrona to the purification of lipoprotein lipase from bovine milk (60), and purifications from a variety of tissues in a number of species have since been reported (see 61,62). Purification of the enzymc from post-heparin plasma initially proved more difficult because of the presence therein of antithrombin and of the distinct lipase that is released into the blood from the liver following heparin injection (*see above*). Both of these proteins also bind ionically to heparin and methods therefore had to be devised to exploit differences in the relative binding affinities. The problems have now been overcome (58,63,64), and both tissue and plasma enzyme can be readily prepared in high purity and yield. The availability of the tissue enzyme in particular in a highly-purified

*There are exceptions to the general rule. Thus, the enzyme is present in the milk of many species (35) and its is also synthesized and secreted by macrophages in culture (90,91). In both these cases there is no self-evident binding to endothelial cells; but also, as yet, no clear physiological function. Again it has been suggested that the enzyme may, in particular situations, be active on stored triglycerides within the parenchymal cells in which it is synthesized. However, such proposals have not received wide support.

form has undoubtedly acted as a tremendous stimulus to molecular studies. Thus, in addition to the enzyme's association with its substrate at the active site, distinct domains have been shown to be involved in its binding at the lipid interface, and in its interactions with lipoprotein apoproteins, with heparin (and similar polyanions), and with fatty acids and detergents. Specific proposals have been advanced for the binding of the active dimeric form of the enzyme, both to its lipid substrate and to heparan sulphate at the endothelial cell surface, and a much fuller understanding generally of the major kinetic features of the enzyme's activity has been achieved (see 35,61,62).

The Future

The various contributions to the present text amply demonstrate the very considerable understanding of the properties, the actions, and the significance of lipoprotein lipase which we now possess. Nevertheless, major questions remain for the future. For example:

a) *Do different tissues contain identical or distinct molecular forms of lipoprotein lipase?* Some workers have reported differences in molecular weight (see 49,61), in kinetic properties (65), and in thermolability (66) between the enzyme in adipose tissue and in heart muscle, but there is also evidence to the contrary and the case remains unproven (67). The issue is an important one that needs to be settled. Thus, the various tissue-specific changes in the enzyme's activity that have been described could be accounted for by the presence in different tissues of distinct structural genes producing distinct molecular forms of the enzyme. Alternatively, they could be explained in terms of transcriptional, translational, or post-translational control of the activity of a single enzyme form which could operate to different extents in different tissues—for example, through variations from one tissue to another in hormone receptor number or function.

b) *How is lipoprotein lipase transferred from its site of synthesis to its functional site?* The general assumption with respect to the initial stages of the transport of lipoprotein lipase following its synthesis in the parenchymal cell, is that the enzyme moves directionally within a variety of closed membrane structures from the cisternae of the endoplasmic reticulum through the Golgi complex to the cell plasma membrane. Many details of both the biochemistry and the cell biology of this transport process remain to be clarified, however.

For example, lipoprotein lipase is a glycosylated protein and recent studies have shown that, when glycosylation is inhibited, the enzyme continues to be synthesized but in an inactive form (68, see also 69,70). While this clearly suggests that its activity is dependent on its glycosylation, it is not known whether the activation occurs cotranslationally—that is, during core glycosylation—or, as earlier work would suggest (71–73), post-translationally during remodelling of the polysaccharide moiety of the enzyme as it passes through the Golgi complex. Again, the intracellular transport pathway for lipoprotein lipase within the parenchymal cell presumably ends *in vivo* with the fusion of exocytotic vesicles containing the enzyme with the plasma membrane. However, it has recently been shown that a substantial proportion of the enzyme that is synthesized during incubations of adipose tissue *in vitro* is rapidly degraded again (74). Rapid degradation also occurs when preadipocytes are cultured under conditions where the enzyme is not released into the culture medium (70). In the light of these findings, the possibility that degradation within the parenchymal cell may be an alternative to release from it, is one that needs to be investigated further (*see below*).

Considerable uncertainty also surrounds the final stages of the transport process—namely the movement of the enzyme to the luminal surface of the capillary endothelial cell. On one view, the enzyme is secreted from the parenchymal cell into the extracellular fluid and is then bound by heparan sulphate residues on the surface of adjacent endothelial cells. In support of this are the results of a number of studies showing that lipoprotein lipase in solution associates with endothelial cells in a specific, saturable fashion (75—77). However, the enzyme could also be transferred directly from the parenchymal to the endothelial cell. Thus, if it were to be already bound to the inner surfaces of the membranes of exocytotic vesicles within the parenchymal cells, it would, following exocytosis, appear on the outside of the plasma membranes thereof. Transfer to the endothelial cell surface could then occur without prior secretion into the medium. The fact that the enzyme is not spontaneously released into the medium when preadipocytes are cultured *in vitro* (70) is consistent with this possibility.

Whatever the precise mechanism of the transfer from the parenchymal cell to the endothelial cell may be, it will presumably result in the enzyme being bound initially at a site on the endothelial cell's plasma membrane that is facing the parenchymal cell. It will still not be able to express its activity, however, since it will not have access to the chylomicron and very low density lipoprotein triglycerides in the plasma. In order to gain such access, it will have to move to the luminal surface of the endothelial cell. Whether such movement occurs in the plane of the plasma membrane, or whether the enzyme is carried across the endothelial cell within membrane-bound vesicles, is also completely unknown.

c) *How is lipoprotein lipase activity regulated?* The specific action of insulin and glucocorticoids in promoting lipoprotein lipase synthesis in adipose tissue *in vitro* (51—53) suggests that transcriptional or translational control by these and other hormones could be of major importance in regulating the enzyme's activity *in vivo*. However, the promptness of response, in terms of a change in functional activity, to an alteration in the enzyme's rate of synthesis will depend on both the time of transit from the endoplasmic reticulum of the parenchymal cell to the luminal surface of the endothelial cell, and the half-life of the enzyme in the tissue. While the latter appears to be of the order of only 1 to 2 hours *in vivo* (67,78), the former remains difficult to estimate on present evidence.

Hormonal effects exerted at a stage subsequent to the enzyme's synthesis would be more rapidly effective in changing the activity at the endothelial cell surface. We have, therefore, been particularly intrigued to find that the progressive and rapid decline in lipoprotein lipase activity which occurs when adipose tissue is incubated in the presence of adrenaline *in vitro* is accompanied not only by a fall in the rate of synthesis of the enzyme, but also by a further substantial increase in the rate of its degradation (54). We do not yet know whether similar effects of adrenaline are observable *in vivo;* nor do we know whether the enhanced degradation occurs before or after the release of lipoprotein lipase from the adipocyte. However, there is already convincing evidence that the effects of adrenaline on the enzyme's activity are mediated by cyclic AMP (47,79), even though they do not seem to involve the direct protein kinase-mediated phosphorylation of the enzyme protein (80). The possibility of a protein kinase-dependent increase in the rate of the enzyme's degradation needs to be considered, therefore. It could, of course, be either direct or indirect—perhaps even mediated via a change in the intracellular free fatty acid concentration, as first proposed several years ago (81).

Additional possibilities for indirect control of the enzyme's activity through effects on its degradation can also be envisaged. For example, if the transfer of lipoprotein lipase from the parenchymal cell to the endothelial cell does indeed depend on the availability of suitable enzyme binding sites on the plasma membrane of the endothelial cell, then, if these were limiting, there could be an increase in the extent of endocytosis and lysosomal breakdown of the enzyme by the parenchymal cell (82). Again, it has been known for many years that there is a release of lipoprotein lipase into the blood from the luminal surfaces of the endothelial cells *in vivo* (27). Moreover, much of the released enzyme is taken up and degraded in the liver and this process may, therefore, contribute significantly to the overall rate of turnover of the enzyme (83,84). Since the release into the blood is probably accounted for by the ability of chylomicrons and very low density lipoproteins to combine with the enzyme in competition with heparan sulphate binding sites on the endothelial cells, the loss of enzyme from the endothelial cell surface is likely to vary with the plasma triglyceride concentration (83,84). Thus, changes in the functional activity could ultimately occur through either dietary or hormonal effects on the rate of influx of triglycerides into the bloodstream.

Finally, there are several ways whereby the expressed activity of lipoprotein lipase could alter even without a change in the concentration of enzyme at the endothelial cell surface (49,50,61,62). For example, whereas the CII apoprotein is essential for optimal activity of the enzyme on its triglyceride substrates, other lipoprotein apoproteins appear to inhibit that activity. Alterations in the apoprotein composition of the lipoproteins could therefore affect the rate of plasma triglyceride hydrolysis. Again, changes in the relative proportions of cholesterol ester and of triglyceride in the core of a plasma lipoprotein could substantially alter its suitability as a substrate. It has also been argued that, if different molecular species of the enzyme with different kinetic properties exist, their particular tissue distribution *in vivo* could influence the sites of uptake of the plasma triglyceride fatty acids. Alternatively, it has been suggested that, if the proportions of active dimer and inactive monomer forms of the enzyme differed from one tissue to another and from one physiological situation to another, this could have a similar controlling effect on the tissue sites of removal. Clearly, it will be a substantial future challenge to determine the true significance *in vivo* of such a variety of potential regulatory factors.

d) *What is the pathological significance of disturbed lipoprotein lipase function?* Our knowledge of the cellular and molecular biology of lipoprotein lipase seems likely to increase dramatically in the near future through application of the techniques of cellular immunology and genetic analysis. Such work, and further intensive investigation of the hormonal regulation of the enzyme, can be fully justified simply in terms of its central physiological role in controlling the tissue distribution of the plasma triglyceride fatty acids. However, there is also the possibility that abnormalities in the enzyme's function could have significant implications in relation to the development of a variety of disease states in man. For example, there is evidence that increased adipose tissue lipoprotein lipase activity may characterize the obese state, at least in some experimental situations (85). Again, the enzyme's action in hydrolysing chylomicron and very low density lipoprotein triglycerides leads, through a complex pattern of cholesterol, phospholipid and apoprotein transfers, to the formation of remnant and intermediate density lipoproteins and, eventually, of low density lipoproteins that serve to regulate the supply of cholesterol both to the hepatic and extrahepatic tissues (see 86). The sequence of events also involves the plasma high density lipoproteins, both as a reservoir of the enzyme's CII apoprotein co-factor and as an acceptor of lipids and of apoproteins released during the breakdown of the triglyceride-rich lipoprotein substrates of the enzyme (see 87). Changes in the enzyme's activity due to genetic, hormonal or dietary factors may therefore cause alterations in the distribution of the lipoproteins and their constituents that could, for example, significantly affect the risk of ischaemic heart disease in the human population (30,88,89).

A major difficulty in assessing the significance of changes in lipoprotein lipase activity in particular clinical situations is, however, the uncertainty that exists as to how the true functional enzyme level can best be determined. The usual method that is employed is to measure the enzyme activity that appears in the plasma after the injection of heparin. However, the procedure has never been properly standardized with respect to nutritional status, heparin dosage, time of blood sampling after heparin injection, assay method, etc. and, moreover, it gives little or no information about the tissue distribution of the enzyme.

In particular clinical situations, it has been feasible also to determine the tissue enzyme activity in adipose tissue or muscle biopsy samples. However, there is again no general agreement as to how the functional enzyme should be assayed in such tissue samples. Most of the techniques employed seek to measure the enzyme activity that is released through incubation of the tissue in a medium containing heparin, but factors such as the accessibility of heparin to the tissue binding site of the enzyme, the optimum heparin concentration, and the possible loss of released activity during the incubation period, are rarely seriously considered. Clearly, further attention needs to be given to this important problem.

Conclusion

It has been a privilege to introduce the first text to be concerned exclusively with lipoprotein lipase. The enzyme has been my major research interest for over thirty years and it has, therefore, been a particular pleasure to identify some of the major landmarks in its study in a more leisurely fashion than publishers and editors normally allow. At first sight, the intensive study of an enzyme that simply hydrolyses triglyceride ester bonds might not seem to offer much interest and excitement to the active investigator. The example of lipoprotein lipase surely belies this, however, whether considered with respect to the complexity of its molecular interactions, its cell biology, its hormonal control, or its physiological functions. Long may it continue to puzzle and intrigue us!

Colleagues too numerous to mention by name have contributed immeasurably over the years to my pleasure in working on and thinking about lipoprotein lipase. Their names frequently appear as the senior authors of my various publications on the enzyme. However, I should particularly like to thank here my colleague, Dr. B. K. Speake, for his help and advice in the writing of this brief overview of the enzyme: and the Medical Research Council for their ongoing support of my research.

References

1. Hahn, P. F. 1943. *Science.* 98:19–20.
2. Anderson, N. G., and B. Fawcett. 1950. *Proc. Soc. Exp. Biol. Med.* 74:768–771.
3. Anfinsen, C. B., E. Boyle, and R. K. Brown. 1952. *Science.* 115:583–586.
4. Brown, R. K., E. Boyle, and C. B. Anfinsen. 1953. *J. Biol. Chem.* 204:423–434.
5. Gordon, R. S., E. Boyle, R. K. Brown, A. Cherkes, and C. B. Anfinsen. 1953. *Proc. Soc. Exp. Biol. Med.* 84:168–170.
6. Robinson, D. S., and J. E. French. 1953. *Q. J. Exp. Physiol.* 38:233–239.
7. Shore, B., A. V. Nichols, and N. K. Freeman. 1953. *Proc. Soc. Exp. Biol. Med.* 83:216–220.
8. Korn, E. D. 1955. *J. Biol. Chem.* 215:1–14.
9. Korn, E. D. 1955. *J. Biol. Chem.* 215:15–26.

10. Korn, E. D., and T. W. Quigley. 1955. *Biochim. Biophys. Acta* 18:143—145.
11. Scanu, A. 1966. *Science* 153:640—641.
12. LaRosa, J. C., R. I. Levy, P. Herbert, S. E. Lux, and D. S. Frederickson. 1970. *Biochem. Biophys. Res. Commun.* 41:57—62.
13. Havel, R. J. 1973. *Circ. Res.* 27:595—600.
14. Kinnunen, P. K. J. 1983. *In*: Lipases. B. Borgstrom and H. L. Brockman, editors. Elsevier, Amsterdam, New York and Oxford. 307—328.
15. Gofman, J. W., H. B. Jones, F. T. Lindgren, T. P. Lyon, H. A. Elliott, and B. Strisower. 1950. *Circulation* 2:161—178.
16. Graham, D. M., T. P. Lyon, J. W. Gofman, H. B. Jones, A. Yankley, J. Simonton, and S. White. 1951. *Circulation* 4:666—673.
17. Robinson, D. S., J. E. French, and P. M. Harris. 1956. *In*: The Blood Lipids and the Clearing Factor. Proceedings of the Third International Conference on Biochemical Problems of Lipids. Paleis der Academien, Brussels. 310.
18. Frederickson, D. S., and R. S. Gordon. 1958. *Physiol. Rev.* 38:585—630.
19. Havel, R. J., and R. S. Gordon. 1960. *J. Clin. Invest.* 39:1777—1790.
20. Borgstrom, B., and P. Jordan. 1959. *Acta Soc. Med. Upsalien.* 64:185—193.
21. Olivecrona, T. 1962. *J. Lipid Res.* 3:439—444.
22. Robinson, D. S., and P. M. Harris. 1959. *Q. J. Exp. Physiol.* 44:80—90.
23. Robinson, D. S., P. M. Harris, and C. R. Ricketts. 1959. *Biochem. J.* 71:286—292.
24. Robinson, D. S., and J. E. French. 1957. *Q. J. Exp. Physiol.* 38:233—239.
25. Havel, R. J. 1958. *Am. J. Clin. Nutr.* 6:662—668.
26. Robinson, D. S., and J. E. French. 1960. *Pharmacol. Rev.* 12:241—261.
27. Robinson, D. S. 1963. *Adv. Lipid Res.* 1:133—182.
28. Kompiang, I. P., A. Bensadoun, and M. W. W. Yang. 1976. *J. Lipid Res.* 17:498—505.
29. Schotz, M. C., J. -S. Twu, M. E. Pedersen, C. -H. Chen, A. S. Garfinkel, and J. Borensztajn. 1977. *Biochim. Biophys. Acta* 489:214—220.
30. Brunzell, J. D., A. Chait, and E. L. Bierman. 1978. *Metabolism* 27:1109—1127.
31. Breckenridge, W. C., J. A. Little, P. Alaupovic, D. Cox, F. T. Lindgren, and A. Kuksis. 1983. *In*: The Adipocyte and Obesity. Cellular & Molecular Mechanisms. A. Angel, C. H. Hollenberg & A. K. Roncari, editors. Raven Press, New York. 137—147.
32. Schoefl, G. I., and J. E. French. 1968. *Proc. Roy. Soc. B.* 169:153—165.
33. Scow, R. O., E. J. Blanchette-Mackie, and L. C. Smith. 1976. *Circ. Res.* 39:149—160.
34. Olivecrona, T., G. Bengtsson, S. -E. Marklund, U. Lindahl, and M. Hook. 1977. *Federation Proc.* 36:60—65.
35. Olivecrona, T., and G. Bengtsson. 1983. *In*: Lipases. B. Borgstrom and H. L. Brockman, editors. Elsevier, Amsterdam, New York and Oxford. 205—261.
36. Hollenberg, C. H. 1959. *Amer. J. Physiol.* 197:667—670.
37. Cherkes, A., and R. S. Gordon. 1960. *J. Lipid Res.* 1:97—101.
38. Robinson, D. S. 1960. *J. Lipid Res.* 1:332—338.
39. Hollenberg, C. H. 1960. *J. Clin. Invest.* 39:1282—1287.
40. Alousi, A. A., and S. Mallov. 1964. *Amer. J. Physiol.* 206:603—609.
41. Kessler, J. I. 1963. *J. Clin. Invest.* 42:362—367.
42. Nikkilä, E. A., P. Torsti, and O. Penttila. 1963. *Metabolism* 12:863—865.
43. McBride, O. W., and E. D. Korn. 1963. *J. Lipid Res.* 4:17—20.
44. Robinson, D. S. 1963. *J. Lipid Res.* 4:21—23.
45. Barry, J. M., W. Bartley, J. L. Linzell, and D. S. Robinson. 1963. *Biochem. J.* 89:6—11.
46. Rodbell, M. 1964. *J. Biol. Chem.* 239:753—755.
47. Robinson, D. S., and D. R. Wing. 1970. *In*: Adipose Tissue, Regulation and Metabolic Functions. B. Jean Renaud and D. Hepp, editors. Acad. Press, New York and London. 41—46.
48. Robinson, D. S. 1970. *Compr. Biochem.* 18:51—116.
49. Nilsson-Ehle, P., A. S. Garfinkel, and M. C. Schotz. 1980. *Annu. Rev. Biochem.* 49:667—693.

50. Cryer, A. 1981. *Int. J. Biochem.* 13:525–541.
51. Vydelingum, N., R. L. Drake, J. Etienne, and A. H. Kissebah. 1983. *Amer. J. Physiol.* 245:E121–131.
52. Speake, B. K., C. Parkinson, and D. S. Robinson. 1985. *Horm. Metab. Res.* 17:637–640.
53. Speake, B. K., S. M. Parkin, and D. S. Robinson. 1986. *Biochim. Biophys. Acta* 881:155–157.
54. Ball, K. L., B. K. Speake, and D. S. Robinson. 1986. *Biochim. Biophys. Acta* 877:399–405.
55. Borensztajn, J., S. Otway, and D. S. Robinson. 1970. *J. Lipid Res.* 11:102–110.
56. Guidicelli, H., and J. Boyer. 1973. *J. Lipid Res.* 14:592–594.
57. Kinnunen, P. K. J. 1977. *Med. Biol.* 55:187–191.
58. Becht, I., O. Schrecker, G. Klose, and H. Greten. 1980. *Biochim. Biophys. Acta* 620:583–591.
59. Olivecrona, T., T. Egelrud, P. -H. Iverius, and U. Lindahl. 1971. *Biochem. Biophys. Res. Commun.* 43:524–529.
60. Egelrud, T., and T. Olivecrona. 1972. *J. Biol. Chem.* 247:6212–6217.
61. Smith, L. C., and H. J. Pownall. 1983. *In*: Lipases. B. Borgstrom and H. L. Brockman, editors. Elsevier, Amsterdam, New York and Oxford. 263–305.
62. Quinn, D., K. Shirai, and R. J. Jackson. 1983. *Prog. Lipid Res.* 22:35–78.
63. Ostlund-Lindqvist, A. -M., and J. Boberg. 1977. *FEBS Lett.* 83:231–236.
64. Ostlund-Lindqvist, A. -M. 1979. *Biochem. J.* 179:555–559.
65. Fielding, C. J. 1976. *Biochemistry.* 15:879–884.
66. Ben-Zeev, O., A. J. Lusii, R. C. LeBoeuf, J. Nikazy, and M. C. Schotz. 1983. *J. Biol. Chem.* 258:13632–13636.
67. Speake, B. S., S. M. Parkin, and D. S. Robinson. 1985. *Biochem. Soc. Trans.* 13:29–31.
68. Chajek-Shaul, T., G. Friedman, H. Knobler, O. Stein, J. Etienne, and Y. Stein. 1985. *Biochim. Biophys. Acta* 837:123–134.
69. Olivecrona, T., S. S. Chernick, G. Bengtsson-Olivecrona, J. E. Paterniti, W. V. Brown, and R. O. Scow. 1985. *J. Biol. Chem.* 260:2552–2553.
70. Vannier, C., E. -Z. Amri, J. Etienne, R. Negrel, and G. Ailhaud. 1985. *J. Biol. Chem.* 260:4424–4431.
71. Ashby, P., D. P. Bennett, I. M. Spencer, and D. S. Robinson. 1978. *Biochem J.* 176:865–872.
72. Spooner, P. M., S. S. Chernick, M. M. Garrison, and R. O. Scow. 1979. *J. Biol. Chem.* 254:10021–10029.
73. Parkin, S. M., K. Walker, P. Ashby, and D. S. Robinson. 1980. *Biochem. J.* 188:193–199.
74. Speake, B. K., S. M. Parkin, and D. S. Robinson. 1985. *Biochim. Biophys. Acta* 840:419–422.
75. Shimada, K., P. Jo Gill, J. E. Silbert, W. H. J. Douglas, and B. L. Fanburg. 1981. *J. Clin. Invest.* 68:995–1002.
76. Cheng, C. -F., G. M. Oosta, A. Bensadoun, and R. D. Rosenberg. 1981. *J. Biol. Chem.* 256:12893–12898.
77. Williams, M. P., H. B. Streeter, F. S. Wusteman, and A. Cryer. 1983. *Biochim. Biophys. Acta* 756:83–91.
78. Wing, D. R., C. J. Fielding, and D. S. Robinson. 1967. *Biochem. J.* 104:45c–46c.
79. Friedman, G., T. Chajek-Shaul, O. Stein, and Y. Stein. 1983. *Biochim. Biophys. Acta* 752:106–117.
80. Steinberg, D., and J. C. Khoo. 1977. *Federation Proc.* 36:1986–1990.
81. Nikkilä, E. A., and O. Pykalisto. 1968. *Life Sci.* 7:1303–1309.
82. Friedman, G., T. Chajek-Shaul, T. Olivecrona, O. Stein, and Y. Stein. 1982. *Biochim. Biophys. Acta* 711:114–122.
83. Chajek-Shaul, T., G. Friedman, O. Stein, J. Etienne, and Y. Stein. 1985. *Biochim. Biophys. Acta* 837:271–278.
84. Peterson, J., T. Olivecrona, and G. Bengtsson-Olivecrona. 1985. *Biochim. Biophys. Acta* 837:262–270.

85. Greenwood, M. R. C. 1985. *Int. J. Obesity.* 9:Suppl. 1, 67–70.
86. Havel, R. J. 1984. *J. Lipid Res.* 25:1570–1576.
87. Eisenberg, S. 1984. *J. Lipid Res.* 25:1017–1058.
88. Grundy, S. M. 1984. *J. Lipid Res.* 25:1611–1618.
89. Zilversmit, D. B. 1979. *Circulation* 60:473–485.
90. Khoo, J. C., E. M. Mahoney, and J. L. Witztum. 1981. *J. Biol. Chem.* 256:7105–7108.
91. Lindqvist, P., A. -M. Ostlund-Lindqvist, J. L. Witztum, and D. Steinberg. 1983. *J. Biol. Chem.* 258:9086–9092.

Chapter 2

LIPOPROTEIN LIPASE FROM MILK—THE MODEL ENZYME IN LIPOPROTEIN LIPASE RESEARCH

Thomas Olivecrona and Gunilla Bengtsson—Olivecrona

Twenty years ago it had become apparent that a major step in the metabolism of plasma lipoproteins is hydrolysis of their triglycerides by an endothelial-bound lipase (1,2). To probe the biochemistry of the system one

---

ABBREVIATIONS USED apo-CII: human apolipoprotein CII; DFP: diisopropylfluorophosphate; DIP: diisopropylphosphoryl; DMPC: dimyristoylphosphatidylcholine; ELISA: enzyme-linked immunoassay; HDL: high density lipoproteins; LCAT: lecithin cholesterol acyl transferase; LDL: low density lipoproteins; PAGE: polyacrylamide gel electrophoresis; PC: phosphatidylcholine; PMSF: phenylmethylsulfonylfluoride; SDS: sodium dodecyl sulfate; VLDL: very low density lipoproteins

of us set out to purify this enzyme. This was a disheartening endeavor as long as the classical methods of protein purification were used and the starting material was animal tissues. Two events were required to break the impasse. One came from a collaborative study with Dr. Ulf Lindahl on the relation between LPL and heparin (3). This led to the demonstration, together with Drs. T. Egelrud and P. -H. Iverius, of a strong, specific interaction (4) which opened the way for affinity purification (5). The other event was the good advice of Dr. Edward Korn to use bovine milk as the starting material. Milk contains as much (or more) LPL on a weight basis as other tissues do (6,7). It is possible to obtain almost a milligram of pure LPL from one liter of bovine milk. To obtain the same amount of enzyme one would have to process more than a kg of hearts or of adipose tissue.

LPL from milk has become a model enzyme used in many studies on the structural and kinetic properties of LPL. It is also used for *in vitro* studies on lipoprotein transformation, as well as for studies on the turnover of the enzyme itself and for studies on the effects of LPL in tissue culture systems. Antibodies raised against the milk enzyme are used for immunoinhibition, immunoassay and immunoprecipitation of LPLs from other tissues.

In this Chapter we will review the studies that have been carried out with LPL from milk. We have been asked to review also the activator protein and its role in LPL action. We will only briefly discuss the relation between LPL in milk and LPL in other tissues. There is no compelling evidence that there are major differences. The recent advances in knowledge of the protein structure and the physical properties of milk LPL together with the cloning of its cDNA (8) will undoubtedly lead to rapid progress in understanding the relation between milk LPL and LPL in other tissues.

Why and in What State is LPL Present in Milk?

The functional role of LPL in milk is not known. Until recently, the major hypothesis was that the enzyme leaks out from the mammary gland where it is produced in abundance (9). This hypothesis is now in question. Mehta et al. (10) studied the appearance of LPL in human milk. They collected milk from one breast by a pump, and also collected the milk which simultaneously dripped from the other breast. Several intracellular enzymes were present in higher amounts in the pumped milk. LPL activity was, however, higher in the drip milk. This argues against the idea that LPL appears in milk because of tissue damage. In guinea-pigs, LPL accounts for about the same proportion of the protein in milk (0.1%) (11) as of protein synthesis in the mammary gland (12). This suggests that LPL is secreted into milk as efficiently as other milk proteins are.

There is a large literature on LPL activity in bovine milk as a function of the stage of lactation, nutrition, etc. Freshly drawn bovine milk contains less than 0.5 μmol free fatty acids per ml. If the milking and storage procedures are appropriate, the milk can be kept for several days with little further development of free fatty acids. If this were not so, the modern dairy industry could not exist. Hydrolysis of as little as 1–2% of the milk triglycerides gives the milk a rancid or "lipolyzed" flavor, and makes it unpalatable. Although very little lipolysis occurs in normal milk, some cows produce milk with significant lipolysis. Lipolysis can also be induced by rough mechanical treatment of the milk. Because of the economic importance, much effort has been spent in dairy research to understand the process of lipolysis and the factors which influence it. This information is summarized in a report prepared for the International Dairy Federation (13), and in some review articles (14,15). The rapid development in the biochemistry of LPL is now being put to use in studies on lipolysis in milk (16).

In bovine (16) and in guinea pig milk (11) about 80% of the LPL is associated with the casein micelles. This binding has been studied in some detail (17). The casein micelles are large aggregates of phosphoproteins held together by Ca^{++} bridges and by hydrophobic interactions. The aggregates are disrupted into smaller "soluble" protein complexes when Ca^{++} is removed by dialysis or by addition of a Ca^{++} chelator. This brings LPL into solution. The lipase can also be released from the casein micelles by increasing the salt concentration or by addition of heparin. This indicates that the binding is primarily electrostatic. In human milk, a significant fraction of the LPL is associated with the fat globules (18). This may relate to the much lower amount of casein in human that in bovine milk.

Bovine milk is usually drawn at intervals of 8–16 hours. At body temperature the lipase loses activity in milk with a half-life of about 4 hours (Figure 1). Some of this may be ascribed to proteolysis, but most of the inactivation occurs by other mechanisms. This is evident from the experiment in Figure 1. Lipase activity decreased about 70% in 6 hours, but there was no loss of enzyme protein as measured by an immunoassay. Milk thus contains a mixture of active and inactive LPL (19). Fortunately, the inactive lipase does not bind well to heparin-Sepharose and is therefore removed in most purification procedures.

Purification of LPL From Milk

All procedures for purification of milk LPL are based on the enzyme's affinity for heparin. The first step is usually a batch adsorption to heparin-agarose. The gel is washed and the enzyme is eluted by 1.5–2 M NaCl. It is then further purified by readsorption to heparin-agarose followed by gradient elution (7). This basic procedure has been modified and other steps have been added. Examples are the use of nonionic detergents to decrease non-specific binding (20,21), absorption of the enzyme to calcium phosphate or C–γ–alumina gel (22,23), use of dextran-agarose instead of heparin-agarose (24), additional purification by chromatography on hydroxylapatite (25) or by gel filtration (26).

Posner et al. (27) have introduced an alternative first step based on the procedure that Fielding (28) developed for purification of LPL from post-

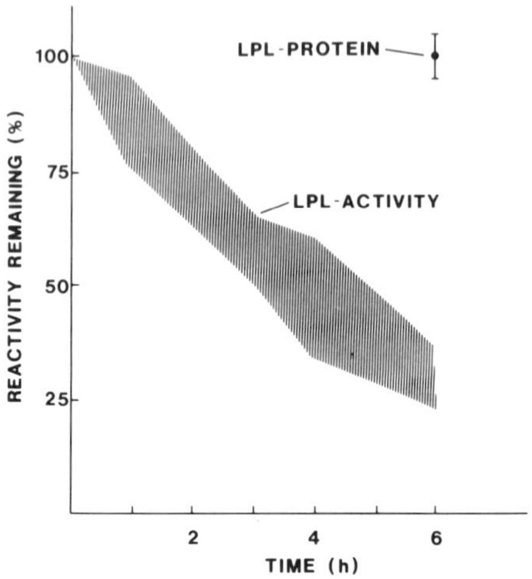

FIGURE 1 *Inactivation of LPL in bovine milk.* Milk samples were obtained from 10 cows and were kept at 37°C. Samples were taken for assay of LPl activity and for radioimmunoassay of LPL protein at the indicated times. The first samples (time 0) were taken with 2 hours after milking. Values are expressed as percent of initial. The hatched area is the range within which values for LPL activity fell.

heparin plasma. In this method, Intralipid is added to skim milk and an Intralipid-LPL complex is collected by centrifugation. Delipidation of the complex yields a powder which can be stored for long times at −20°C. This powder is a convenient source of crude LPL and a good starting material for further purification.

Socorro et al. (21,29) advocates the use of 1 mM phenylmethylsulfonylfluoride (PMSF) to prevent proteolysis during purification. The same group has, however, reported that 1 mM PMSF reacts with and inactivates LPL (30–32).

The ability to bind to heparin is not unique for LPL but is shared by several plasma proteins (reviewed in 33), such as antithrombin (34), complement factors (35), lipoproteins containing apolipoprotein B and/or E (36,37) as well as many intracellular proteins with binding sites for nucleotides, e.g. RNA (38) and DNA polymerases (39). This makes it unlikely that chromatography on heparin-agarose would be sufficient to purify LPL from tissue sources. The situation is more advantageous with milk where the main task is to separate the lipase from casein and other milk secretory proteins. In human milk, there are two proteins which have a relatively high affinity for heparin, namely lactoferrin (40) and the bile salt stimulated lipase (41). A major difficulty in the purification of LPL from blood plasma has been to separate the lipase from antithrombin (42,43). In the bovine milk used in our laboratory the content of antithrombin is usually low. Occasional batches do, however, contain significant amounts of antithrombin. On gradient elution, this protein elutes slightly before LPL and can give rise to either a double peak of protein or a skewed protein peak (see SDS/PAGE, Figure 2). The fractions most likely to be free of antithrombin are from the trailing portion of the peak of lipase activity. Alternatively, one can rechromatograph the preparation on heparin which has been N-desulfated and then acetylated. This results in a much reduced affinity for antithrombin (7, see also below). With guinea pig milk, this is the only way to obtain pure LPL (11).

Molecular Aspects

Physical properties

LPL from bovine milk is a noncovalent dimer of two indentical subunits. The first indication of this structure was provided by Iverius and Östlund-Lindqvist (22). They studied the size of the enzyme by ultracentrifugation at pH 7.4 in 0.15 M NaCl. Under these "physiological" conditions, the enzyme is not stable but tends to aggregate. Therefore, they could not carry centrifugation to equilibrium but had to base their conclusions on extrapolation of the initial sedimentation velocity. More recently, the sedimentation of milk LPL was analyzed in buffers where the enzyme is more stable (44). The results show that the preparations contained a complex mixture of dimers and both reversibly and irreversibly aggregated higher oligomers. When the profile of enzyme activity was determined across the tube, it became evident that the dimer was the active species (44). The size

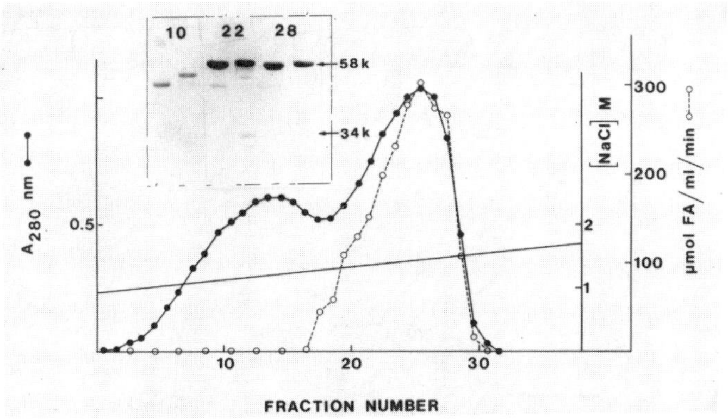

FIGURE 2 *Partial separation of LPL from antithrombin by chromatography on heparin-agarose.* This was an unusual batch of bovine milk which contained antithrombin. The protein peak preceding and partly overlapping the peak of LPL activity was collected and further analyzed. Its N-terminal amino acid sequence (20 residues determined in collaboration with prof. Hans Jörnvall, Stockholm) showed homologies to human antithrombin. (●) A_{280}, (O) LPL activity. The inset shows an SDS/PAGE on fractions from the column. In each pair, the sample to the right was reduced before electrophoresis.

of the enzyme in complex with various ligands has been studied by target analysis (radiation inactivation) (45). These studies showed that the enzyme remains dimeric when it is in complex with heparin, when it is bound to lipid with or without apo-CII present, and when it is in complex with detergents.

Osborne it al. (44) explored if the enzyme can be dissociated into active monomers. For this, 0.75 M guanidinium chloride was used. Sedimentation velocity measurements demonstrated that this treatment led to dissociation of the lipase protein into monomers. Concomitant with dissociation, there was an irreversible loss of catalytic activity and a moderate change in secondary structure as detected by circular dicroism. The rate of inactivation increased with decreasing concentration of active lipase, but the addition of inactive lipase protein did not slow down the inactivation. This indicates that reversible interaction between active species precede the irreversible loss of activity. The implication is that dissociation initially leads to a monomer form which is in reversible equilibrium with the active dimer, but which decays rapidly into an inactive form (Figure 3), and is therefore not detected as a stable component in the system. The dimeric structure is thus required to maintain conformational stability. It is not known if any of the other functions of LPL depend on its dimeric structure. Each subunit has a heparin-binding site, and a heparin chain of sufficient length can simultaneously satisfy both sites on the dimer (24). This results in cooperative binding with enhanced affinity. There is also an apo-CII binding site on each subunit, but in this case two apo-CII molecules are needed to satisfy

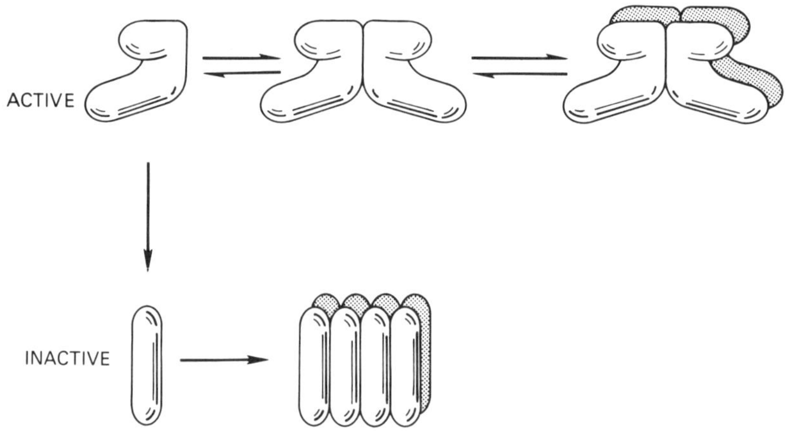

FIGURE 3 *Mechanism for inactivation of LPL, as deduced from the effects of low concentrations of guanidinium chloride.* Active LPL is a dimer of two identical subunits. This dimer is in rapid, reversible equilibrium with a monomer, which is, however, prone to undergo an essentially irreversible change in conformation. Inactive monomers can, in turn, aggregate to higher oligomers. Active dimeric lipase can also (reversibly) form higher oligomers. Based on data from ref. 44.

the sites, and there is no cooperation between them (46). It is not known whether there is one or two active sites in the dimer. The recent demonstration that reaction with DFP results in stoichiometric incorporation of one DIP per subunit (47) implies that each subunit has a functional active site.

The instability of LPL makes studies on its properties and its interactions difficult. The rate of inactivation depends on the pH, the salt concentration, and the temperature (7). LPL is also unstable under physiological conditions (48). Thus, it appears that the LPL molecule has a built-in mechanism to self-destruct. This may be an important property for an enzyme whose activity should decrease rapidly on the appropriate hormonal signal, even though the enzyme is secreted into the extracellular space from the hormone-sensitive cells.

Subunit structure and domain subdivisions

The subunit size of LPL from bovine milk, as determined by sedimentation equilibrium centrifugation, is 41.7 kDa (49). Of this, 8% is carbohydrate (22). The primary structure is known in part. Ben-Avram et al. (50) have published partial sequences for 13 tryptic peptides. Several of these showed homology to porcine pancreatic lipase. Based on this homology, a tentative alignment of the LPL peptides could be made. The DIP-containing peptide studied by Reddy et al. (47) also displayed some homology to pancreatic lipase. Further sequence information has come from a study on domain borders in LPL (51). Adding up the published information, more than half of the primary structure of bovine LPL is now known. cDNA clones corresponding to its mRNA are being studied in several laboratories. This work should reveal the complete sequence within the near future.

The structure of LPLs from human and guinea-pig milk have recently been compared to that of the bovine enzyme (51). There were strong homologies in the N-terminal sequences, but there were also interesting differences. For instance, bovine LPL has two additional N-terminal amino acids as compared to the guinea-pig and human lipases. A direct comparison of the mobilities on SDS/PAGE suggested that the human subunit is slightly larger than the bovine or guinea-pig subunits. Hayashi et al. (52) recently compared the properties of LPL from human postheparin plasma with the enzyme from bovine milk. They also found that the human enzyme is slightly larger as evaluated by SDS-PAGE.

We noticed several years ago that trypsin cleaves bovine LPL into two fragments of about equal size (53). The two fragments are held together by disulfide bonds. There is no detectable change in molecular size and only a small change in conformation (49). The enzyme retains all its functional regions apparently intact, i.e., the heparin-binding site, the site for adsorption to lipid-water interfaces, the active site as well as the site for interaction with activator protein. The only marked change is a decrease in activity against lipoprotein triglycerides and emulsions of long-chain triglycerides

(53). This has been interpreted as due to disrupted connection between the lipid binding site and the active site of the enzyme. Recently, the cleavage has been studied in more detail (51). Trypsin produced three main fragments (T1, T2a, and T2b) suggesting cleavage at an exposed segment delineating domain borders (see also Figure 4). Time studies gave no evidence for precursor-product relationships between the fragments, and prolonged incubations did not lead to further cleavage. Fragments T2a and T2b had the same N-terminal sequence as intact lipase. Fragment T1 revealed a new sequence and represents the C-terminal half of the molecule. Tryptic cleavage of guinea-pig LPL yielded two fragments. One had the same size as bovine fragment T2b; the other had a similar size as bovine fragment T1, and a N-terminal sequence homologous with that of T1. Thus, trypsin recognizes the same unique site in guinea-pig LPL as in the bovine enzyme. This confirms the conclusion that this segment is the border between two domains in the subunit. Chymotrypsin was found to cleave off a relatively small fragment from the C-terminal end of the molecule, after which exposure to trypsin still resulted in cleavage at the same sites as in intact lipase. Thus, chymotrypsin may recognize another domain border (Figure 4).

LPL retains its ability to bind heparin after SDS/PAGE and transfer to nitrocellulose. This made it possible to localize the heparin-binding region to the C-terminal domain. Furthermore, heparin-binding was retained also after chymotryptic cleavage which indicates that the binding region is localized to the N-terminal part of the C-terminal domain, i.e. the middle domain (Figure 4). Analysis of cDNA for LPL from guinea-pig milk (8) has recently shown that there is a cluster of positively charged amino acids in this part of the molecule, which may form the heparin-binding site.

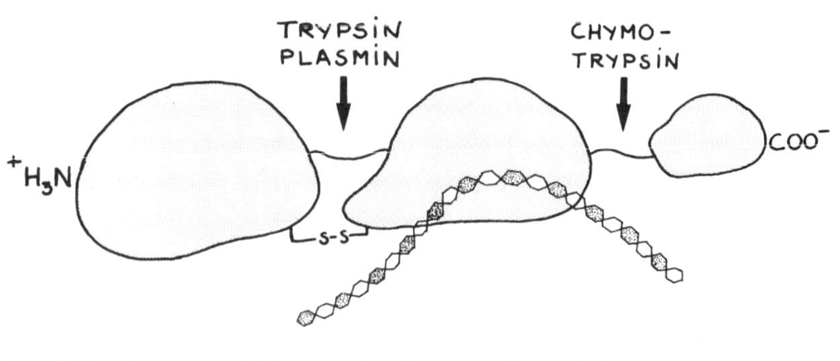

FIGURE 4 *Domains of LPL as deduced from studies with limited proteolysis.* This schematic figure shows the two exposed segments in the bovine LPL subunit which are attacked by certain proteases. The fragments which are generated by trypsin and plasmin are held together by disulfide bonds. A heparan sulfate chain is illustrated as a string of saccharide units to show that its binding site is on the middle domain. Based on data from ref. 51.

None of the other functional sites in the lipase molecule can as yet be definitely assigned. It can be inferred from the homology to pancreatic lipase in combination with the cDNA data that the putative active site peptide Reddy et al. (47) have isolated from bovine LPL is localized in the N-terminal part of the molecule. This is in accord with the observation that binding of heparin to the enzyme does not markedly change the efficiency of the active site (54,55), as expected if the two functions reside on separately folded domains.

Protein components similar in size to the fragments produced by trypsin are present in most preparations of LPL from bovine milk (5,7). We found several years ago that an antiserum raised against these components reacted with LPL, demonstrating that they are proteolytic degradation products (53). More recently, Socorro and Jackson (29) have demonstrated that monoclonal antibodies recognize both intact LPL and several proteolytic fragments which are present in milk or are produced during purification.

Immunochemistry

Milk LPL has proven to be a good antigen to produce poly- and monoclonal antibodies for immunochemical studies. Such antibodies have been used for selective determination of LPL in other tissues (56,57) and in plasma (58) by immunoinhibition, for immunoprecipitation of the lipase in studies of its synthesis and turnover (12,56,59), for immunolocalization (60,61), for immunoassay (56,62) and for indentification of cDNA clones (8). Antisera raised against LPL from guinea-pig milk fully inhibit LPL activity in a variety of guinea pig tissues (11). On immunoprecipitation of ^{35}S-labeled guinea-pig tissue proteins, they detect a single component which has the same apparent molecular size as the milk enzyme (Figure 5) (12,59). This suggests that the milk enzyme is similar to, or perhaps identical with, LPL in other tissues. Some rabbit antisera against bovine milk LPL also inhibit human (52,63,64) and porcine LPL (64,65). Chicken antisera against bovine milk LPL show wider cross-reactivity; they recognize also the rat and the mouse enzyme (56,62). A monoclonal antibody raised against bovine milk LPL was found to react with LPL from human postheparin plasma, and with LPL from a mouse cell line (66). These observations indicate that there is substantial homology between LPL in different species.

We found that *Fab* fragments prepared from a rabbit antiserum blocked binding of the enzyme to triglyceride/phospholipid droplets but had no effect on the hydrolysis of water-soluble substrates (62). Shirai et al. (64) had previously reported that monovalent *Fab*-fragments prepared from a rabbit antiserum retained their ability to inhibit LPL. Thus, the inhibition was not contingent on precipitation of the enzyme but must have been a direct consequence of binding of the antibody. Lipid droplets partially protected the enzyme against the inhibition. Apo-CII enhanced this protection, but had no effect in the absence of lipid. They concluded that interaction with

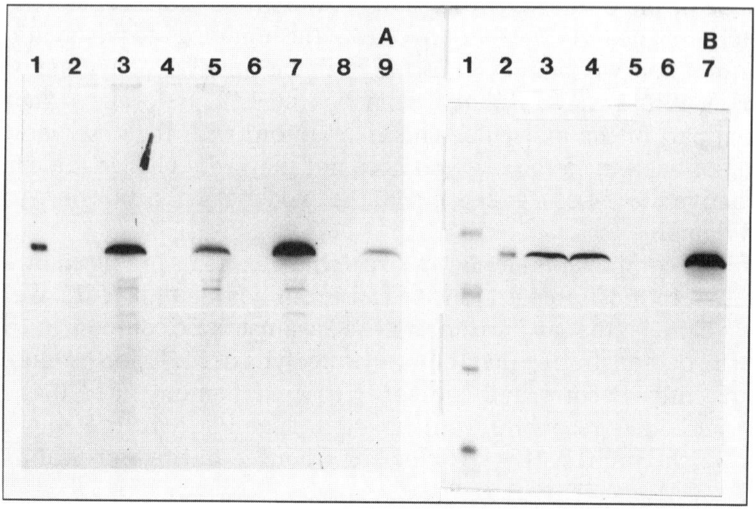

FIGURE 5 *Immunoprecipitates of LPL from guinea pig tissues labeled with ^{35}S-methionine.* In A, tissue pieces from a lactating guinea pig (6 days after delivery) were incubated in medium with ^{35}S-methionine for 45 min. In B, guinea-pig hearts were perfused with a medium containing ^{35}S-methionine for 15 min (heart 1) and 10 min (heart 2), respectively. LPL was immunoprecipitated using a rabbit antiserum raised against LPL purified from guinea-pig milk. The immunoprecipitates were separated by SDS/PAGE and displayed by fluorography. A. Lane 1: ^{125}I-labeled bovine LPL. Lanes 3, 5, 7, and 9: Immunoprecipitates from mammary gland, lung, periovarial adipose tissue, and diaphragm muscle. Lanes 2, 4, 6, 8: Controls with nonimmune serum, corresponding to lanes 3, 5, 7, and 9. B. Lane 1: molecular weight markers (serum albumin, ovalbumin, carbonic anhydrase, lactoglobulin A). Lane 2: ^{125}I-labeled bovine LPL. Lanes 3, 4: Immunoprecipitates from hearts 1 and 2, respectively. Lanes 5, 6: Controls corresponding to lanes 4 and 7. Lane 7: Immunoprecipitate from adipocytes (from the epididymal adipose tissue of a fed guinea-pig) labeled for 15 min. From ref. 12 by permission.

lipid and with apo-CII caused conformational changes in the enzyme molecule which impeded its reaction with the antibodies.

Voyta et al. (66) have described an interesting monoclonal antibody to LPL from bovine milk. It inhibited completely the apo-CII dependent hydrolysis of a triglyceride/phospholipid emulsion, but had no effect on the hydrolysis of water-soluble substrates. When the enzyme was preincubated with apo-CII, four times more antibody was required to achieve 50% inactivation of the enzyme activity. Furthermore, the antibody disrupted binding of dansylated apo-CII peptides to LPL both in the presence and absence of lipid. This antibody thus appears to recognize the apo-CII binding site on LPL.

The reaction of milk LPL with its antibodies is conformation-dependent. Voyta et al. (66) raised ten murine monoclonal antibodies against bovine LPL. All of these antibodies showed immunoreactivity toward the purified lipase by ELISA and were able to remove enzyme activity from solution using indirect immunoprecipitation. However, only two of the ten antibodies recognized the enzyme on Western blot analysis. We have studied about 30 rabbit and hen antisera (62). Most of these were more reactive towards denatured than towards native LPL, but a few of the antisera were more reactive against the native form. Denatured LPL does not compete effectively with the native enzyme for those antibodies in polyclonal sera which inhibit the enzyme's activity (62,67).

The observation that the reaction of LPL with its antibodies is conformation-dependent has important consequences for immunoassay of the enzyme. We have found it necessary to ensure that all materials, tracer, standard as well as samples, are in their denatured form (56,62). This can be achieved by heating the materials in SDS, which is then diluted with a nonionic detergent so that it does not inhibit the immunoreaction. This approach has the additional advantage that it will dissociate and bring into solution LPL associated with cell membranes, lipoproteins or otherwise complexed in biological samples.

Interactions with heparin-like polysaccharides

The ability to bind to heparin appears to be a general property of LPLs (68,69) but details of this interaction have been studied primarily with the enzyme from bovine milk.

Clarke et al. (24) studied the interaction between heparin and milk LPL using fluorescence polarization spectroscopy. They found that the type of complex formed depended on the chain length of the heparin. With excess heparin of $M_r > 10000$, one heparin chain formed a very stable complex with the dimeric protein molecule. With shorter heparins (M_r 6600–8000) the complexes contained 2 heparin chains per protein dimer. At 0.2 M NaCl Kd values of 4×10^{-8} M and 6×10^{-9} M were assigned to the 2:1 and 1:1 complexes, respectively. These results suggest that there is a heparin-binding site on each subunit of the dimeric enzyme and that a single heparin chain of $M_r > 10000$ can satisfy both sites. Smaller heparin chains are unable to span the sites, and two chains must interact with each enzyme molecule. The Stoke's radius of LPL is reported to be 4.4 nm (22). Since a heparin molecule of M_r 10000 is about 12.5 nm, it can interact simultaneously with heparin binding sites on opposite sides of the dimer. This model is supported by the observation that the inactive monomeric form of LPL binds to heparin with lower affinity than the dimeric enzyme does (48). The model provides a ready explanation for the stabilizing effect that heparin has on the enzyme (48,70). It appears that inactivation proceeds via dissociation of the dimeric enzyme followed by re-folding of the monomer to a catalytically inactive form (44, Figure 3). Under conditions where dissociation of the dimer is the rate determining step, heparin could stabilize the enzyme by decreasing the dissociation.

Heparin preparations are polydisperse both in size and in chemical composition (33,71). This polydispersity is evident in its interaction with LPL (72–75). Heparin elutes from LPL-Sepharose over a wide range of salt concentrations (72,73). Re-chromatography of heparin fractions eluted at low and high salt concentrations, respectively, yield clearly separated elution profiles. When presented with an excess of heparin, LPL-Sepharose binds those heparin molecules which have the highest affinity for the enzyme (72–74). The bound fraction elutes as a sharp peak at high salt concentration. By this method a heparin subfraction with high affinity for LPL can be prepared.

The structure in heparin required for binding of LPL has been studied in some detail. Heparin can be separated into two fractions with high and with low affinity for antithrombin (76), but these two fractions do not differ in their affinity for LPL (77). Partially N-desulfated heparin is unable to bind LPL, but this ability is restored by re-N-sulfation or by acetylation of the free amino groups (78). This acetylated derivative of heparin is a useful affinity ligand for isolation of LPL in situations where antithrombin is a major contaminant (11). The minimal sized heparin fragments with a definite ability to interact with LPL are octasaccharides (78). This may indicate the size of the heparin binding site on each subunit of the enzyme.

The heparin binding site on LPL can accommodate other polyanions also. Of particular interest is that the enzyme binds to heparan sulfate (69,78). Based on the amounts of heparin and of heparan sulfate required to release the enzyme from a Sepharose-bound heparan sulfate, the difference in affinity was about 40-fold (78). Clarke et al. (24) studied the interaction of milk LPL with a heparan sulfate of M_r 17000. Only one type of complex was demonstrated. This had a 1:1 stoichiometry, i.e. one enzyme dimer per haparan sulfate chain. The Kd at 0.2 M NaCl was 1.6×10^{-7} M, i.e. the affinity was about 30 times lower than for a heparin of similar molecular weight.

The rather high affinity of LPL for heparan sulfate and the specificity of the binding attracted Klinger et al. (79) to use the enzyme as an affinity ligand for isolation of heparan sulfate proteoglycan from brain. This had previously not been possible due to considerable similarities with respect to size, charge, and density of the heparan sulfate to the much larger amounts of accompanying chondroitin sulfate proteoglycan. When low sample loads were applied, both types of proteoglycan bound and were only partially resolved. However, when the column was "overloaded," the specificity for binding of heparan sulfate became apparent and a very good separation was obtained. Thus, LPL can recognize rather subtle differences in the carbohydrate structure.

The finding that LPL binds tightly to heparan sulfate, and considerations of the known properties of the enzyme at the vascular endothelium, led us and others to suggest that the enzyme is attached at the endothelium via interaction with membrane-bound heparan sulfate (2,69). The validity of this hypothesis has since been tested in experiments with cultured endothelial cells. Shimada et al. (80) studied the binding of LPL from bovine milk to bovine endothelial cells. The enzyme retained its catalytic activity while bound to the endothelial cells and was almost quantitatively released by heparin. Thus, the binding had the same characteristics as *in vivo.* Removal of heparan sulfate from the endothelial cells by purified heparinase totally inhibited the binding, but the removal of chondroitin sulfate by chondroitin ABC-lyase had no effect on the binding. In a similar study with endothelial cells isolated from the vein of human umbilical cords, Wang-Iversen et al. (81) confirmed the result of Shimada et al. (80). Cheng et al. (82) have obtained similar results using avian LPL. In all three studies, the LPL concentration at half maximal binding was between 0.14 and 0.52 μM.

Williams et al. (83) have studied the binding of LPL to aortic endothelium. They made interesting calculations on the number of LPL molecules and heparan sulfate proteoglycans per endothelial cell. This group has also discussed the properties of endothelial-bound LPL in detail (84,85). It has recently been shown that the concentration of LPL in plasma of rats and humans is about 1 nM (58,86). If the dissociation constants measured in the studies with cultured endothelial cells are applicable *in vivo,* receptor occupancy must be low, only about 1%. This is plausible since the *in vitro* studies showed that the binding capacity is high.

Lipoprotein lipase is not the only protein that binds to heparan sulfate at the vascular endothelium. Other proteins for which a similar mode of attachment seems likely include antithrombin (87), a diamine oxidase (88), a superoxide dismutase (89), and thrombin (90). There may be many more. General aspects of the functions of heparan sulfate proteoglycans have recently been reviewed (33, 71,91).

The model for binding of LPL to endothelial heparan sulfate was originally proposed to unify a number of disparate experimental observations into a rational picture (69). It has more recently been discussed in detail by Cryer (84) (see also Chapter 11). One important aspect is that it puts the enzyme some distance out from the membrane (Figure 6). A lipoprotein particle which approaches an endothelial cell will see only its glycocalyx, and would have difficulty reaching a lipase integrated in the plasma membrane proper. Heparan sulfate chains protrude further out from the membrane than most other components in the glycocalyx, and an enzyme located on these chains would have a much improved ability to interact with plasma lipoproteins. Recent studies have shown that the LDL receptor has a domain with a cluster of negatively charged O-linked glycan chains (92). It seems likely that this domain spans the glycocalyx and therefore puts the ligand binding domain outside this layer (Figure 6). Thus, the two main receptors for large lipoproteins may both reside in the outer layer of the glycocalyx, where it is easy for lipoprotein particles in blood to reach them.

Interaction with substrate lipoproteins may be facilitated by the heparan sulfate. To attact the lipoprotein particles, a long-range force is needed. This

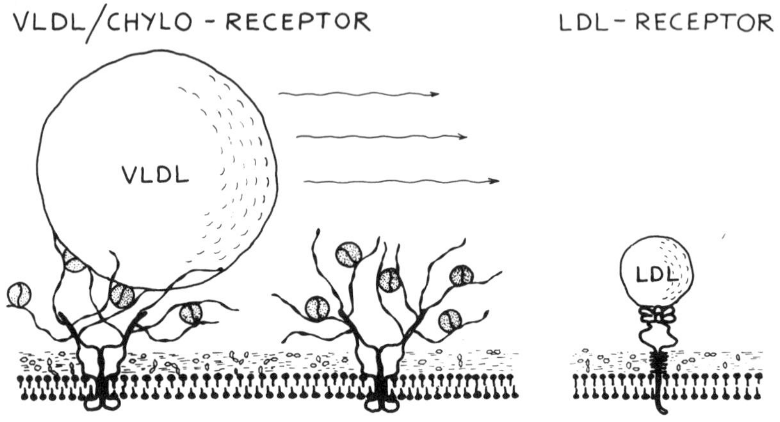

FIGURE 6 *Schematic view of how lipoproteins interact with their receptors.* Left panel. Heparan sulfate proteoglycans are intercalated in the plasma membrane of an endothelial cell. Each core protein of the proteoglycan carries several polysaccharide chains which protrude further out from the cell surface than other components of the glycocalyx (see ref. 33 for a detailed discussion of heparan sulfate proteoglycans). This puts the attached LPL molecules (dotted, small spheres) in a position where they can freely interact with VLDL and chylomicra. Several important aspects are not illustrated in this simplified drawing:

- other enzymes may be bound to the heparan sulfate chains: antithrombin, diamine oxidase, a superoxide dismutase, etc.
- apolipoproteins B and E on the lipoprotein also bind to the heparan sulfate chains
- chylomicra are much larger than VLDL and probably interact simultaneously with several heparan sulfate proteoglycans.

Right panel. The LDL receptor may also have its ligand binding domain outside the glycocalyx. This is accomplished by a domain with 0-linked glycan chains, which spans the glycocalyx.

could be provided by electrostatic interaction between the clusters of positive charges on apolipoproteins B and E on the one hand, and the negative charge on heparan sulfate on the other hand. Evidence in support of this has been provided by Clark and Quarfordt (93). They studied hydrolysis of triglycerides in model emulsions, and in rat chylomicra, by bovine milk LPL bound to heparin-Sepharose. Addition of apo E to the emulsion resulted in a 7-fold lowering of the K_m for triglyceride with no change in V_{max}. In addition, increased binding of triglyceride to the heparin-Sepharose-enzyme complex was directly demonstrated.

There are a number of disparate reports on effects of heparin on the catalytic efficiency of LPL. Both stimulation and inhibition has been observed. Examples are enumerated and discussed elsewhere (55,69,75,94,95). The activity of bovine milk LPL against simple substrates is not markedly changed by heparin (54,55). This indicates that binding of heparin has little or no effect on the active site itself. In crude systems, for instance tissue homogenates, heparin can solubilize the enzyme and cause an apparent increase in enzyme activity. Under other circumstances, the primary effect of heparin can be to stabilize the enzyme. In fact heparin is often included in assay media for this purpose (e.g. 96). There are reports that heparin may impede binding of LPL to lipids (94,97), but it has been directly shown that the enzyme can bind heparin while it remains bound to phospholipid liposomes (97). As discussed above, interaction with apolipoprotein E (or B) may actually enhance binding of lipoproteins to a heparan sulfate-LPL complex at the endothelium (93). There are reports that heparin interferes in a competitive manner with the interaction of LPL with apo-CII (27,94). Clarke et al. (24) found that heparin weakens the interaction between LPL and apo-CII in solution. In the presence of lipid, however, the LPL-apo-CII interaction was much tighter and was insensitive to heparin. It has been directly demonstrated that LPL immobilized on heparin-Sepharose can be stimulated by apo-CII (55,93). Thus, model studies with the bovine milk enzyme indicate that a LPL-heparan sulfate complex would be able to fulfill the biological functions of the enzyme, lending support to the proposed model for endothelial attachment. It has also been directly demonstrated that the enzyme can hydrolyze lipoprotein lipids while it is bound to cultured endothelial cells (98).

Binding to detergents, fatty acids and interfaces

LPLs from a variety of sources are stabilized by detergents and by fatty acids (99,100). Using deoxycholate as a model substance, we have demonstrated, by equilibrium dialysis and by charge shift electrophoresis, that milk LPL binds detergent (101). The enzyme retained its catalytic activity, indicating that the detergent bound to the native form of the enzyme. Target analysis showed that the enzyme remained dimeric in detergent solution (45). Helenius and Simons (102) have demonstrated that deoxycholate does not bind to the native form of most water-soluble proteins, but it binds to proteins with lipid-binding regions such as membrane proteins and some apolipoproteins. Thus, the binding of deoxycholate to LPL signifies that this protein has a lipid binding region. This may be the same region as that involved in binding to lipid/water interfaces.

The binding of deoxycholate has several effects on LPL; it increases its solubility (101), it desorbs the enzyme from lipid droplets (54); and enhances its stability (101). Long chain fatty acids also have these effects. The stabilization by detergents or detergent-fatty acid mixtures is useful for studies of LPL, e.g. for extraction of the enzyme from tissues (23,56,59) for purification of the enzyme (103) and during immunotitration experiments (62). The binding of fatty acids to LPL is of particular interest because of its possible relation to product inhibition of the enzyme (104,105). LPL stabilized by long chain fatty acids is destabilized when sufficient amounts of albumin are added (104). Apparently, albumin has about 7 binding sites with an affinity for fatty acids which is higher than that of LPL for fatty acids. This observation parallels that on hydrolysis of triglycerides in media with limited albumin; when the molar ratio of fatty acids to albumin exceeds 6–7, further hydrolysis is inhibited (105).

Binding of LPL to lipid-water interfaces also stabilizes the enzyme (106). This suggests, but does not prove, that the same region on the enzyme molecule is involved in this binding as in binding to detergents/fatty acids. The stabilization is quite dramatic as illustrated in Figure 7. When LPL is incubated in an assay system without any lipid present, the enzyme rapidly loses activity. In contrast, when lipid is included in the assay system, enzyme activity is retained. This is why it is possible to obtain linear release of fatty acids during assay of LPL activity.

LPL binds avidly to lipid-water interfaces. Binding which is tight enough so that LPL-lipid complexes can be isolated by centrifugation or gel filtration has been demonstrated with chylomicrons and chylomicron remnants (107), remnants of VLDL (108), phospholipid-triglyceride droplets (109), other types of tryglyceride droplets (110–111), milk fat globules (16,112), and phospholipid liposomes (97,113,114). McLean and Jackson (114) have determined the dissociation constant for interaction of LPL with sonicated vesicles of a nonhydrolyzable phosphatidylcholine analogue. LPL-lipid com-

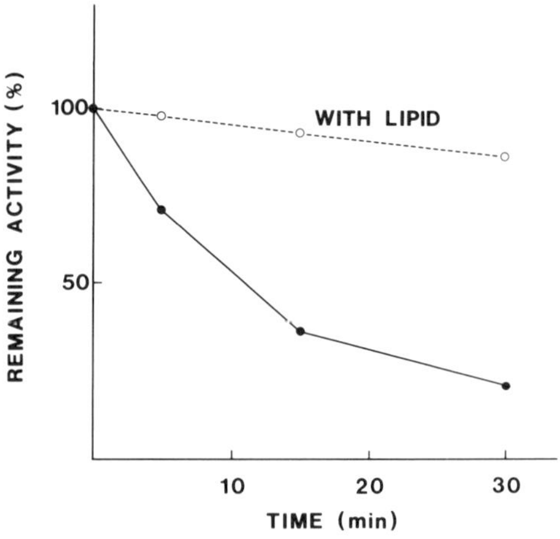

FIGURE 7 *Effect of lipid substrate on the stability of LPL.* LPL (from bovine milk, 10 μg/ml) was incubated in 0.1 M Tris-Cl, 0.1 M NaCl containing 60 mg bovine serum albumin per ml at pH 8.5, with (○) or without (●) Intralipid added (5 mg triglyceride/ml). The temperature was 37°C. These conditions are often used for assay of LPL. Remaining LPL activity was determined at a series of times by incubation of aliquots in regular assay medium containing radioactive triglyceride substrate. Note that in the absence of lipid the enzyme rapidly loses catalytic activity. It is only because binding to the substrate droplets stabilizes the enzyme that release of fatty acids progresses linearly under assay conditions.

plexes with a stoichiometry of one molecule LPL per 320 molecules of phospholipid were isolated by density gradient ultracentrifugation. The dissociation constant for the complex was 43 nM. In assay systems using phospholipid stabilized emulsions of triglycerides, a typical concentration for phospholipid is 100 μM. If the dissociation constant determined with the sonicated vesicles is relevant for the emulsion systems, essentially all LPL should be on the droplets. This is in accord with actual measurements; 80–90% of the LPL floats with the emulsion droplets on centrifugation (109).

For many proteins, binding to lipid causes a major rearrangement in the secondary structure. Binding of LPL to phosphatidylcholine vesicles does not, however, cause any significant change in its circular dicroic spectrum (113). This rules out major refolding of the molecule, but does not rule out some re-arrangement since only a small portion of the protein may bind to lipid. The binding was associated with an increase in blue shift of fluorescence suggesting that at least one of the tryptophan residues in LPL was transferred to a more hydrophobic environment.

The catalytic rates for pancreatic lipase and for pancreatic phospholipase A_2 increase several hundred or thousand fold when these enzymes bind to interfaces. This is called "surface activation" and is presumably caused by conformational changes in the enzyme molecules (115). Shirai and Jackson (96) have found that the V_{max} of LPL against the soluble substrate p-nitrophenylbutyrate is increased up to 8 fold on interaction with phospholipid liposomes. Their interpretation was that on binding to lipid, there is a conformational change in the LPL molecule causing a favorable realignment of the active site residues. The same group has, however, also reported that there is no evidence of surface activation of LPL in its action on lipids located in the interface. This conclusion comes from studies with short-chain phosphatidylcholines (116,117). Such substrates have been used to study surface activation of phospholipase A_2, which hydrolyzes them much more rapidly when they are presented as micelles than when they are monomeric. With LPL there was no difference in catalytic rate above or below the critical micellar concentration of the two phosphatidylcholines studied (116,117). Thus, it remains unclear whether LPL undergoes surface activation. In comparison to surface activation of pancreatic lipase and pancreatic phospholipase A_2 the effect is, in any case, small.

Binding of LPL to substrate droplets is a rapid process (25,118). Hydrolysis usually starts immediately on addition of the enzyme and an appreciable "lag-time" has only been reported in a few studies (46,119). The binding is also rapidly reversible. The enzyme distributes without any discernable lag-time to new lipid droplets which are added to a reaction that is already in full progress (25,118). A corollary of this is that even when there is less than one enzyme molecule per substrate particle, all particles will be degraded in parallel if they are physically equivalent.

Kinetic Properties

Nature of the active site

Earlier data on the active site mechanism have been summarized and discussed in a review by Quinn et al. (30). They concluded that the most likely mechanism is nucleophilic attack by an active site serine resulting in formation of a transient fatty acyl enzyme. Their two main arguments were (a) that LPL is inhibited by some serine esterase and protease inhibitors and (b) consideration of the pH profile for LPL activity. Solvent isotope effects (120) and the fact that the enzyme is inhibited by benzene boronic acid (121) (a transition state analogue), also support this type of mechanism. These arguments are, however, open to discussion.

LPL is inhibited by DFP (47), by dietyl-p-nitrophenyl phosphate (122), and by PMSF (30–32), but the concentrations needed are much higher than for most other serine hydrolases. The reactions are stoichiometric. The putative active site peptide has been isolated by two groups (32,47), and sequenced by one (47). It shows a certain degree of homology to residues 101–117 in porcine pancreatic lipase. However, as pointed out by Reddy et al. (47), treatment of pancreatic lipase with DFP leads to no loss of activity but results in modification of a nonessential tyrosine. Diethyl-p-nitrophenylphosphate reacts with serine 152 in pancreatic lipase. This leads to loss of activity against emulsified substrates, but activity against soluble substrates is retained (see ref. 123 for discussion). Thus, although this is not the active site, the segment appears to be involved in lipid binding. Homologous sequences are found in pregastric lipase (124), in LCAT (125), in LPL (50), and in hepatic lipase (50).

The second argument for a serine esterase type of active site is that LPL shows a bell-shaped profile for activity versus pH with optimum between 8 and 9. There are, however, also reports that the activity continues to rise with pH to at least 10.5 with no evidence of any break in the curve at the classical "pH optimum" around 8.5. This was first reported in 1973 for a deoxycholate-monoglyceride system (126) and was later also demonstrated with tributyrin (54) and Intralipid (106,127). The implication is that the decrease in activity at higher pH is due to some factor other than the active site reaction. This was explored using milk fat globules as the substrate (127). Binding of LPL to the lipid droplets was found to be a pH-dependent process with optimum around pH 8. The active site reaction increased continuously with pH over the range 6–10.5. The pH-activity curve was a composite of the pH effect on the binding step and the pH effect on the active site reaction. This resulted in a "typical" bell-shaped curve. Parallel experiments were carried out with Intralipid as substrate. Under the conditions used, there was essentially complete binding of the lipase to these droplets, and a continuous rise in reaction rate.

LPL shows many similarities in its kinetic properties to pancreatic lipase and to the hepatic heparin-releasable lipase (128) suggesting that they have the same active site mechanism, and may have evolved from a common ancestral gene. The recent demonstration that there are sequence homologies (47,50) between the enzymes verify this hypothesis. The details of the active site mechanism are still somewhat unclear for all three enzymes.

Substrate specificity

LPL shows a rather low degree of chemical substrate specificity; it can hydrolyze long- and short chain triglycerides (54,126), diglycerides (109,129), monoglycerides (126,129,130), long- and short-chain phosphatidylcholines (116,117,131–135), p-nitrophenylesters (31,96,126), and Tween (126). Like pancreatic lipase and hepatic lipase, LPL hydrolyzes preferentially the primary ester bonds in triglycerides generating sn-2 monoglycerides and free fatty acids as the principal products (129). The sn-1 position is hydrolyzed at a higher rate than the sn-3 position (136–138). Monoglycerides are hydrolyzed at high rates only after isomerization to the sn-1(3) derivatives (129). Thus, the predominant pathway for complete hydrolysis of a triglyceride is via isomerization of the initially formed 2-monoglyceride to the 1(3)-isomer.

The rates observed with different substrates vary greatly (Table 1). Phosphatidylcholines are hydrolyzed at only a small percent of the rate at which triglycerides are hydrolyzed. The soluble substrate p-nitrophenyl butyrate,

TABLE 1 Comparison of the rates at which LPL hydrolyzes some different substrates.

	Rate of hydrolysis (μmol/min $\times$ mg LPL)		
Substrate	*−apo-CII*	*+apo-CII*	*Reference*
Human VLDL[a]		400[b]	109
Intralipid triglycerides[a]	81	490	109
Triolein-gum arabic[a]	480	730	109
Triolein-Triton X-100[a]	450	710	109
Tributyrin-gum arabic[a]	450	425	54
Diolein-gum arabic[a]	[c]	1500	109
Monolein-Triton x-100[a]	20	400	130
Sonicated rat liver PC[a,d]	1.4	8.9	109
Sonicated DMPC[e,f]	0.3	5.8	134
DMPC-Triton X-100[e,f]	0.7	7.8	134
p-nitrophenylbutyrate[g]	6.7	1.3[h]	31
p-nitrophenylacetate[g]	2.0	0.4[h]	31

[a]pH 8.5, 25°C.
[b]No extra apo-CII was added.
[c]No data are given for pH 8.5. At pH 7.3 apo-CII caused a 1.5-fold stimulation.
[d]PC = phosphatidylcholine
[e]DMPC = dimyristoylphosphatidylcholine
[f]pH 8.0, 37°C
[g]pH 7.25, 25°C
[h]Estimated from the statement that high concentrations of apo-CII caused a maximal 70–90% inhibition.

which has been much used in kinetic studies, is hydrolyzed at less than 2% of the rate observed with tributyrin. Since the same fatty acid is released with both substrates, it is clear that some step other than hydrolysis of an acyl-enzyme intermediate must be rate-limiting, at least for hydrolysis of p-nitrophenyl butyrate. This is an important point to note when one extrapolates conclusions reached from kinetic experiments with soluble substrates to the action of LPL on lipoproteins. It is not clear that the same step is rate limiting in the two cases.

Jackson and his collaborators have studied the chain length dependency of the LPL-catalyzed hydrolysis of phosphatidylcholine (134,135). For this they have used phosphatidylcholines presented to the enzyme as detergent complexes or as monolayers. In the absence of apo-CII, LPL activity decreased with increasing fatty acyl chain length. Phospholipids containing unsaturated fatty acyl chains were hydrolyzed at rates 5–10 times faster than were saturated lipids. No simple relation was apparent between the absolute rates of hydrolysis and the fatty acid chain length or the physical property of the phospholipid. With triglycerides as the substrate, the fatty acid chain length seems to be of only minor importance for the reaction rate. Thus, the rate of tributyrin hydrolysis is about 0.6, and that of trioctanoin hydrolysis is about 1.3 of that for triolein (Table 1). Again, it is important to note that these rates are in general about 100 times faster than the rates for corresponding phosphatidylcholines, demonstrating that factors other than the nature of the fatty acid are the main determinants for the reaction rate.

Comparisons of maximal rates and relative affinities for different lipid substrates should be interpreted with caution. Differences in aggregation, hydration and interfacial orientation are major determinants and often difficult to evaluate. This can be illustrated by the action of LPL on monoglycerides. It was earlier thought that LPL hydrolyses 1(3)monoglyceride much slower than tri- and diglycerides. The basis for this was the observation that monoglycerides in deoxycholate solution were hydrolyzed slowly (126), and that monoglycerides accumulated in the system during hydrolysis of triglycerides (129). Both of these observations have been found to reflect an unfavorable physical state of the monoglycerides rather than an intrinsically low ability of the enzyme to hydrolyze them. The slow rate of hydrolysis in the presence of deoxycholate was found to be due primarily to the fact that this detergent abolishes the effect of activator protein (130). When monoglycerides were dispersed in Triton instead, the rate was enhanced about 20-fold by activator and became almost as high as the rates reported for triglyceride hydrolysis (130, see Table 1). That monoglycerides accumulate during hydrolysis of lipoproteins is due in part to slow isomerization of the sn-2 to the sn-1(3) isomers. In addition, however, the monoglycerides are bound by albumin (105) and/or high density lipoproteins (139), if present in the system, and are thereby removed from the site of lipolysis. When the reactions are carried out with limited albumin so that the monoglyceride remains with the enzyme, there is little or no accumulation of monoglycerides (105).

LPL catalyzes not only cleavage of ester bonds, but also their formation; it is a transacylase (104,140). In this reaction, mono- and diglycerides are efficient acyl acceptors, but glycerol is not. It is not known whether lysophospholipids can be acylated. Fatty acids, which are added to the system, can be used as a substrate by the enzyme, as shown by incorporation of labeled oleate into di- and triglycerides (104). LPL shares the ability to transacylate with pancreatic lipase and with hepatic lipase. The acylation is very prominent under conditions when there is an insufficient amount of fatty acid acceptor in the system. Under such conditions, an equilibrium between the forward and reverse reactions can be reached, and the net reaction becomes dependent on the rate at which monoglycerides are hydrolyzed to give free glycerol.

Action of lipoproteins and other insoluble substrates

When absorbed to a lipoprotein or a lipid droplet, LPL will only see the lipid molecules that are located at the interface. Hamilton and Small (141) have demonstrated that up to about 2.8% triolein can be solubilized in bilayers of egg yolk phosphatidylcholine. A similar amount of triglyceride is probably present in the surface layer on lipoproteins and on phosphatidylcholine-triglyceride droplets. All three acyl chains are extended toward the interior with the conformation such that the primary carbonyls are closer to the aqueous medium than the secondary carbonyl. Thus, the triglycerides are present in the phospholipid layer in an orientation appropriate for enzymatic hydrolysis, and with the second substrate (water) in close proximity.

Several studies have shown that phospholipids and triglycerides are hydrolyzed in parallel by the enzyme, both on natural lipoproteins (131,142,143) and on synthetic emulsions (109,133). The rate of phospholipid hydrolysis is much slower than that of triglyceride hydrolysis, only one or a few percent. It appears that phospholipid and triglyceride hydrolysis are independent processes which are governed by the orientation of the enzyme's active site with respect to the interface, by the enzyme's affinity for the molecular species involved, and by their relative concentrations in the surface layer on the particle. Studies with monolayer systems (119,144–150) have shown that the activity of LPL is critically dependent on how the substrate molecules are organized at the lipid-water interface; the activity varies profoundly with the surface pressure, as well as with the composition of the film.

Foster and Berman (151) developed a mathematical model for LPL-catalyzed hydrolysis of chylomicron glycerides based on data from a study by Scow and Olivecrona (105). One noteworthy feature was that they found it necessary to include a direct pathway from triglyceride to monoglyceride to account for the data. The implication is that most of the diglycerides formed never leave the site of lipolysis but are further hydrolyzed to monoglyceride without mixing back into the bulk of glycerides. This is reasonable since diglycerides are more surface active than triglycerides and will therefore tend to remain in the surface layer of the particle.

LPL is an efficient enzyme with a turnover number of about 1000. The lipoprotein particles that it acts on are, however, large aggregates on the molecular scale. A chylomicron may contain 10^6 triglyceride molecules. Hydrolysis to monoglycerides and fatty acids would require 2×10^6 hydrolytic events. To account for chylomicron turnover *in vivo*, there must be a way to accomplish this hydrolysis in less than 10 minutes. This would require the continuous action of 3–4 LPL molecules, but the particle spends much of its time in the circulating blood. The conclusion is that *in vivo*, many LPL molecules act simultaneously on chylomicra while they are at the endothelium. This must result in a cooperative binding of the lipoprotein particle and may actually hold the chylomicron at the endothelium for a relatively long time, contributing to the efficient metabolism of these particles (compare Figure 6). In contrast, VLDL are much smaller particles and are turned over less rapidly *in vivo*. Their triglycerides could be degraded by a single LPL molecule in one minute. This is a much shorter time than the *in vivo* turnover time which is several hours. Thus, in contrast to the situation with chylomicra, turnover of VLDL can easily be accomplished by a limited number of short interactions with single LPL molecules.

Activator Proteins

Properties

Human apo-CII is a single chain polypeptide of 79 residues (152,153). It is present on plasma chylomicra and on VLDL (154). Thus, the activator is provided together with the lipid substrate, and its interaction with LPL presumably takes place with, or after, binding of the lipoprotein particle to the enzyme. There is no evidence that activation by soluble apo-CII would precede binding of the lipoprotein particle to LPL at the vascular endothelium, or that apo-CII would remain with the enzyme when the lipoprotein particle detaches after a round of lipolysis. As the core of the lipoprotein is depleted of triglyceride, excess surface material is shed from the particle and taken up into the HDL fraction (154). These lipoproteins thus serve as a reservoir of apo-CII from which the activator can move to newly secreted chylomicra/VLDL. In this way the activator is re-used many times.

Individuals with genetic defect of apo-CII, have the clinical syndrome of Type I hyperlipoproteinemia (155), characterized by a massive accumulation of triglyceride-rich lipoproteins in plasma. Another illustration of the importance of apo-CII for LPL action is provided by milk. Milk fat globules can be considered as a type of triglyceride-rich lipoproteins. Although milk contains high levels of LPL, the enzyme can apparently not attack these lipoproteins. If apo-CII is added, lipolysis starts immediately (112).

Jackson et al. (156) have estimated that levels of apo-CII corresponding to only 10% of normal would be sufficient for maximal rate of LPL action. This comes from *in vitro* studies on the action of LPL from bovine milk on model lipid emulsions and on lipoproteins obtained from patients with apo-CII-deficiency. Administration of only a small volume of normal serum to a patient with apo-CII deficiency resulted in a profound lowering of the plasma triglyceride level (155). It has been suggested that the biological role of apo-CII is to serve as a recognition signal for the lipase (7,157). According to this hypothesis, the need for apo-CII restricts the action of LPL to lipoproteins and prevents it from hydrolyzing other lipid droplets, such as milk fat globules. A corollary is that at the levels prevailing in normal plasma apo-CII is probably not a rate limiting factor.

Activator proteins are present on plasma lipoproteins in most mammals (158–164) and on plasma lipoproteins and egg yolk lipoproteins in birds (165–166). There does not seem to be any strict species specificity in the interaction of the lipase with its activator protein. Thus, LPLs from such different sources as chicken adipose tissue (68,167,168), rat heart (169), guinea pig milk (11) and bovine milk (159) are stimulated by human serum, and activator protein from hen's egg yolk lipoproteins can fully stimulate bovine and human LPLs (166). Posner et al. (170) compared the activation of LPLs from human and bovine milk by human apo-CII, and Hayashi et al. (52) made a similar comparison for LPL from human postheparin plasma and LPL from bovine milk. In both studies the K_m for apo-CII was found to be somewhat lower with the bovine than with the human enzyme. In another study, the dose-response relation for activation by human apo-CII was found to be similar for LPLs from bovine milk, guinea pig milk and human postheparin plasma (11). Posner et al. (170) reported that the activity of human LPL was very low in the absence of apo-CII. In the other two studies, the stimulation factor was found to be higher with the human than with the bovine enzyme. Thus, more apo-CII may be needed for optimal action of human LPL than was estimated from model studies with LPL from bovine milk.

Havel et al. (171) reported that there are two common genetic variants of apo-CII in humans. Fojo et al. (172) have shown that there are 4 isoforms of apo-CII in human plasma. Two of these are glycosylated and contain sialic acid. The major isoform is the 79 amino acid, unglycosylated protein previously identified. They designated this isoform proapo-CII. It can undergo proteolytic cleavage of a 6 amino acids peptide from its N-terminal. This cleavage is analogous to that involved in maturation of proapo-AI. They suggest that apo-CII is secreted as a carbohydrate containing proprotein which then undergoes deglycosylation and proteolytic cleavage to generate mature apo-CII, a minor isoform in plasma. The relative effectiveness of the various isoforms as activators of LPL is unknown. In bovine plasma there are also several variants of the activator (164). In hen's egg yolk there are two activator proteins of different sizes (165). The smaller one contains only about 43 amino acid residues. Both of these exist in several charge variants.

In addition to human apo-CII, activator proteins have been purified from porcine serum (173), bovine serum (162,164), and from hen's egg yolk (165). The pig activator is similar to human apo-CII in many respects but does not crossreact immunologically and is inactive after isolation (173). The hen activators differ from apo-CII both in size and in composition (165). Thus, there is a fairly large variation in overall structure between the known activators. Presumably, there are sequence homologies within the molecules, corresponding to a common structure mediating the activation. This hypothesis has received support from studies on the bovine activator (174). This protein is quite different from human apo-CII in amino acid composition and in electrophoretic behavior. However, sequence studies have demonstrated that it is highly homologous to human apo-CII.

The primary structure of apo-CII was first determined by Jackson et al. (152). Some corrections to this structure were later made by Hospattankar et al. (153). In the first structure, one of the residues was not detected. The amino acid sequence number in earlier publications should therefore be increased by one after residue 25. The functional roles of different parts of the molecule have been explored by the use of fragments obtained by selective cleavage of the apolipoprotein (175,176,177) or by solid phase synthesis (144,145,150,176,178,179). These studies indicate that the molecule has two functional parts (180, Figure 8). Residues *1–52*, corresponding to the N-terminal ⅔ of the molecule, appear to be involved with binding to lipoproteins through interaction with surface phospholipids. Modelling, according to Chou and Fassman rules suggested that this region contains three amphipathic helixes, similar in structure to those found in several other apolipoproteins (180,181). The C-terminal third of apo-CII is suggested to be involved with binding to and activation of LPL. This part of the molecule is predicted to contain a β-sheet structure between residues *62–75*. Earlier studies with apo-CII peptides indicated that this part of the molecule was sufficient for activation of LPL (144,176,178,180). In more recent studies using monolayer systems, Vainio et al. (144) and Jackson et al. (150,179) found that at high surface pressures, the apo-CII fragment 51–79 or shorter, were not able to activate. Residues *44–49* were required. The N-α-palmitoyl derivative of apo-CII fragment 56–79 was also active, suggesting that it is the lipid-binding property that is required (179).

cDNA clones corresponding to apo-CII mRNA have been obtained in several laboratories (182,183). The gene structure has also been determined (184). In humans, the gene is on chromosome 19 (183,184). It contains four exons separated by three intervening sequences. This is similar to the organization of the genes for several other apolipoproteins (184). The structure predicted from the nucleic acid sequences indicate that apo-CII, as synthesized, contains a signal peptide preceding the structure of the secreted protein.

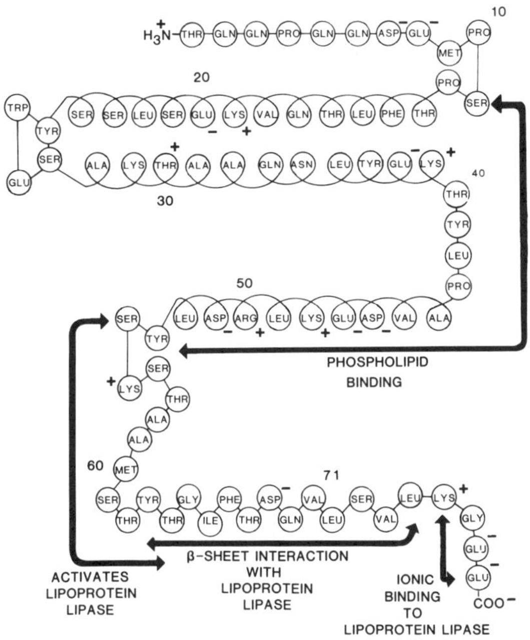

FIGURE 8 *Functional regions of human apolipoprotein CII.* From ref. 180 by permission.

Studies on the physical properties and lipid binding properties of apo-CII indicate that it behaves similarly to other C-apolipoproteins (181,185). In solution, apo-CII tends to aggregate to dimers and possibly higher oligomers. Apo-CII binds avidly to lipid/water interfaces, be they provided as emulsion particles, liposomes, or as a monolayer. The binding is associated with an increase in helical content, presumably signaling formation of the predicted amphipathic helixes (181). The dissociation constant for apo-CII bound to phospholipid stabilized triolein emulsions was found to be 0.45–1.07 μM (186), similar to the dissociation constants for apo-AII and apo-CIII. The maximum binding level was similar for each of these apolipoproteins. Binding of apo-CII to liposomes has also been studied. Dissociation constants of 3 μM and 6.5 μM were obtained with vesicles of dimyristoyl- and dipalmitoyl-phosphatidylcholine, respectively (114,187).

LPL-apo-CII interactions

Clarke and Holbrook (46) studied the interaction of dansylated human apo-CII with LPL from bovine milk. They found that each subunit of the dimeric enzyme binds a single activator molecule with a dissociation constant of 0.2 μM. There was no cooperative effect, i.e. binding of apo-CII to one of the subunits did not change the affinity of the other subunit for apo-

CII. Studies on the effects of apo-CII on LPL activity have generally been interpreted in terms of a 1:1 stoichiometry (25–27,30,130).

Voyta et al. (188) studied the interaction of synthetic apo-CII peptides with LPL. They found significant binding apo-CII fragment 65–79. This peptide does not activate LPL. They concluded that separate sites may be required for binding and for activation (Figure 8). Extension of the peptide with 4 amino acid residues to apo-CII fragment 61–79 resulted in a 10-fold increase in binding affinity. This peptide caused some activation of LPL. Further extension of the peptide did not result in significant increase in binding affinity, but resulted in large increases in the ability to activate the lipase. With the longest peptide studied, apo-CII fragment 44–79 the dissociation constant for interaction with LPL was 2 μM. From a study on hydrolysis of a soluble substrate, Quinn et al. (31) calculated dissociation constants of 0.26–0.83 μM, similar to the value obtained by Clarke and Holbrook (46), 0.2 μM. These studies demonstrate that LPL and apo-CII interact in solution (pathway IV in Figure 9), albeit rather weakly. In the presence of lipid emulsions or lipoproteins, apo-CII will bind to the particles (pathway I), and its concentration in solution will be far too low to drive formation of soluble apo-CII-LPL complexes.

Voyta et al. (188) did not find any effect of high salt concentration on the LPL-apo-CII interaction. In contrast, Clarke and Holbrook (46) found that interaction in solution was weakened by raising the salt concentration and by binding heparin to the enzyme. In the presence of lipid, however, there were no marked effects of salt or of heparin on the LPL-apo-CII interaction.

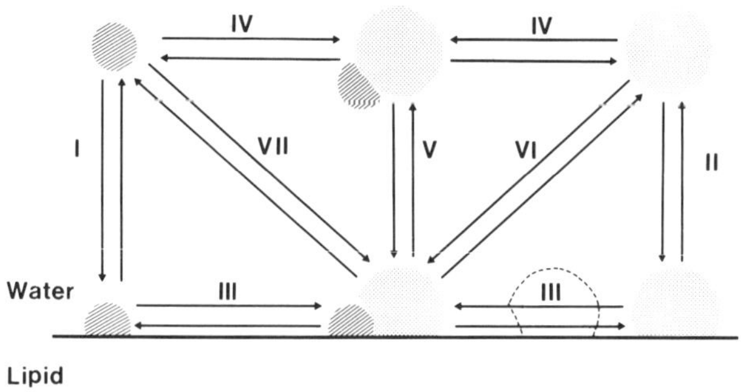

FIGURE 9 *Schematic illustration of the pathways for interaction between LPL, its activator protein, and a lipid-water interface.* The lipase is represented by the larger dotted sphere, the activator by the smaller hatched sphere. The possibility that there is a conformational change in LPL on binding to lipid which enhances its interaction with the activator is illustrated in the lower right part of the figure by a dashed enzyme symbol on pathway III. The figure is not intended to illustrate the interactions of the active site with single substrate molecules, only the overall interactions of the protein molecules. From ref. 7 by permission.

The association of apo-CII with LPL is much tighter in the presence of lipid (pathway III in Figure 9). Voyta et al. (188) determined the dissociation constant for the apo-CII fragment 44–79 to be 50 nM in the presence of lipid. This represented a more than 40-fold increase in affinity over the interaction in solution. Clarke and Holbrook (46) obtained values of 7–10 nM. The interaction between apo-CII and milk LPL has also been estimated from kinetic data. With Intralipid, figures of 40–70 nM (26,130,159) have been reported. Posner et al. (27) reported values around 50 nM. It is of interest to note, however, that not all lipid substrates cause this increase in apparent affinity. The amount of apo-CII required for half-maximal stimulation of hydrolysis of monoolein dispersed in Triton X-100 was 0.34 μM (130), a value similar to that for LPL-apo-CII interaction in solution.

Tajima et al. (25) have studied the interaction between LPL and apo-CII in the presence of phospholipid/triglyceride droplets. The amount of apo-CII needed for half maximal stimulation varied with the size of the lipid droplets and with the concentration of lipid in the system. However, when analyzed in terms of surface density of apo-CII on the particles, the "K_m" values became similar. This suggests that in their system, the main pathway to the complex is that apo-CII and LPL bind independently to the lipid-water interface (pathways I and II in Figure 9), and then use two-dimensional diffusion to find each other (pathway III).

Mechanism of activation

Two main mechanisms have been proposed for this activation. One is that apo-CII induces a conformational change in the lipase, or changes its orientation at the lipid-water interface. There appears to be general agreement that this type of mechanism operates. Another mechanism that has been proposed is that the activator also enhances binding of the lipase to the interface. This is the dominant mechanism for activation of pancreatic lipase by colipase (123,189). Its application to the LPL-apo-CII system is, however, controversial. It is clear that this mechanism does not always come into play, although some investigators claim that it can be of major importance. Jackson and his collaborators, on the other hand, have repeatedly stated that it never operates in the LPL-apo-CII system (30,142,190). We expect that this dispute will turn out to be one of degree and emphasis. This is what has happened to theories on the activation of pancreatic lipase by colipase. Early studies led to the view that the only effect of colipase was to enhance binding of the lipase to the interface. In more recent studies, however, it has become apparent that colipase also enhances the catalytic efficiency of interface-located lipase (123,189). In the following, we will focus on evidence for and against the two types of mechanisms for activation of LPL by apo-CII. Other aspects of the activation have been discussed in a number of recent reviews on LPL (7,30,190,191). More general reviews on enzyme kinetics of lipolysis are also available (115,192).

It is clear that in some systems LPL binds to the substrate droplets without any need for apo-CII. The first direct demonstration that apo-CII can accelerate hydrolysis in such systems was with Intralipid as the substrate (109). More than 90% of the lipase adsorbed to the substrate droplets even in the absence of activator, but the addition of activator accelerated hydrolysis 6-fold. This could not have been accomplished by bringing more enzyme to the interface. Posner and his collaborators reached the same conclusion in studies with another type of triglyceride emulsion (111). Activation of LPL independent of an effect on adsorption to the lipid-water interface has also been demonstrated in monolayer systems. By the use of ^{125}I-labeled LPL, it was possible to simultaneously measure adsorption of LPL to the monolayer, and hydrolysis of lipids in the monolayer. Jackson et al. (119) found that apo-CII decreased the amount of LPL adsorbed to the monolayer, but at the same time increased the rate of hydrolysis. Vainio et al. (144,145) found that over the range of surface pressures they explored, apo-CII did not much change the amount of LPL adsorbed to the monolayer, but increased the rate of hydrolysis. With films of 1,2-didodecanoyl-sn-glycerol-3-phosphoglycerol, apo-CII increased the turnover number for LPL 4-fold at surface pressures below 20 dyn x cm^{-1}. This effect was also obtained with non-lipid binding fragments, e.g. apo-CII fragment 56–79. At higher surface pressures, apo-CII activated in an all-or-none manner. The presence of the phospholipid-binding residues *44–51* in apo-CII fragments was needed for this effect. Similar results on the effects of different apo-CII fragments have subsequently been published by Jackson and his collaborators (150,179).

McLean and Jackson (114) have compared the binding of LPL and of apo-CII to sonicated vesicles of a nonhydrolyzable phosphatidylcholine analogue. The dissociation constant for LPL-lipid complexes was 43 nM, while that for apo-CII-lipid complexes was 3 μM. These data thus suggest that LPL binds more strongly than apo-CII to phosphatidylcholine-water interfaces. Cooperation between the four lipid binding sites on a complex between dimeric LPL and two molecules of apo-CII could, however, result in enhanced binding of the complex to lipid. There may also be conformational changes on formation of LPL-apo-CII complexes, which enhance the binding to lipid.

There is direct evidence that in some systems apo-CII is important for binding of LPL to the substrate droplets. Posner and his collaborators (110,191), studied the action of LPL on triolein in a protein stabilized emulsion. They found that LPL itself was unable to bind to these droplets, and hence it did not hydrolyze the lipids. When apo-CII was added, however, the lipase bound to the droplets and hydrolyzed their triglycerides. We have made similar observations using milk fat globules as the substrate (112,127).

In most studies, however, binding of LPL to the lipid/water interface has not been measured. Interpretation relies on determination of apparent K_m and apparent V_{max}. Depending on the system studied, the results have varied from effects of apo-CII on the K_m with no effect on V_{max}, to effect on V_{max} with no effect on K_m. In some studies apo-CII was found to affect both parameters. Recently, two groups published a collaborative study in which experiments were carried out with different substrates under otherwise identical conditions (156). With a phosphatidylcholine stabilized emulsion of triolein, the effect of apo-CII was almost exclusively on V_{max}, with only a minor change of K_m, whereas in parallel experiments with VLDL from a patient with genetic deficiency of apo-CII the effect of the apo-CII was on K_m with no significant change in V_{max}. It is apparent that one major reason for the discrepancy in previous results relates to differences in the substrates used. It follows that the effect of apo-CII can be manifested in different ways.

Effects of apo-CII on V_{max} have been given two types of interpretation which are not mutually exclusive. One is that the interaction modulates the conformation of the enzyme's active site. Arguments in favor of this comes from detailed analyses of the effects of apo-CII on LPL-catalyzed hydrolysis of soluble substrates (31,193). On the other hand, one must account for the fact that almost as high rates of hydrolysis can be obtained without as with apo-CII (e.g. with trioctanoin or diolein as substrate, see Table 1). Apo-CII may also increase the catalytic efficiency of LPL by changing the orientation of its active site with respect to the interface (7,109,111,144). This is so because the substrate molecules have limited mobilities, except within the interface. This restriction is, however, not the same for all molecules (192). For instance, short-chain triglycerides have more mobility perpendicular to the interface than long-chain triglycerides. The effect of apo-CII is most marked in systems where the substrate molecules are strictly confined to the interface. The effect is pronounced for triolein in phospholipid stabilized droplets, it is less pronounced for diolein, small for trioctanoin, and almost nonexistent for tributyrin (see Table 1). Shinomiya et al. (134,135) have shown that for saturated diacylphosphatidylcholines, the activation factor increases logarithmically with the fatty acyl chain length of the substrate.

It is particularly important to understand the mechanism of activation in systems where the main effect of apo-CII is to lower the apparent K_m of LPL for the lipid substrate, since this appears to be the case with natural lipoproteins (142,156,194–196). The most direct interpretation of a decrease in apparent K_m is that apo-CII enhances binding of LPL to the substrate droplets. The basis for this is that the substrate concentration governing the formation of molecular enzyme-substrate complexes is the two-dimensional concentration of substrate molecules at the lipid-water interface. This quantity does not change when the number of lipid droplets in the system is changed. What may change is the fraction of enzyme adsorbed at the interface. Jackson and his collaborators interpret K_m in a different way (30,142,190). According to their analysis a major determinant for the apparent K_m is the active site occupation factor, i.e. the fraction of the interface-located lipase molecules which are actively engaged in hydrolysis. There seems to be rather general agreement that apo-CII can enhance the catalytic efficiency of LPL by increasing the active site occupation factor. This is implied in the hypotheses that apo-CII brings the active site of the enzyme into its proper orientation at the interface, as related above. The question is whether this would show up in the apparent K_m for emulsified substrates and lipoproteins. Clarke and Holbrook (46) have pointed out that this would require that dissociation from the lipid surface is an obligatory step in each catalytic cycle. In a typical experiment, the molar concentration of lipid particles is 10^{-8}M, and the rate of hydrolysis is 100–1000 molecules of fatty acid per enzyme molecule per second. To satisfy the equation defining K_m the "on-rate" (k_1) must be $10^9 - 10^{10}\ M^{-1} \times s^{-1}$. This rate is unacceptably rapid, since the fastest diffusion-controlled "on-rates" in enzymic reactions, even for small substrates, are of the order of $10^8\ M^{-1} \times s^{-1}$. In order to support the rate of product formation, the enzyme must complete many catalytic cycles before it detaches from the substrate surface. From this, Clarke and Holbrook (46) conclude that any effect of apo-CII on "K_m" must be achieved by altering the affinity of the enzyme for the lipid-water interface. If apo-CII were to influence any other step in the mechanism, a change would occur in the value of V_{max} not K_m.

A unifying hypothesis would be that the role of apo-CII is to ensure that LPL gets into the right orientation at the interface so that its active site has ready access to substrate molecules. This is accomplished by formation of an apo-CII-LPL complex at the lipid-water interface. In some systems, the enzyme itself binds to the interface but does not adequately reach the substrate molecules. The role of apo-CII here is to bring the enzyme into the right orientation. How stringent the requirement is for precise orientation depends on the physical properties of the interface and of the substrate molecules. In other systems, the enzyme itself does not bind to the interface, and the primary role of apo-CII is to bring the enzyme to the interface. Combinations of these situations could explain why activation varies so much with the system studied.

A third possible mechanism for the activation is that the activator changes the organization of the lipid substrate. This is the case for some activators of sphingolipid hydrolyzing enzymes (197), for the activation of bee venom phospholipase by mellitin (198), and for the activation of LCAT by certain apolipoproteins (199). In contrast, there is evidence that the lipid binding portion of apo-CII does not activate LPL (177,180). It has been reported that some apolipoproteins including apo-CII stimulate the activity of snake venom phospholipase against liposomes of dimyristoylphosphatidylcholine (200). Since specific interactions between this enzyme and the apolipoproteins are unlikely, the stimulation is probably due to a perturbing action of the proteins on the lipid packing, analogous to the well known effects of detergents in this and similar systems (115,201). Whether this effect of apo-CII is relevant to its stimulation of LPL activity is not known. A novel type of mechanism which also emphasizes the interaction of apo-CII with the lipid rather than with the enzyme has been proposed by Kinnunen and coworkers (202). In their model, apo-CII acts as an acyl acceptor, facilitating removal of fatty acids from the site of lipolysis. Their evidence is that apo-CII can catalyze hydrolysis of certain water-soluble fatty acid esters and that this action is abolished when serine-61 is blocked by chemical modification. This modification also impedes the effect of apo-CII in the LPL system (144). The rates reported for apo-CII hydrolysis of fatty acid esters are slow, however, 2–3 orders of magnitude lower than the rates for LPL hydrolysis. Furthermore, other apolipoproteins, which do not stimulate LPL, hydrolyze the same fatty acid esters. This proposed mechanism has neither been supported nor refuted by studies in other laboratories.

Other Factors Which Influence LPL Action

Regulation by lipolytic products

Compared to other lipases, LPL seems to be unusually sensitive to product inhibition (7,104). Studies using LPL from milk have shown that several factors contribute to the inhibition, some of which are general for lipases while others are more specific for LPL (104).

The fatty acids and the monoglycerides produced are sparingly water soluble and tend to remain at the surface of the lipid particle, if there is no fatty acid acceptor in the medium (105,203). Thus, a surface layer of fatty acids and monoglycerides (together with phospholipids if originally present on the particle), will be formed. Scow and his collaborators (203) have shown that the lipolytic products can in fact extend the surface of chylomicra into bilayer protrusions. It is not known what the solubility of triglycerides is in such a surface layer. Since the lipolytic products are more surface active the concentration of triglycerides is probably low. Both the fatty acids and the monoglycerides are substrates for the enzyme and compete for its active site (104). Thus, the inhibition can be seen as a change in composition of the interface from predominantly triglycerides (or a mixture of triglycerides and phospholipids) to predominantly fatty acids and monoglycerides. This factor should be operative in product inhibition of other lipases also, but its severity must be related to the enzyme's affinity for the different substrates available at the interface. By inference, LPL may have a relatively high affinity for monoglycerides and fatty acids.

When the fatty acids are not removed from the site of lipolysis, LPL will catalyze the "reverse reaction," i.e. formation of tri- and diglycerides from fatty acids and monoglycerides (104,129,140). Even though it remains catalytically fully competent, the enzyme will spend its time in the non-productive pursuit of hydrolyzing and then reforming glycerides. At pH 8.5, the reverse reaction is almost nonexistent. LPL is, however, strongly inhibited by its products also at this pH (104). Thus, reverse reaction is not the only cause of product inhibition.

As discussed above, LPL binds fatty acids. Formation of enzyme-fatty acid complexes has at least two effects relevant to the product inhibition:

1. Fatty acids interfere with binding of the enzyme to the lipid droplets (104). Less lipase will be associated with the droplets and much of the lipase which remains with the droplets may be sequestered in complex with fatty acids in the surface film or in bilayer extensions of the surface film. It is of interest to note that hydrolysis of monoglycerides is much less sensitive to inhibition by fatty acids than hydrolysis of triglycerides (130). Monoglycerides probably mix freely with the fatty acids and thereby remain accessible to the enzyme.

2. Fatty acids abolish the effects of the activator protein. This occurs both with emulsions of long chain triglycerides (104) and with dispersions of monoglycerides (130).

Product inhibition may be an efficient mechanism for control of LPL action *in vivo* so that products are not formed more rapidly than they can be taken up by the tissue (105,157,203). As soon as fatty acids accumulate, hydrolysis of the lipoprotein lipids slows down, primarily because the lipolysis-promoting effects of the activator protein are abolished. The interaction between LPL and the lipoprotein particle is weakened (104). Consequently, the lipoprotein particle may detach and go back into circulation. Fatty acids also weaken the interaction of LPL with heparin (204). Thus, dissociation of LPL from its endothelial site may be a further adaptation when the tissue can not use fatty acids as quickly as LPL can provide them.

Effects of other proteins

The activity of LPL is inhibited by a variety of proteins. The mechanism of this inhibition has not been explored in detail. It is probably non-specific since inhibition is seen with many different proteins (166). In no case has a specific protein-protein interaction between the lipase and an inhibitory protein been demonstrated. The common denominator seems to be that the proteins bind to the surface of the substrate droplets.

Some proteins, e.g. apolipoproteins, bind reversibly to lipid-water interfaces. Other proteins undergo an irreversible surface denaturation and become unfolded at the interface. This process is favored at high interfacial energy. Thus, it will occur when lipids are emulsified with the protein ("protein stabilized emulsion") or when the lipid is dispersed with emulsifyers with relatively low surface activity, (e.g. gum-arabic), and the emulsion is then incubated with proteins. An example of triglyceride droplets coated with denatured protein that has been used in LPL research is the albumin stabilized emulsion introduced by Posner and his collaborators (94,100,111). Much less unfolding of non-specific proteins takes place at the surface of phospholipid covered triglyceride droplets, since the phospholipids cause a large decrease in surface energy. Binding to such droplets requires specific properties in the protein such as the lipid binding sites on apolipoproteins.

Pancreatic lipase is inhibited by a variety of proteins (205,206). In this case, the inhibitory proteins have been shown to impede binding of the lipase to the lipid droplets. In a study with the hepatic (heparin-releasable) lipase, a similar mechanism was inferred for the inhibition by apolipoproteins AI and AII (207). The binding of these proteins to the lipid emulsion was determined, and the remaining free area at the droplet surface was calculated. It could be shown that the relation between enzyme activity and substrate concentration remained the same if the substrate concentration was expressed in terms of free area available for binding of lipase. It is possible that the inhibition of LPL can be explained at least in part by a similar mechanism. There are reports that the inhibition can be relieved by increasing the amount of lipid substrate, and/or activator protein (166).

Inhibition of LPL by other apolipoproteins is of particular interest because of its possible relevance to lipoprotein metabolism. Jackson et al. (156) have recently studied the mechanism of this inhibition. For this they used a phospholipid stabilized triolein emulsion and LPL from bovine milk. Addition of apo-CIII could cause more than 95% inhibition of the apo-CII stimulated lipolysis. This was found to correlate closely to displacement of apo-CII from the lipid droplets. They point out that previous studies have shown that apo-CII and apo-CIII have similar affinities for phospholipid surfaces (186,187). In their system, a more than 20-fold excess of apo-CIII over apo-CII was required for substantial inhibition. This is far outside the physiological range.

A special case of other proteins is albumin, which is usually added in large amounts to assay systems as fatty acid acceptor. Typically, the system contains less than a microgram of LPL per ml, but 10–100 mg of albumin, a molar ratio of at least 10^4. In unpublished experiments, we have found that preincubation of a gum arabic-trioleoylglycerol emulsion with albumin before LPL is added can cause marked inhibition. This is seen with all albumin preparations and is associated with binding of albumin to the triglyceride droplets. The inhibition increases with the time of preincubation and is promoted by higher temperature, e.g. 37°C compared to 25°C. Like inhibition by other proteins, it is relieved by activator protein, particularly if the activator is added before or with the albumin. Some albumin preparations contain apolipoproteins and phospholipids as contaminants (208). These contaminants have pronounced effects on the lipase reaction in model systems. They have also been a source of complication in studies on *in vitro* transformations of lipoproteins (209).

Inhibition by inorganic salts

One of the first characteristics noted for LPL was that its activity is inhibited by high salt concentration. This property has been used to differentiate LPL from other tissue lipases as well as from the hepatic (heparin-releasable) lipase in post-heparin plasma. However, as discussed by Riley and Robinson (210), there is considerable variation in the extent of inhibition obtained between different laboratories and also in the same laboratory using different assay conditions, different enzyme sources, or enzyme from the same source but at different degrees of purity.

More recently, systems have been described where the activity of LPL is not inhibited by salt, e.g. with a tributyrin emulsion (54), with monolayers of didecanoin (119), with liposomes of dimyristoyl phosphatidylcholine (132) and, under certain conditions, with Intralipid (109,127,166). Thus, the salt inhibition is not exerted directly on the active site reaction. An alternative mechanism was suggested by Fielding and Fielding (211), namely that salt interferes with the enzyme-activator interaction. More recently, however, it has been shown that apo-CII interacts with LPL even at high salt concentration (156,188). Furthermore, apo-CII can stimulate LPL activity at high salt concentration (109,127). These studies suggest that the effect of salt is exerted directly on the enzyme molecule. That the structure of LPL is sensitive to salt is apparent from the rather dramatic changes in its stability and its solubility that result from changes in buffer composition (7).

Considerations of the effect of salt on LPL activity have taken a prominent place in mechanistic discussions of its kinetic properties and its interaction with activator protein. It now appears that the effect of salt is not exerted at this level but rather on the physical state of the enzyme molecule.

Use of LPL From Milk in Studies on the Physiology of the Enzyme and Its Action

In vitro *studies on lipoprotein transformations*

The milk enzyme has been extensively used for *in vitro* studies on the pathways of lipoprotein degradation. The initial studies posed the question: what happens to the surface components on VLDL and chylomicra when the core of the particle is depleted of triglycerides through the action of LPL? The results showed that surface components are shed from the particles (212,213). This includes phospholipids, free cholesterol and the lower molecular weight apolipoproteins (apo-C, apo-E, and in the case of chylomicra also apo-A). The surface components will fuse with HDL particles, if present in the system (214). The surface components will, however, be transferred to the HDL and LDL density ranges even in the absence of acceptor particles (212,213). Thus, acceptor lipoproteins are not required for lipolysis to proceed. The *in vitro* systems made it possible to study the products formed from different subfractions of VLDL (215) to delineate in what proportions, and at what stages of lipolysis, the different surface components leave the lipoprotein (216,217), and to study the relative rates at which individual lipid components are being hydrolyzed as the degradation proceeds from a large triglyceride-rich particle to a remnant (218–220). It has also been used to assess the relative rates at which triglycerides are hydrolyzed in lipoproteins from normal and from hypertriglyceridemic subjects (221,222), and to produce remnant particles for *in vivo* studies (223).

The final products formed *in vitro* from VLDL by LPL alone resembled in many ways native LDL and HDL (214,224). Closer analysis revealed, however, that there were important differences. One important point was that human VLDL usually contain more cholesteryl ester molecules than do LDL particles (225). Since LPL does not hydrolyze cholesteryl esters (218) some other pathway must account for their removal. Model experiments showed that this could be accomplished by coupled core lipid exchange and lipolysis. LDL-like particles obtained by in vitro degradation of human VLDL, or native human LDL, were incubated with lipid transfer protein and with triglyceride-rich particles (225). This resulted in exchange of cholesteryl esters for triglycerides. A second round of lipolysis then removed the triglycerides. This provides a pathway for the LDL-like particles to lose cholesteryl esters. It also points to an important aspect of the system. Since triglycerides are relatively rapidly removed by lipolysis, the size of long-lived lipoprotein particles such as LDL and HDL is to a large extent governed by the amount of cholesteryl esters they contain. This concept has been applied to HDL interconversions (226–230). HDL can gain in size by addition of cholesteryl esters to their core through the LCAT reaction, whereas exchange of cholesteryl esters for triglyceride, followed by lipase action will decrease the size of the particles. Thus, there is a dynamic equilibrium in plasma where triglyceride metabolism has an important role in regulating the size and composition of long-lived cholesterol-rich lipoproteins (228,231). Studies *in vitro* using purified lipases, LCAT, lipid transfer proteins, and other components have thus been able to add to the understanding of the pathways of lipoprotein transformation, and of the interrelationship between different classes of plasma lipoproteins. For a more detailed discussion, the reader is referred to current literature on lipoprotein metabolism.

Lipid transfer activity

Y. and O. Stein and their collaborators studied the transfer of cholesteryl esters from plasma lipoproteins to cells. They noted that cells which produce LPL were more active in this transfer than other cells. To study the role of the lipase, they turned to model experiments where bovine milk LPL was added to cell cultures (232). This addition caused a dramatic increase in the rate of cholesteryl ester transfer; more than 100-fold with some cell types. Further studies have led to the hypothesis that the lipase acts as a cellular receptor for the lipoprotein (233), binding it in the same way as during hydrolysis of lipoprotein triglycerides. Hydrolysis is, however, not a prerequisite for cholesteryl ester transfer which occurs also from chylomicron remnants and from liposomes prepared from non-hydrolyzable analogues of phospholipids (234). Traber et al. (235) have studied a similar process; the transfer of tocopherol from chylomicra to human fibroblasts. In their experiments, addition of bovine milk LPL resulted in hydrolysis of chylomicron triglycerides and transfer of both fatty acids and tocopherol to the cells. In the absence of LPL, no increase in cellular tocopherol was detectable. Heparin abrogated the transfer of tocopherol to fibroblasts without altering the rate of triglyceride hydrolysis, indicating that binding of the lipase to the cells was necessary for transfer. In these studies, the transfer resulted in a many fold increase in cellular tocopherol, as determined by chemical analysis.

It has also been demonstrated that milk LPL enhances the transfer of cholesterol ester from HDL to VLDL which is mediated by cholesteryl ester transfer protein (236). In a similar manner, LPL can cooperate with plasma phospholipid transfer protein to enhance transfer and exchange of phospholipids between VLDL and HDL during lipolysis (237).

Turnover of LPL

The model for binding of LPL at the capillary endothelium via noncovalent interaction with heparan sulfate predicts that there should be some LPL in the circulating blood. This is in fact so. The concentration is about 1 nM (58, 86). To explore the fate of this lipase, we prepared ^{125}I-labeled bovine LPL and injected it intravenously in rats (238). The lipase disappeared within minutes from the blood due to uptake both in the liver (about 50% of the injected dose) and in extrahepatic tissues. Lipase enzyme activity disappeared in parallel to the ^{125}I-radioactivity. Thus, there was no inactivation of LPL in the circulating blood. By use of supradiaphragmatic rats, it could be shown that the extrahepatic uptake was saturable, but that the amount of lipase that could be bound far exceeded the amounts of endogeneous lipase expected to be at the endothelium. When lipase was denatured before injection, its removal in supradiaphragmatic rats became slower, and, in intact rats, the fraction of the uptake that occurred in extrahepatic tissues was much decreased. This suggests that recognition by the extraheptic receptors depends on the native conformation of LPL. The extrahepatic uptake was impeded by injection of heparin prior to injection of the lipase and the uptake could to a large extent be reversed by injection of heparin after the lipase. Even after one hour, LPL that had been taken up by extrahepatic tissues reappeared immediately in the blood on injection of heparin. This was true both for enzyme activity and for enzyme radioactivity. Thus, internalization-inactivation-degradation occurred only slowly in extrahepatic tissues. It seem possible that the extrahepatic binding occurs to the enzyme's physiological receptors. In contrast, the hepatic uptake was not dependent on the native conformation of the lipase, was less sensitive to heparin, and was not saturable. The enzyme was not rapidly inactivated after uptake, its activity could be detected in liver homogenates even after two hours. Degradation to acid soluble products in the liver was relatively slow; the $t_{1/2}$ for native LPL was about one hour. In comparison, asialofetuin was degraded with a $t_{1/2}$ of about 15 minutes. These experiments suggest two important processes (Figure 10). Active lipase may spread throughout the vascular tree from the sites where it is synthesized, but avid uptake in the liver keeps the concentration of LPL low in the circulating blood and, consequently, also in tissues where LPL is not made.

The metabolism of bovine LPL has also been studied in tissue culture (239). Several different types of cells were found to bind the enzyme and

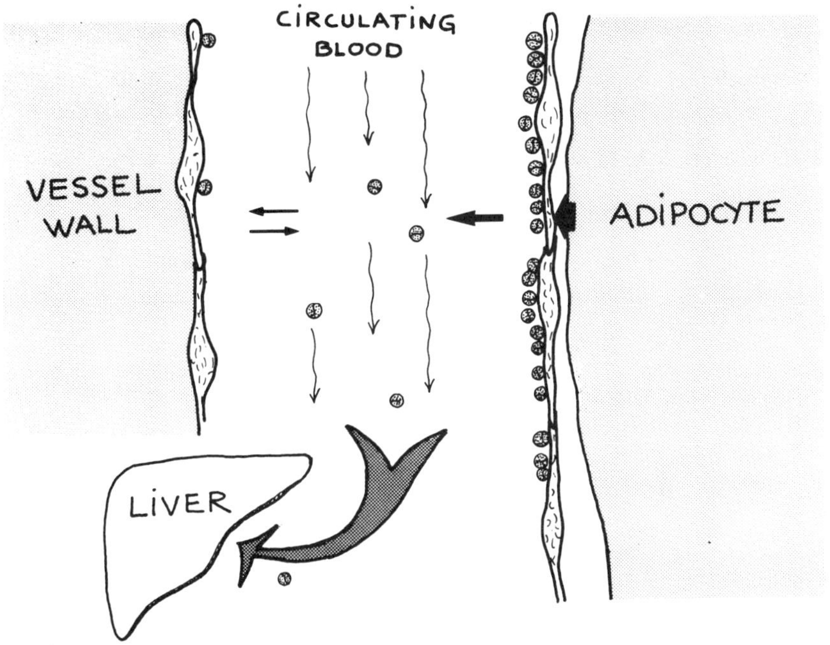

FIGURE 10 *Turnover of LPL.* LPL is produced in parenchymal cells, illustrated here by an adipocyte to the right. The enzyme is then released and transferred to the endothelium where it acts (small, dotted spheres). From here, LPL can dissociate into the blood and then bind to endothelial sites in other tissues as illustrated in the left part of the figure. However, avid uptake by the liver keeps the concentration of LPL low in the blood.

then internalize and degrade it. Interestingly, cells which themselves produce LPL appear to be particularly active in this process. Of the cell types studied thus far, it is only blood cells which do not bind LPL (Bengtsson-Olivecrona, unpublished).

Excellent secretarial assistance by Mrs. Marianne Lundberg is gratefully acknowledged. The original work reported in this review was supported by the Swedish Medical Research Council (grant No. 13X–727).

References

1. Olivecrona, T. 1962. *J. Lipid Res.* 3:439–444.
2. Robinson, D. S. 1963. *Adv. Lipid Res.* 1:133–182.
3. Olivecrona, T., and U. Lindahl. 1969. *Acta Chem. Scand.* 23:3587–3589.
4. Olivecrona, T., T. Egelrud, P. -H. Iverius, and U. Lindahl. 1971. *Biochem. Biophys. Res. Commun.* 43:524–529.
5. Egelrud, T. and T. Olivecrona. 1972. *J. Biol. Chem.* 247:6212–6217

6. Korn, E. D. 1962. *J. Lipid Res.* 3:246–250.
7. Olivecrona, T., and G. Bengtsson. 1984. In "Lipases." B. Borgström and H. Brockman, editors. Elsevier, Amsterdam, 206–261.
8. Enerbäck, S., H. Semb, G. Bengtsson-Olivecrona, P. Carlsson, M. L. Hermanson, T. Olivecrona and G. Bjursell. In preparation.
9. Scow, R. O. and S. S. Chernick. 1986. This book, Chapter 6.
10. Mehta, N. R., J. B. Jones, and M. Hamosh. 1982. *J. Pediatr. Gastroenterol. Nutr.* 1:317–326.
11. Wallinder, L., G. Bengtsson, and T. Olivecrona. 1982. *Biochim. Biophys. Acta* 711:107–113.
12. Semb, H., and T. Olivecrona. 1986. *Biochim. Biophys. Acta.* 878:330–337.
13. Olivecrona, T. 1980. *Int. Dairy Fed. Doc.* 118:19–25.
14. Jensen, R. G., and R. E. Pitas. 1976. *J. Dairy Sci.* 59:1203–1214.
15. Chilliard, Y. 1982. *Le Lait* 62:1–31 and 126–154.
16. Sundheim, G. and G. Bengtsson-Olivecrona. 1986. *J. Dairy Sci.* 69:1776–1783.
17. Downey, W. K., and R. F. Murphy. 1975. *Int. Dairy Fed. Doc.* 86:19–23.
18. Hernell, O., and T. Olivecrona. 1974. *J. Lipid Res.* 15:367–374.
19. Bengtsson-Olivecrona, G., and T. Olivecrona. In preparation.
20. Kinnunen, P. K. J. 1977. *Med. Biol.* 55:187–191.
21. Socorro, L., C. C. Green, and R. L. Jackson. 1985. *Prep. Biochem* 15:133–143.
22. Iverius, P. -H., and A. -M. Östlund-Lindqvist. 1976. *J. Biol. Chem.* 251:7791–7795.
23. Iverius, P. -H., and A. -M. Östlund-Lindqvist. 1986. *Methods Enzymol.* 129:691–704.
24. Clarke, A. R., M. Luscombe, and J. J. Holbrook. 1983. *Biochim. Biophys. Acta* 747:130–137.
25. Tajima, S., S. Yokoyama, and A. Yamamoto. 1984. *J. Biochem.* 96:1753–1767.
26. Havel, R. J., C. J. Fielding, T. Olivecrona, V. G. Shore, P. E. Fielding, and T. Egelrud. 1973. *Biochemistry* 12:1828–1833.
27. Posner, I., C. -S. Wang, and W. J. McConathy. 1983. *Arch. Biochem. Biophys.* 226:306–316.
28. Fielding, C. J. 1969. *Biochim. Biophys. Acta* 178:499–507.
29. Socorro, L., and R. L. Jackson. 1985. *J. Biol. Chem.* 260:6324–6328.
30. Quinn, D., K. Shirai, and R. L. Jackson. 1983. *Prog. Lipid Res.* 22:35–78.
31. Quinn, D. M., K. Shirai, R. L. Jackson, and J. A. K. Harmony. 1982. *Biochemistry* 21:6872–6879.
32. Socorro, L., D. M. Quinn, and R. L. Jackson. 1983. *Arteriosclerosis* 3:494a (abstract).
33. Fransson, L.-Å. 1985. In "The polysaccharides Vol VII." G. O. Aspinall, editor. Academic Press, New York. 337–415.
34. Miller-Andersson, M., H. Borg, and L. -O. Andersson. 1974. *Thromb. Res.* 5:439–452.
35. McKay, E. J., A. B. Laurell, U. Maartensson, and A. G. Sjoeholm. 1981. *Mol. Immunol.* 18:349–357.
36. Iverius, P. -H. 1972. *J. Biol. Chem.* 247:2607–2613.
37. Quarfordt, S. H., R. S. Jain, L. Jakoi, S. Robinson, and F. Shelburne. 1978. *Biochem. Biophys. Res. Commun.* 83:786–793.
38. Sternbach, H., R. Engelhardt, and A. G. Lezius. 1975. *Eur. J. Biochem.* 60:51–55.
39. Brennessel, B. A., D. P. Buhrer, and A. A. Gottlieb. 1978. *Anal. Biochem.* 87:411–417.
40. Bläckberg, L., and O. Hernell. 1980. *FEBS Lett.* 109:180–184.
41. Bläckberg, L., and O. Hernell. 1981. *Eur. J. Biochem.* 116:221–225.
42. Thim, L. 1978. *Scand. J. Clin. Lab. Invest.* 38:71–81.
43. Östlund-Lindqvist, A. -M., and J. Boberg. 1977. *FEBS Lett.* 82:231–236.
44. Osborne, J. C. Jr., G. Bengtsson-Olivecrona, N. Lee, and T. Olivecrona. 1985. *Biochemistry* 24:5606–5611.
45. Olivecrona, T., G. Bengtsson-Olivecrona, J. C. Osborne Jr., and E. S. Kempner. 1985. *J. Biol. Chem.* 260:6888–6891.
46. Clarke, A. R., and J. J. Holbrook. 1985. *Biochim. Biophys. Acta* 827:358–368.

47. Reddy, M. N., J. M. Maraganore, S. C. Meredith, R. Heinrikson, and F. J. Kezdy. 1986. *J. Biol. Chem.* 261:9678–9683.
48. Bengtsson-Olivecrona, G., and T. Olivecrona. 1985. *Biochem. J.* 226:409–413.
49. Olivecrona, T., G. Bengtsson, and J. C. Osborne Jr. 1982. *Eur. J. Biochem.* 124:629–633.
50. Ben-Avram, C. M., O. Ben-Zeev, T. D. Lee, K. Haaga, J. E. Shively, J. Goers, M. E. Pedersen, J. R. Reeve Jr., and M. C. Schotz. 1986. *Proc. Natl. Acad. Sci. USA* 83:4185–4189.
51. Bengtsson-Olivecrona, G., T. Olivecrona, and H. Jörnvall. 1986. *Eur. J. Biochem.* 161:281–288.
52. Hayashi, R., S. Tajima, and A. Yamamoto. 1986. *J. Biochem.* (*Tokyo*) 100:319–331.
53. Bengtsson, G., and T. Olivecrona. 1981. *Eur. J. Biochem.* 113:547–554.
54. Rapp, D., and T. Olivecrona. 1978. *Eur. J. Biochem.* 91:379–385.
55. Bengtsson, G., and T. Olivecrona. 1981. *FEBS Lett.* 128:9–12.
56. Olivecrona, T., S. S. Chernick, G. Bengtsson-Olivecrona, J. R. Paterniti Jr., V. W. Brown, and R. O. Scow. 1985. *J. Biol. Chem.* 260:2552–2557.
57. Semb, H., J. Peterson, J. Tavernier, and T. Olivecrona. 1987. *J. Biol. Chem.* In press.
58. Peterson, J., T. Olivecrona, and G. Bengtsson-Olivecrona. 1985. *Biochim. Biophys. Acta* 837:262–270.
59. Semb, H., and T. Olivecrona. 1986. *Biochim. Biophys. Acta* 876:249–255.
60. Jonasson, L., G. K. Hansson, G. Bondjers, G. Bengtsson, and T. Olivecrona. 1984. *Atherosclerosis* 51:313–326.
61. Blanchette-Mackie, E. J., T. Olivecrona, N. K. Dwyer and R. O. Scow. 1985. *J. Cell Biol.* 441a (abstract).
62. Olivecrona, T., and G. Bengtsson. 1983. *Biochim. Biophys. Acta* 752:38–45.
63. Hernell, O., T. Egelrud, and T. Olivecrona. 1975 *Biochim. Biophys. Acta* 381:233–241.
64. Shirai, K., D. A. Wisner, J. D. Johnson, L. S. Srivastava, and R. L. Jackson. 1982. *Biochim. Biophys. Acta* 712:10–20.
65. Enholm, C., P. K. J. Kinnunen, J. K. Huttunen, E. A. Nikkilä, and M. Ohta. 1975. *Biochem. J.* 149:649–655.
66. Voyta, J. C., D. P. Via, P. K. J. Kinnunen, J. T. Sparrow, A. M. Gotto Jr., and L. C. Smith. 1985. *J. Biol. Chem.* 260:893–898.
67. Vannier, C., E. -Z. Amir, J. Etienne, R. Negrel, and G. Ailhaud. 1985. *J. Biol. Chem.* 260:4424–4431.
68. Egelrud, T. 1973. *Biochim. Biophys. Acta* 296:124–129.
69. Olivecrona, T., G. Bengtsson, S. E. Marklund, U. Lindahl, and M. Höök. 1977. *Fed. Proc.* 36:60–65.
70. Iverius, P.-H., U. Lindahl, T. Egelrud, and T. Olivecrona. 1972. *J. Biol. Chem.* 247:6610–6616.
71. Lindahl, U., and M. Höök. 1978. *Ann. Rev. Biochem.* 47:385–417.
72. Bengtsson, G., and T. Olivecrona. 1977. *Biochem. J.* 167:109–119.
73. Olivecrona, T., and G. Bengtsson. 1978. In "International Conference on Atherosclerosis." L. A. Carlson, editor. Raven Press, New York. 153–157.
74. Jackson, R. L., L. Socorro, G. M. Fletcher, and A. D. Cardin. 1985. *FEBS Lett.* 190:297–300.
75. Shirai, K., N. Matsuoka, and R. L. Jackson. 1981. In "Chemistry and Biology of Heparin." R. L. Lundblad, W. V. Brown and H. R. Roberts, editors. Elsevier, Amsterdam. 195–205.
76. Höök, M., I. Björk, J. Hopwood, and U. Lindahl. 1976. *FEBS Lett.* 66:90–93.
77. Bengtsson, G., T. Olivecrona, M. Höök, and U. Lindahl. 1977. *FEBS Lett.* 79:59–63.
78. Bengtsson, G., T. Olivecrona, M. Höök, J. Riesenfeld, and U. Lindahl. 1980. *Biochem. J.* 189:625–633.
79. Klinger, M. M., R. U. Margolis, and R. K. Margolis. 1985. *J. Biol. Chem.* 260:4082–4090.
80. Shimada, K., P. -J. Gill, J. E. Silbert, W. H. J. Douglas, and B. L. Fanburg. 1981. *J. Clin. Invest.* 68:995–1002.
81. Wang-Iverson, P., and W. V. Brown. 1982. *Ann. New York Acad. Sci.* 401:92–101.

82. Cheng, C. -F., G. M. Oosta, A. Bensadoun, and R. D. Rosenberg. 1981. *J. Biol. Chem.* 256:12893–12898.
83. Williams, M. P., H. B. Streeter, F. S. Wusteman, and A. Cryer. 1983. *Biochim. Biophys. Acta* 756:83–91.
84. Cryer, A. 1983. In "Biochemical Interactions at the endothelium." A. Cryer, editor. Elsevier, Amsterdam. 245–247.
85. Cryer, A. 1985. *Biochem. Soc. Trans.* 13:27–28.
86. Chajek-Shaul, T., G. Friedman, O. Stein, J. Etienne, and Y. Stein. 1985. *Biochim. Biophys. Acta* 837:271–278.
87. Marcum, J. A., D. A. Atha, L. M. S. Fritze, P. Nawroth, D. Stern, and R. D. Rosenberg. 1986. *J. Biol. Chem.* 261:7507–7517.
88. Robinson-White, A., S. B. Baylin, T. Olivecrona, and M. A. Beaven. 1985. *J. Clin. Invest.* 76:93–100.
89. Marklund, S., and K. Karlsson. 1987. *Biochem. J.* In press.
90. Shimada, K. and T. Ozawa. 1985. *J. Clin. Invest.* 75:1308–1316.
91. Fransson, L.- Å., I. Carlstedt, L. Cöster, and A. Malmström. 1986. In preparation.
92. Yamamoto, T., C. G. Davis, M. S. Brown, W. J. Schneider, M. L. Casey, J. L. Goldstein, and D. W. Russell. 1984. *Cell* 39:27–38.
93. Clark, A. B., and S. H. Quarfordt. 1985. *J. Biol. Chem.* 260:4778–4783.
94. Posner, I., and A. D. Morrison. 1979. *Acta Cient. Venezolana* 30:152–161.
95. Brown, W. V., P. Wang-Iverson, and J. R. Paterniti. 1981. In "Chemistry and Biology of Heparin." R. L. Lundblad, W. V. Brown, K. G. Mann and H. R. Roberts, editors. Elsevier/North-Holland, New York. 175–185.
96. Shirai, K., and R. L. Jackson. 1982. *J. Biol. Chem.* 257:1253–1258.
97. Shirai, K., N. Matsuoka, and R. L. Jackson. 1981. *Biochim. Biophys. Acta* 665:504–510.
98. Wang-Iverson, P., E. A. Jaffe, and W. V. Brown. 1980. In "Atherosclerosis V." A. M. Gotto, L. C. Smith and B. Allen, editors. Springer-Verlag, New York, 375–378.
99. Fielding, C. J. 1968. *Biochim. Biophys. Acta* 159:94–102.
100. Baginsky, M. L., and W. V. Brown. 1977. *J. Lipid Res.* 18:423–437.
101. Bengtsson, G., and T. Olivecrona. 1979. *Biochim. Biophys. Acta* 575:471–474.
102. Helenius, A., and K. Simons. 1977. *Proc. Natl. Acad. Sci. USA* 74:529–532.
103. Parkin, S. M., B. K. Speake, and D. S. Robinson. 1982. *Biochem. J.* 207:485–495.
104. Bengtsson, G., and T. Olivecrona. 1980. *Eur. J. Biochem* 106:557–562.
105. Scow, R. O., and T. Olivecrona. 1977. *Biochim. Biophys. Acta* 487:472–486.
106. Bengtsson, G., and T. Olivecrona. 1982. *Biochim. Biophys. Acta* 712:196–199.
107. El-Magrabi, M. R., M. Waite, L. L. Rudel, and P. Sisson. 1978. *J. Biol. Chem.* 253:947–981.
108. Jackson, R. L., N. Matsuoka, and J. A. K. Harmony. 1979. *FEBS Lett.* 105:53–57.
109. Bengtsson, G., and T. Olivecrona. 1980. *Eur. J. Biochem.* 106:549–555.
110. Posner, I., and A. D. Morrison. 1979. *Acta Cient. Venezolana* 30:143–151.
111. Posner, I. 1980. *Acta Cient. Venezolana* 31:318–323.
112. Bengtsson, G., and T. Olivecrona. 1982. *FEBS Lett.* 147:183–187.
113. McLean, L. R., W. J. Larsen, and R. L. Jackson. 1986. *Biochemistry* 25:873–878.
114. McLean, L. R., and R. L. Jackson. 1985. *Biochemistry* 24:4196–4201.
115. Verger, R. 1980. *Methods Enzymol.* 64:340–392.
116. Shinomiya, M. and R. L. Jackson. 1983. *Biochim. Biophys. Res. Commun.* 113:811–816.
117. Wittenauer, L. A., K. Shirai, R. L. Jackson, and J. D. Johnson. 1984. *Biochem. Biophys. Res. Commun.* 118:894–901.
118. Bengtsson, G., and T. Olivecrona. 1983. *FEBS Lett.* 154:211–213.
119. Jackson, R. L., F. Pattus, and G. De Haas. 1980. *Biochemistry* 19:373–378.
120. Quinn, D. M. 1985. *Biochemistry* 24:3144–3149.
121. Vainio, P., J. A. Virtanen, and P. K. J. Kinnunen. 1982. *Biochim. Biophys. Acta* 711:386–390.
122. Puinn, D. M. 1985. *Biochim. Biophys. Acta* 834:267–271.

123. Verger, R. 1984. In "Lipases." B. Borgstöm and H. Brockman, editors. Elsevier, Amsterdam. 83–184.
124. Docherty, A. J. P., M. Bodmer, S. Angal, R. Verger, C. Riviere, P. Lowe, A. Lyons, J. Emtage, and T. Harris. 1985. *Nucleic Acids Res.* 13:1891–1903.
125. McLean, J., C. Fielding, D. Drayna, H. Dieplinger, B. Baer, W. Kohr, W. Henzel, and R. Lawn. 1986. *Proc. Natl. Acad. Sci. USA* 83:2335–2339.
126. Egelrud, T. and T. Olivecrona. 1973. *Biochim. Biophys. Acta* 306:115–127.
127. Bengtsson, G., and T. Olivecrona. 1983. *Biochim. Biophys. Acta* 751:254–259.
128. Olivecrona, T., and G. Bengtsson-Olivecrona. 1986. In "Atherosclerosis VII." N. H. Fidge and P. J. Nestel, editors. Elsevier, Amsterdam. 201–204.
129. Nilsson-Ehle, P., T. Egelrud, P. Belfrage, T. Olivecrona, and B. Borgström. 1973. *J. Biol. Chem.* 248:6734–6737.
130. Bengtsson, G., and T. Olivecrona. 1979. *FEBS Lett.* 106:345–348.
131. Scow, R. O., and T. Egelrud. 1976. *Biochim. Biophys. Acta* 431:538–549.
132. Muntz, H. G., N. Matsuoka, and R. L. Jackson. 1979. *Biochem. Biophys. Res. Commun.* 90:15–21.
133. Stocks, J., and D. Galton. 1980. *Lipids* 15:186–190.
134. Shinomiya, M., L. R. McLean, and R. L. Jackson. 1983. *J. Biol. Chem.* 258:14178–14180.
135. Shinomiya, M., R. L. Jackson, and L. R. McLean. 1984. *J. Biol. Chem.* 259:8724–8728.
136. Morely, N., and A. Kuksis. 1972. *J. Biol. Chem.* 247:6389–6393.
137. Paltauf, F., F. Esfandi, and A. Holasek. 1974. *FEBS Lett.* 40:119–123.
138. Åkesson, B., S. Gronowitz, B. Herslöf, P. Michelsen, and T. Olivecrona. 1983. *Lipids* 18:313–318.
139. El- Magrabi, R., M. Waite, and L. L. Rudel. 1978. *Biochem. Biophys. Res. Commun.* 81:82–88.
140. Borgström, B., and L. A. Carlson. 1957. *Biochim. Biophys. Acta* 24:638–639.
141. Hamilton, J. A., and D. M. Small. 1981. *Proc. Natl. Acad. Sci. USA* 78:6878–6882.
142. Fitzharris, T. J., D. M. Quinn, E. H. Goh, J. D. Johnson, M. L. Kashyap, L. S. Srivastava, R. L. Jackson, and J. A. K. Harmony. 1981. *J. Lipid Res.* 22:921–933.
143. Eisenberg, S., and D. Shurr. 1976. *J. Lipid Res.* 17:578–587.
144. Vainio, P., J. A. Virtanen, P. K. J. Kinnunen, J. C. Voyta, L. C. Smith, A. M. Gotto Jr., J. T. Sparrow, F. Pattus, and R. Verger. 1983. *Biochemistry* 22:2270–2275.
145. Vainio, P., J. A. Virtanen, P. K. J. Kinnunen, A. M. Gotto, J. T. Sparrow, F. Pattus, P. Bougis, and R. Verger. 1983. *J. Biol. Chem.* 258:5477–5482.
146. Demel, R. A., K. Shirai, and R. L. Jackson. 1982. *Biochim. Biophys. Acta* 713:629–637.
147. Demel, R. A., P. J. Dings, and R. L. Jackson. 1984. *Biochim. Biophys. Acta* 793:399–407.
148. Demel, R. A., and R. L. Jackson. 1985. *J. Biol. Chem.* 260:9589–9592.
149. Jackson, R. L., and R. A. Demel. 1985. *Biochem. Biophys. Res. Commun.* 128:670–675.
150. Jackson, R. L., A. Balasubramaniam, R. F. Murphy, and R. A. Demel. 1986. *Biochim. Biophys. Acta* 875:203–210.
151. Foster, D. M., and M. Berman. 1981. *J. Lipid Res.* 22:506–513.
152. Jackson, R. L., H. N. Baker, E. B. Gilliam, and A. M. Gotto. 1977. *Proc. Natl. Acad. Sci. USA* 74:1942–1945.
153. Hospattankar, A. V., T. Fairwell, R. Ronan, and H. B. Brewer Jr. 1984. *J. Biol. Chem.* 259:318–322.
154. Havel, R. J., J. P. Kane, and M. L. Kashyap. 1973. *J. Clin. Invest.* 52:32–38.
155. Breckenridge, W. C., J. A. Little, G. Steiner, A. Chow, and M. Poapst. 1978. *N. Engl. J. Med.* 298:1265–1273.
156. Jackson, R. L., S. Tajima, T. Yamamura, S. Yokoyama, and A. Yamamoto. 1986. *Biochim. Biophys. Acta* 875:211–219.
157. Olivecrona, T., and G. Bengtsson-Olivecrona. 1987. In "The Biology and Clinical Science of Atherosclerosis." A. Olsson, editor. Churchill Livingstone, London. In press.
158. LaRosa, J. C., R. I. Levy, P. Herbert, S. E. Lux, and D. S. Fredrickson. 1970. *Biochem. Biophys. Res. Commun.* 41:57–62.

159. Havel, R. J., V. G. Shore, B. Shore, and D. M. Bier. 1970. *Circulat. Res.* 27:595–600.
160. Herbert, P. N., H. B. Windmueller, T. P. Bersot, and R. S. Shulman. 1974. *J. Biol. Chem.* 249:5718–5724.
161. Knipping, G. M., G. M. Kostner, and A. Holasek. 1975. *Biochim. Biophys. Acta* 393:88–99.
162. Lim, C. T., and A. M. Scanu. 1976. *Artery* 2:483–496.
163. Clegg, R. A. 1978. *Biochem. Soc. Trans.* 6:1207–1210.
164. Astrup, H. N., and G. Bengtsson. 1982. *Comp. Biochem. Physiol.* 72B:487–491.
165. Bengtsson, G., S. -E. Marklund, and T. Olivecrona. 1977. *Eur. J. Biochem.* 79:211–223.
166. Bengtsson, G., and T. Olivecrona. 1977. *Eur. J. Biochem.* 79:225–231.
167. Korn, E. D., and T. W. Quigley. 1957. *J. Biol. Chem.* 226:833–839.
168. Gershenwald, J. E., A. Bensadoun, and A. Saluja. 1985. *Biochim. Biophys. Acta* 836:286–295.
169. Twu, J. S., A. S. Garfinkel, and M. C. Schotz. 1975. *Atherosclerosis* 22:463–472.
170. Posner, I., C. -S. Wang, and W. J. McConathy. 1985. *Comp. Biochem. Physiol.* 80B:171–174.
171. Havel, R. J., L. Kotile, and J. P. Kane. 1979. *Biochem. Med.* 21:121–128.
172. Fojo S. S., L. Taam, T. Fairwell, R. Ronan, C. Bishop, M. S. Meng, J. M. Hoeg, D. L. Sprecher, and H. B. Brewer, Jr. 1986. *J. Biol. Chem.* 261:9591–9594.
173. Jackson, R. L., B. H. Chung, L. C. Smith, and O. D. Taunton. 1977. *Biochim. Biophys. Acta* 490:385–394.
174. Bengtsson-Olivecrona, G., and K. Sletten. In preparation.
175. Musliner, T. A., E. C. Church, P. N. Herbert, M. J. Kingston, and R. S. Shulman. 1977. *Proc. Natl. Acad. Sci. USA* 74:5358–5362.
176. Kinnunen, P. K. J., R. L. Jackson, L. C. Smith, A. M. Gotto, and J. T. Sparrow. 1977. *Proc. Natl. Acad. Sci. USA* 74:4848–4851.
177. Musliner, T. A., P. N. Herbert, and E. C. Church. 1979. *Biochim. Biophys. Acta* 573:501–509.
178. Catapano, A. L., P. K. J. Kinnunen, W. C. Breckenridge, A. M. Gotto, R. L. Jackson, J. A. Little, L. C. Smith, and J. T. Sparrow. 1979. *Biochem. Biophys. Res. Commun.* 89:951–957.
179. Balasubramaniam, A., A. Rechtin, L. R. McLean, and R. L. Jackson. 1986. *Biochem. Biophys. Res. Commun.* 137:1041–1048.
180. Smith, L. C. and H. J. Pownall. 1984. In "Lipases" B. Borgström and H. L. Brockman, editors. Elsevier, Amsterdam. 263–305.
181. Mantulin, W. W., M. F. Rohde, A. M. Gotto Jr., and H. J. Pownall. 1980. *J. Biol. Chem.* 255:8185–8191.
182. Myklebost, O., B. Williamson, A. F. Markham, S. R. Myklebost, J. Rogers, D. E. Woods, and S. E. Humphries. 1984. *J. Biol. Chem.* 259:4401–4404.
183. Jackson, C. L., G. A. P. Bruns, and J. L. Breslow. 1984. *Proc. Natl. Acad. Sci. USA* 81:2945–2949.
184. Wei, C. -F., Y. -K. Tsao, D. L. Robberson, A. M. Gotto Jr., K. Brown, and L. Chan. 1985. *J. Biol. Chem.* 260:15211–15221.
185. Tajima, S., S. Yokoyama, Y. Kawai, and A. J. Yamamoto. 1982. *J. Biochem* 91:1273–1279.
186. Tajima, S., S. Yokoyama, and A. Yamamoto. 1983. *J. Biol. Chem.* 258:10073–10082.
187. Cardin, A. D., R. L. Jackson and J. D. Johnson. 1982. *J. Biol. Chem.* 257:4987–4992.
188. Voyta, J. C., P. Vainio, P. K. J. Kinnunen, A. M. Gotto Jr., J. T. Sparrow, and L. C. Smith. 1983. *J. Biol. Chem.* 258:2934–2939.
189. Borgström, B., and C. Erlanson-Albertsson. 1984. In "Lipases." B. Borgström and H. L. Brockman, editors. Elsevier, Amsterdam. 131–184.
190. McLean, L. R., R. A. Demel, L. Socorro, M. Shinomiya, and R. L. Jackson. 1986. *Methods in Enzymology* 129:738–763.
191. Posner, I. 1982. *Atheroscler. Rev.* 9:123–156.

192. Brockman, H. L. 1984. In "Lipases," B. Borgström and H. L. Brockman, editors. Elsevier, Amsterdam. 3–46.
193. Shirai, K., R. L. Jackson, and D. M. Quinn. 1982. *J. Biol. Chem.* 257:10200–10203.
194. Shirai, K., T. J. Fitzharris, M. Shinomiya, H. G. Muntz, J. A. K. Harmony. R. L. Jackson, and D. M. Quinn. 1983. *J. Lipid Res.* 24:721–730.
195. Matsuoka, N., K. Shirai, J. D. Johnson, M. L. Kashyap, L. S. Srivastava, T. Yamamura, A. Yamamoto, Y. Saito, A. Kumagai, and R. L. Jackson. 1981. *Metabolism* 30:818–824.
196. Catapano, A. L., P. K. J. Kinnunen, and A. Capurso. 1982. Abstr.21 W, "6th Int. Symp. Atherosclerosis, Berlin."
197. Li, S. -C., and Y. -T. Li. 1976. *J. Biol. Chem.* 251:1159–1163.
198. Mollay, C., G. Kreil and H. Berger. 1976. *Biochim. Biophys. Acta* 426:317–324.
199. Jonas, A. 1986. *J. Lipid Res.* 27:689–698.
200. Bengtsson, G., and T. Olivecrona. 1982. *FEBS Lett.* 140:135–138.
201. Verheij, A. M., A. J. Slotboom, and G.H. de Haas. 1981. *Rev. Physiol. Biochem. Pharmacol.* 91:91–203.
202. Kinnunen, P. K. J., J. A. Virtanen, and P. Vainio. 1983. *Atherosclerosis Reviews* 11:65–105.
203. Scow, R. O., and J. Blanchette-Mackie. 1985. *Prog. Lipid Res.* 24:197–241.
204. Olivecrona, T., and G. Bengtsson-Olivecrona. 1985. In "Atheroma and Thrombosis." V. V. Kakkar, editor. Pitman, London. 250–256.
205. Borgström, B., and C. Erlanson. 1978. *Gastroenterology* 75:382–386.
206. Gargouri, Y., G. Pieroni, C. Riviére, A. Sugihara, L. Sarda, and R. Verger. 1985. *J. Biol. Chem.* 260:2268–2273.
207. Kubo, M., Y. Matsuzawa, S. Yokoyama, S. Tajima, K. Ishikawa, A. Yamamoto, and S. Tarui. 1982. *J. Biochem.* 92:865–870.
208. Fainaru, M., and R. J. Deckelbaum. 1979. *FEBS Lett.* 97:171–174.
209. Deckelbaum, R. J., T. Olivecrona, and M. Fainaru. 1980. *J. Lipid Res.* 21:425–434.
210. Riley, S. E., and D. S. Robinson. 1974. *Biochim. Biophys. Acta* 369:371–386.
211. Fielding, C. J., and P. E. Fielding. 1976. *J. Lipid Res.* 17:248–256.
212. Glangeauld, M. C., S. Eisenberg, and T. Olivecrona. 1977. *Biochim. Biophys. Acta* 486:23–35.
213. Schaefer, E. J., M. G. Wetzel, G. Bengtsson-Olivecrona, R. O. Scow, H. B. Brewer, and T. Olivecrona. 1982. *J. Lipid Res.* 23:1259–1273.
214. Patsch, J. R., A. M. Gotto, T. Olivecrona, and S. Eisenberg. 1978. *Proc. Natl. Acad. Sci. USA* 75:4519–4523.
215. Oschry, T., T. Olivecrona, R. J. Deckelbaum, and S. Eisenberg. 1985. *J. Lipid Res.* 26:158–167.
216. Eisenberg, S., and T. Olivecrona. 1979. *J. Lipid Res.* 20:614–623.
217. Eisenberg, S., J. R. Patsch, J. T. Sparrow, A. M. Gotto, and T. Olivecrona. 1979. *J. Biol. Chem.* 254:12603–12608.
218. Wang, C. -S., D. Weiser, P. Alaupovic, and W. J. McConathy. 1982. *Arch. Biochem. Biophys.* 214:26–34.
219. Deckelbaum, R. J. In preparation.
220. Nilsson, Å., B. Landin, and M. C. Schotz. In preparation.
221. Taskinen, M. -R., J. D. Johnson, M. L. Kashyap, K. Shirai, C. J. Glueck, and R. L. Jackson. 1981. *J. Lipid. Res.* 22:382–386.
222. Chung, B. H., and J. P. Segrest. 1986. *Methods Enzymol.* 129:704–716.
223. Chajek-Shaul, T., S. Eisenberg, Y. Oschry, and T. Olivecrona. 1983. *J. Lipid Res.* 24:831–840.
224. Deckelbaum, R. J., S. Eisenberg, M. Fainaru, Y. Barenholz, and T. Olivecrona. 1979. *J. Biol. Chem.* 254:6079–6087.
225. Deckelbaum, R. J., S. Eisenberg, Y. Oschry, E. Butul, I. Sharon, and T. Olivecrona. 1982. *J. Biol. Chem.* 257:6509–6517.

226. Granot, E., R. J. Deckelbaum, S. Eisenberg, Y. Oschry, and G. Bengtsson-Olivecrona. 1985. *Biochim. Biophys. Acta* 833:308–315.
227. Deckelbaum, R. J., S. Eisenberg, Y. Oschry, E. Granot, I. Sharon, and G. Bengtsson-Olivecrona. 1986. *J. Biol. Chem.* 261:5201–5208.
228. Patsch, J., S. Prasad, A. M. Gotto Jr., and G. Bengtsson-Olivecrona. 1984. *J. Clin. Invest.* 74:2017–2023.
229. Barter, P. J., G. J. Hopkins, O. V. Rajaram, and K. -A. Rye. 1986. In "Atherosclerosis VII." N. H. Fidge and P. J. Nestel, editors. Elsevier, Amsterdam. 187–190.
230. Knipping, G., R. Zechner, G. M. Kostner, and A. Holasek. 1985. *Biochim. Biophys. Acta* 835:244–252.
231. Deckelbaum, R. J., T. Olivecrona, and S. Eisenberg. 1984. In "Treatment of Hyperlipoproteinemia." L. A. Carlson and A. G. Olsson, editors. Raven Press, New York. 85–93.
232. Friedman, G., T. Chajek-Shaul, O. Stein, T. Olivecrona, and Y. Stein. 1981. *Biochim. Biophys. Acta* 666:156–164.
233. Chajek-Shaul, T., G. Friedman, O. Stein, T. Olivecrona, and Y. Stein. 1982. *Biochim. Biophys. Acta* 712:200–210.
234. Stein, O., G. Halperin, E. Leitersdorf, T. Olivecrona, and Y. Stein. 1984. *Biochim. Biophys. Acta* 795:47–59.
235. Traber, M. G., T. Olivecrona, and H. J. Kayden. 1985. *J. Clin. Invest.* 75:1729–1734.
236. Tall, A. R., D. Sammett, G. Vita, R. Deckelbaum, and T. Olivecrona. 1984. *J. Biol. Chem.* 259:9587–9594.
237. Tall, A. R., S. Krumholz, T. Olivecrona, and R. J. Deckelbaum. 1985. *J. Lipid Res.* 26:842–851.
238. Wallinder, L., J. Peterson, T. Olivecrona, and G. Bengtsson-Olivecrona. 1984. *Biochim. Biophys. Acta* 795:513–524.
239. Friedman, G., T. Chajek-Shaul, T. Olivecrona, O. Stein, and Y. Stein. 1982. *Biochim. Biophys. Acta* 711:114–122.

Chapter 3

MEASUREMENTS OF LIPOPROTEIN LIPASE ACTIVITY

Peter Nilsson-Ehle

Measurements of lipoprotein lipase (LPL) activity are of interest in numerous contexts, reflecting the various aspects of enzyme function. Besides studies directed primarily towards LPL itself, such as monitoring enzyme activity during purification and studies of the regulation of enzyme activity, assays of LPL activity are widely used in investigations of lipoprotein regulation, dyslipoproteinemias and other metabolic disorders. These situations pose different demands on the method for LPL determination, both with regard to the enzyme source and the enzyme assay. For example, in studies focusing on the role of LPL in lipoprotein regulation, measurements of the enzyme activity in postheparin plasma are relevant; with this enzyme source, the presence of other lipases is a major problem since it may potentially delete the specificity of the LPL assay. In studies of lipid metabolism in tissues, e.g. in relation to obesity, determination of enzyme activity in tissue biopsy specimens is preferable; in such assays, the specificity is generally not a problem, whereas the sensitivity may turn out to be critical. The wide variety of assays published over the last two decades (see 1,2,3,4,5) represent modifications and adaptations to meet these different needs and to increase practicality and speed of operation.

Although modern lipase assays are comparatively easy to carry out, the systems are theoretically quite complex. They are carried out in a two phase oil-in-water emulsion system, stabilized by a detergent; the hydrophobic substrate is degraded in subsequent steps; lipolysis yields several products, some of which are water-soluble and some not; enzyme action depends on a specific activator to interact properly with the enzyme-substrate complex; enzyme activity is highly sensitive to product inhibition by released fatty acid which has to be sequestered during the incubation.

It is obvious that this sequence of events does not conform to the basal rules of enzymology. It is possible, however, to design the assay conditions so that the initial lipolytic step becomes rate-limiting for the whole reaction sequence. This is a prerequisite for a working assay system.

This chapter discusses the major practical problems encountered in assays of LPL and summarizes the advantages and limitations of various published assay systems.

Development of Assay Systems

The first generations of assay systems utilized commercial triglyceride emulsions manufactured for parenteral nutrition, such as Ediol, Lipostrate, Lipomul, Lipophysan, and Intralipid. These are stable emulsions, providing assays with high reproducibility, and especially Intralipid has been reported to share many characteristics with the physiological substrate, chylomicrons, in its interaction with LPL (6). Major disadvantages with these assays are their comparatively low sensitivity, the lack of flexibility, and the cumbersome methods necessary for quantitation of reaction products, i.e. titration or chemical determination of fatty acid or glycerol.

The major criticism, however, concerned the fact that partial glycerides are frequently incorporated as detergents in the preparations. Especially the presence of monoglycerides (7,8), which are excellent substrates for LPL, may critically influence the characteristics of the assay (see below).

The introduction of labeled tracers into the substrate preparations (9,10,11,12,13) eliminated most of these problems. Most notably, the sensitivity of the new techniques was superior and allowed the assay of enzyme activity in minute tissue samples, such as biopsy specimens from adipose tissue and muscle. In combination with simplified systems for isolation of reaction products (14), these substrates allowed rapid, simple and reliable assays with high capacity.

Radiolabeled substrate emulsions are prepared by sonication of the triglyceride in buffer with a suitable detergent. These methods can easily be modified for assay of different lipase activities such as hepatic lipase, hormone-sensitive lipase, pancreatic lipase, and microbial lipases. However, the emulsions have limited stability and need to be prepared daily. Besides the inconvenience of an extra step in the assay, this impairs the reproducibility of the method and necessitates close control of interassay variation.

Attempts to overcome the drawbacks associated with the non-stable emulsions include fixation of a triglyceride film onto Celite particles (15) and preparation of triglyceride droplets coated with gelatine (16). Our experiences with these techniques are mixed and we have had problems with reproducibility between different batches of substrate.

The demonstration that stable emulsions can be prepared by dispersion of triglyceride in glycerol using phospholipids as stabilizer (17) led to the development of stable, radiolabeled substrate stock emulsions (18,19). Probably, the high viscosity of the glycerol medium prevents coalescence of emulsion particles. Assay substrates are prepared by dilution of the stock emulsion in a suitable buffer. These procedures are extremely easy to perform and ensure a high reproducibility. However, just like the commercial emulsions, these substrates cannot easily be modified for assay of other lipases. For example, a triglyceride - lecithin emulsion prepared in glycerol cannot be used for the assay of hepatic lipase (18).

From a theoretical point of view, it is preferable to aim at a certain similarity between the artificial substrate used in an *in vitro* assay and the physiological substrate, i.e. for LPL, chylomicron and VLDL triglyceride. As pointed out above, however, these systems are quite complex and more simple substrates for LPL *in vitro*, such as palmitoyl-CoA (20), and phenyloctanoic acid vinyl ester (21) have been proposed.

LPL has a broad substrate specificity and besides its lipase activity against acylglycerols at oil-water interphases, the enzyme also possesses esterase activity against water-soluble esters (22,23). It is not attractive to use a water-soluble ester as substrate—which would provide an even simpler assay system—because of the widely different characteristics of the LPL reaction with these substrates (22). In practice, such an assay would be useless, since non-specific esterase activities are abundant in essentially all relevant enzyme preparations (7,24,25), thus abolishing the specificity of the LPL assay.

Assay Components

Briefly, a typical LPL assay involves the following steps and components: sonication of triglyceride with a detergent, for example lecithin, to produce a uniform oil-in-water-emulsion; addition of albumin, which acts as a fatty acid acceptor, and serum, which provides the LPL-activator apo CII; incubation of the substrate emulsion with enzyme source; and isolation and quantitation of a reaction product, generally free fatty acid. The concentrations and proportions of the ingredients are interdependent, and if one of the components is exchanged or modified, control experiments for all other components have to be carried out to ensure that the assay operates under optimal conditions. For the same reason, it is not advisable to put together ones own methodology simply by combining steps from different assays.

Substrate

Triolein is the preferred substrate triglyceride because of its suitable physicochemical properties—it is liquid at room temperature and therefore easy to emulsify. Both ^{3}H- and ^{14}C-tracers are commercially available; the tritiated compound is more widely used since it is less expensive. A tracer with the label in the fatty acid moiety is preferable to one with the label in the glycerol moiety since LPL has strict positional specificity for primary ester bonds (26,27); the production of glycerol occurs only after non-enzymatic isomerization of the 2-monoglyceride to 1(3)-monoglyceride. Under extreme conditions, especially with high enzyme activities and short incubations, 2-monoglyceride is indeed the main reaction product and glycerol, the final reaction product, appears only after a considerable lag time (26,27,28).

The most critical part of substrate handling is to ensure the purity of the substrate triglyceride. The radiolabeled tracer is generally kept in a concentrated stock solution and combined with non-labeled triolein to obtain a suitable specific radioactivity for each batch of substrate. During storage, spontaneous degradation results in the formation of partial glycerides and fatty acid. (In the radiolabeled preparations, this phenomenon is more rapid—"radiolysis"—unless stored in a medium, e.g. benzene, which absorbs the radiation energy). The degradation products greatly affect the performance of the assay. The fatty acid impairs enzyme activity by product inhibition; the monoglyceride, on the other hand, is an excellent substrate for LPL, and the enzyme demonstrates in fact a virtually total substrate preference for monoglyceride compared to triglyceride (23). The presence of labeled monoolein, therefore, leads to falsely high enzyme activities (29); in addition, separate monoglyceride hydrolases present in large amounts in post-heparin plasma (7,24) and tissue preparations (27) will also be registered in the assay. As discussed in more detail below, the specificity of the so-called "substrate-specific" assays for determination of LPL and hepatic lipase activities in postheparin plasma is also deleted if labeled monoglyceride is present (29).

Equally important is the purity of the non-labeled triolein. In assays which do not employ labeled tracers, the rapid hydrolysis of monolein will lead to falsely high enzyme activities (7). In the radiolabeled assays, on the other hand, contaminating unlabeled monoglyceride will give falsely low results (29). In this situation, the monoacylglycerol will act as a potent competitive inhibitor for triglyceride hydrolysis; since the assay measures only the release of labeled fatty acid, hydrolysis of non-labeled monoglyceride will not be registered.

Since the LPL assay has to be conducted with low degrees of hydrolysis ($<$ 5–8%) in order to avoid product inhibition, even minor contaminations may give misleading results. The presence of monoglyceride corresponding to 1% of the triglyceride is sufficient to invalidate the data (29). The purity of the labeled and unlabeled triglyceride is most conveniently monitored by thin-layer chromatography on silica gel. A purification procedure must aim at eliminating not only fatty acid, but also partial glycerides. Fatty acid extraction and similar techniques (30,31,32,33) therefore cannot be recommended. We use silicic acid chromatography, which is convenient and efficient in separating partial glycerides; by adding a thin layer of Florisil on top of the column, fatty acid is also removed (19).

Whatever the stated purity of commercial preparations, these generally do not meet the requirements for a lipase assay but have to be purified before use. Spontaneous decomposition of the substrate usually necessitates repurification at 2–4 months intervals.

Emulsifier

The emulsifiers are amphipathic compounds which stabilize the oil-in-water emulsion harboring the substrate triglyceride. In commercial emulsions, the stabilizing agent is generally a phospholipid (e.g. Intralipid) and sometimes a monoglyceride (e.g. Ediol). Radiolabeled substrates can be prepared with synthetic or natural phospholipids (9,11,12,13,34,35), synthetic detergents such as Tween 60 and Triton X-100 (11,12,36), and with polysaccharides such as gum acacia or gum arabic (30,31,37,38,39). The rationale for using phospholipid is that these emulsions closely resemble the physiological substrates, whereas the theoretical advantage with the other alternatives is that these are not, as phospholipids are, potential substrates for LPL.

Optimal proportions between triglyceride and phospholipid are 15–20:1 (molar ratio), whereas Triton X-100 and gum arabic are most frequently used at 0.1% and 0.5%, respectively. There are few directly comparative studies on different detergents. Using a variety of enzyme sources, Blaton et al. (40) demonstrated that soybean phospholipids, which are largely unsaturated, provided higher lipolytic rates than do saturated phospholipids. Using LPL extract from adipose tissue, Chung et al. (41) found that phosphatidylcholine promoted the enzyme reaction better than phosphatidylethanolamine or phosphatidylserine; among the lecithin species, lysolecithin was superior.

We have tried a wide variety of different phospholipids in the assay—egg lecithin, rat liver phospholipids, phosphatidyl choline and lysolecithin from different sources—but with these chemically poorly defined preparations there is considerable variability between batches, and we have therefore changed to dioleoylphosphatidyl choline, which gives satisfactory reproducibility. Lysolecithin has proven an efficient emulsifier, but we have had problems with its solubility during long-term storage in various solvents.

In our own assay system, lecithin-stabilized emulsions give higher enzyme activities than identical systems using Triton X-100 (11). This is presumably due to a direct inhibitory effect of Triton on the enzyme activity, as demonstrated in incubations with VLDL triglyceride (42). Comparisons of lecithin and gum arabic indicate that emulsions with the latter are hydrolyzed more rapidly (43). The systematic difference between assays using these two detergents, however, seems to be of little practical importance since the results with the two methods correlate closely.

The stable trioleoylglycerol emulsions prepared in glycerol utilize phosphatidyl choline (18,19). For unknown reasons, lysolecithin cannot substitute for lecithin in these preparations (19).

Fatty acid acceptor

The high sensitivity of LPL to product inhibition makes it necessary to sequester the fatty acid produced during the incubation to prevent their accumulation at the surface of the emulsion particles. Although early data suggested that both Ca^{2+} and albumin could serve this purpose (44,45), it has now become evident that albumin is a necessary component to obtain maximal enzyme activity. Both the type and the concentration of albumin must be considered.

There are great differences in lipolytic rates obtained with different albumin preparations at comparable concentrations. These differences relate both to the preparation procedure, which may affect the lipid-binding properties of the albumin, and to contaminants present in the final products. Obviously, potentially interfering contaminants include fatty acid, but it has been shown that preparations with similar fatty acid content may differ up to threefold in promoting LPL activity (28), indicating that other factors are also of major importance. Both apolipoprotein AI (46) and C-peptides (47) have been identified in Pentex Albumin type V, which may also contain phospholipid (47). The presence of Apo CII in Sigma Albumin type V has been described (48). Other possibly interfering compounds include metals and organic acids (49,50). Considerable amounts of lipase activity have also been described in one batch of Sigma type V albumin (51). Contaminants may be partly removed by dialysis (50), delipidation, or treatment with active charcoal (52), but such procedures may in turn impair the lipid-binding properties of albumin. The commercially available "fatty-acid poor" or "fatty-acid free" albumin preparations have, at least in our hands, not been particularly efficient.

Only a few comparative studies on different albumin preparations have been published (42,50). Crystalline bovine serum albumin from Sigma emerges as the most efficient preparation, yielding 3–4 times higher LPL activity than other preparations. The crystalline albumin is also comparatively consistent from batch to batch.

The concentration of albumin employed in various assays varies considerably, from about 0.03% (11,12) to at least 5% (6,30). For each assay system, there is an optimal concentration range (19,35), the lower level of which is dependant on the amount of fatty acid released (i.e. mainly determined by the amount of enzyme and the incubation time). Below this level, the rate of lipolysis decreases and the pattern of lipolytic products changes, with a tendency towards accumulation of partial glycerides (53). This critical lower level seems to represent the situation where all available binding sites (6–7 per albumin molecule) are occupied by fatty acid. At high albumin concentrations, the lipolytic rate again seems to decline (53). Probably, two mechanisms contribute: monoglyceride, which is readily bound to albumin, may be sequestered from the enzymic site of action at the oil-water-interphase and thus escape hydrolysis, as evidenced by accumulation of monoglycerides in incubations with excess albumin (53); in addition, albumin may, at these high concentrations, cover the emulsion surface, making the triglyceride less accessible to the enzyme.

The optimal albumin concentration therefore needs to be determined for each assay system and, preferably, for each new batch of bovine serum albumin. The amount of albumin present in the serum generally used to provide apo CII, as well as that added in assays of postheparin plasma, is frequently in the same order of magnitude as that added separately and has to be taken into consideration when optimizing the assay system.

Serum activator

One of the original criteria for LPL activity is its dependence on serum for optimal activity. It has since been conclusively demonstrated that the activating potential resides in apo CII, a 9000 Dalton peptide present mainly in HDL, VLDL and circulating chylomicrons. Although sites responsible for enzyme activation and lipid binding have been identified on the apoprotein, its mode(s) of action have not been defined in detail. Maximal activation by serum or apo CII varies from 2-fold up to 50-fold; this wide range probably reflects the presence of endogenous activator in preparations with little activation.

Although separated VLDL protein (54) or apo CII (34,37) have been employed in routine assay systems, LPL activator is most frequently provided by addition of whole serum. There are considerable differences in activating ability between species: serum from guinea pig contains very little apo CII (55,56), whereas serum from humans, rat, dog, calf and monkey can be used as activator source. It should be pointed out that there are also considerable interindividual variations in activating ability, largely due to variations in VLDL-protein concentration (57). Therefore, pooled serum is preferable to minimize variation between batches. Some authors pretreat the serum with heat (56°C for 1 hour or 62°C for 10 minutes) to abolish endogenous lipase activity (13,18,19,30,58). This seems especially pertinent with dog serum, which in contrast to rat and human serum, contains significant activities of circulating lipase. The serum can be kept at −20°C for at least a year without loss of activating ability.

Optimal serum concentrations vary considerably for different assay systems, from 2.5% (11) to 40% (13). To some extent, the serum requirements reflect the triglyceride concentration of the assay system (3,36,56,59,60), but other factors such as type of emulsifier and ionic strength are also of importance. In most systems, enzyme activity declines considerably if serum concentrations are raised above the optimal range. This may be due to specific interference by other apolipoproteins, for example apo CIII and apo E, which have an inhibitory effect on LPL activity (61), or may represent a more general effect of the high protein concentration on the accessibility of substrate triglyceride on the emulsion surface. In any case, the serum component needs to be carefully calibrated (19,31,35,38,62). As serum activator is of course present in postheparin plasma, assays with this enzyme source (and with varying amounts thereof) have different requirements for exogenous serum than assays with tissue preparations or purified enzymes (62,63).

Other components

With its alkaline pH-optimum, lipoprotein lipase is generally assayed at pH 8-8.6. Ammonium and Tris-HC1 buffers have suitable pK_a values and especially Tris has excellent buffering capacity in this pH range. Optimal ionic strength for the LPL reaction is about 9 mmhos (64). Consequently, 0.1–0.2 M Tris-HCl buffer is a more or less standard incubation medium. Phosphate buffers, which may inhibit LPL (65), should be avoided.

In earlier investigations, heparin was reported to stimulate LPL activity (45) and was included as a standard component in some assays. In subsequent studies, heparin has been demonstrated to activate, to inhibit, or to have no effect on the enzyme reaction. In general terms, stimulatory effects are recorded with low (0.01–5 U/ml) concentrations in assays of crude enzyme preparations (45). The purer the enzyme preparation, the smaller is the heparin stimulation (66,67). Higher concentrations of heparin are generally inhibitory (68). The heparin used as anticoagulant in commercial preheparinized tubes results in heparin concentrations in plasma of 10–50 U/ml, which may greatly inhibit LPL activity (43).

Heparin has high affinity for LPL and evidently, direct effects of heparin on the enzyme are involved in these phenomena. However, the interaction of heparin with lipase assays is more complex and also influenced by the nature of the emulsifier (66). Under otherwise similar conditions, heparin has been reported to stimulate enzyme activity against phospholipid-stabilized emulsions and to inhibit that against Triton X-100-stabilized substrates (6). In another comparative study, we found marked inhibition by heparin on LPL activity towards a phospholipid-stabilized emulsion whereas that towards a gum arabic stabilized emulsion was unaffected (43). Furthermore, the effect of heparin is to some extent modulated by the presence of calcium.

From the practical point of view, these considerations lead to the conclusion that heparin should not be included as a standard component in the assay system. Also, EDTA is a more suitable anticoagulant for collection of blood components for the assay.

Assay Procedures

Substrate preparation

The substrate is presented to the enzyme as an oil-in-water-emulsion, prepared by sonication of triglyceride and emulsifier in buffer. Since the area of the oil-water interphase rather than the molar concentration of triglyceride is relevant for lipolysis, the efficacy of the sonication step and the size of the emulsion particles is of prime importance for the performance of the assay. Morphologic (69) and kinetic (38) data show that total sonication times of 3–4 minutes are generally necessary to ensure uniform particle size and reproducible lipolytic rates. Sonication efficacy is influenced by the sample size, the geometry of the vessel, and the position of the microtip, all of which have to be strictly standardized.

Excavation and deteriorating performance of the microtip, which results in poor emulsification and lower enzyme activities, can be detected by measuring the energy output by registering the gram force on a top-loading balance under standardized conditions (35).

Continuous sonication leads to overheating of the sample with hydrolysis of the triglyceride. Temperatures up to 40°C are acceptable and in fact facilitate emulsification. In our preparation procedure, intermittent sonication (15 seconds bursts) and cooling during the last three minutes of sonication are suitable (35). These emulsions are stable for 6–12 hours. Under the outlined conditions, most (11,35,38) but not all (31) assays demonstrate substrate saturation at triglyceride concentrations of 1–1.5 mmoles/1, similar to those noted with Intralipid as substrate (62).

Albumin and serum can be added to the system before or after sonication. In most systems, the lipolytic activity of LPL is not greatly influenced by these manipulations. However, it is evident that the characteristics of the substrate are altered, since hepatic lipase has virtually no activity against triglyceride-lecithin emulsions which have been sonicated in the absence of protein, and to which albumin and serum are added after the sonication (35). The reason for this selectivity is unknown but probably related to the surface characteristics of the emulsion particles. Likewise, most assays do not employ a preincubation of emulsion and serum before assay. Under some conditions, however, preincubation has been reported to give higher or lower activities depending upon the albumin concentration (30).

The stable triglyceride-lecithin emulsions in glycerol can be prepared only by homogenization, most conveniently by the Polytron, an instrument which combines mechanical shearing action with sonication. From this stock emulsion, which is stable for 6–12 weeks, assay substrates are prepared by dilution in an appropriate buffer. This procedure gives slightly larger emulsion particles, since substrate saturation is reached only at 2.5-5 M triglyceride (18,19). Albumin and serum are added after emulsification, and these substrates are therefore specific for LPL.

Incubation

Incubations are generally started by the addition of substrate emulsion to the enzyme source, suitably diluted, to a final volume of 0.2–0.5 ml. Alternatively, especially with small incubation systems, the reagents can be combined with the incubation tubes kept in an ice bath and the reaction started by transferring the tube rack to a water-bath kept at the incubation temperature. In some assays, shaking during the incubations is recommended. However, with smaller incubation volumes, this is not necessary.

The temperature of incubation is generally 27–37°C. In most assays, linearity is maintained for at least 2 hours at 37°C (11,35,62,63,70). Under some conditions, the rate of lipolysis may decline after 30–60 minutes at 37°C, which may indicate inactivation of the enzyme. To minimize this potential source of error, several assays are conducted at 27°C (36,71), 28°C (38) or 30°C (18).

Extraction and quantitation of reaction products

As stated above, it is preferable to quantitate fatty acid rather than glycerol formed during the incubation. For unlabeled assay systems, extraction according to Dole followed by titration was the standard procedure, although colorimetric or chemical measurement of fatty acid in the heptane extract could also be used. More recently, enzymatic methods for released fatty acid have been described (39,72), some of which do not require separation from other components of the incubation before assay. For specific purposes, such as kinetic studies, continuous registration of fatty acid release by pH-stat titration is feasible (34).

The earliest radioactive assay systems also employed Dole's extraction system or versions thereof (9,12,36,73). Fatty acid can also be separated from the substrate by trichloroaceticacid precipitation of triolein (13) or by extraction of fatty acid onto a cationic exchange resin (20,30,74).

The introduction of one-step liquid-liquid partition systems (14) greatly simplified the extraction step. The reaction is stopped by the addition of a mixture of organic solvents and fatty acid extracted by the sequential addition of an alkaline buffer. Here, the inclusion of chloroform in the organic phase is crucial due to its high density. After partition, the organic solvents (which contain all remaining substrate) will constitute the lower phase, whereas the alkaline aqueous phase (which contains the fatty acid) will be easily available for sampling in the upper phase. In the original report, about 75% of the fatty acid partitioned to the upper phase; with slight modifications even more efficient extraction has been achieved (31,75). Since the aqueous phase also contains methanol, quenching during the scintillation counting has to be monitored. This is most conveniently handled by addition of equilibrated upper phase to all samples, including standards, to obtain uniform counting efficiency. These systems are widely used but do not seem compatible with systems using high detergent and protein concentrations (2,30).

Validation of the Assay

Validation of an assay system requires documentation of precision (intra- and interassay), accuracy, and specificity—the two latter characteristics being closely related. To establish and maintain satisfactory performance from all these points of view, several sets of control experiments must be carried out at regular intervals and documented for the different enzyme sources of interest.

Inter- and intraassay precision is monitored by repeated assays of the same enzyme source (preferably, one with high and one with low enzyme activity) in the same series and on different days. An intraassay imprecision below 3% (coefficient of variation) can easily be obtained, whereas interassay imprecision is usually 5–8%, reflecting the variability of the sonication step (11,35). The stable glycerol-based emulsions give higher reproducibility with an interassay variation only marginally greater than the intrassay variation (19).

Precise quantitation of enzymatic activity relies upon a linear relationship between the amount of enzyme source and the rate of fatty acid release. Deviations from linearity may have several explanations: product inhibition due to excessive lipolysis, instability of the enzyme, insufficient substrate concentration or substrate emulsion area, or suboptimal concentrations of fatty acid acceptor or enzyme activator. In general, the total hydrolysis of the substrate has to be kept below 5–8% by adjustment of incubation time and/or dilution of the enzyme source. Unstable enzyme preparations can be handled by using short incubation times and/or lower incubation temperature.

Specificity of the enzymatic measurement is established by applying the original criteria for LPL activity (45). Thus, quantitative inhibition of the enzyme activity by 1 M NaCl, in combination with serum stimulation and an alkaline pH optimum, strongly indicate that the assay system is specific for LPL. Inhibition of LPL by protamine is variable and therefore less reliable than salt inhibition (6,76). If feasible, specificity should also be checked by immunological inhibition using specific antibodies.

Accuracy, i.e. lack of systematic error so that correct levels of enzyme activity are recorded, is far more difficult to establish since no reference method for LPL has been agreed upon. If possible, a new method should be correlated to an established assay e.g. by exchange of frozen samples. To guard against the occurrence of systematic errors, interassay variation has to be monitored closely. The purity of the substrate triglyceride (29) is particularly critical for maintaining accuracy (see above).

Enzyme Preparations

Postheparin plasma

The injection of heparin into the blood stream leads to the rapid release of several potent lipolytic activities into the circulaton with subsequent hydrolysis of plasma triglyceride; the clearing reaction. Besides LPL, monoglyceride esterase(s) and hepatic lipase contribute to the postheparin lipolytic activity. The amount and time-course of the lipase activities are dependent upon the type and amount of heparin employed (35,36,38,77). With standard heparin preparations (from intestinal mucosa or lung, MW 12000–18000 Dalton), low doses (10–20 U/kg body weight) give a rapid response of LPL within 5–10 minutes, whereafter the enzyme activity declines and disappears within 2 hours. If the dose is increased, enzymatic activity continues to rise up to 15–30 minutes after injection. Maximal response is obtained between 50 and 100 U heparin/kg. With hepatic lipase, maximal response is reached already at 10–20 U/kg; in this case, larger doses essentially prolong the half-life of enzymatic activity. These differences may reflect the release of more or less readily available pools of enzyme, a redistribution of enzyme between circulation and endothelium, or different rates of removal.

If there are no clinical contraindications, a dose of 50–100 U/kg is recommended to give maximal release of postheparin lipases. Sampling at 15–30 minutes after injection is sufficient; samples obtained later do not seem to give additional information on defects in, or regulation of, the lipase activities (70). After heparinization, the enzyme pool at the endothelium is rapidly replenished so that postheparin plasma obtained at 24 hour intervals contain the same amounts of enzyme (36).

There is a considerable biological variation (about 3-fold) for both LPL and hepatic lipase in postheparin plasma. For each individual, on the other hand, the enzyme activities are strikingly reproducible (±10–15%).

Heparin preparations of lower molecular weight, at doses giving equipotent anticoagulation, release considerably lower activities of both LPL and hepatic lipase (78), and are therefore interesting tools for investigations of the turnover and regulation of post-heparin lipase activities. Obviously, they may also be of clinical advantage in conditions requiring long-term anti-coagulation treatment, since intravascular lipolysis and elevated levels of fatty acid and monoglyceride may have adverse effects on cardiac function.

Due to the instability of LPL, samples should be collected as plasma rather than serum to avoid loss of enzyme activity during the time period needed for coagulation. As pointed out above, EDTA is preferable to heparin as anticoagulant. The lipase activites of postheparin plasma are stable for at least one year at −20°C and are suitable as long-term controls for LPL and hepatic lipase assays.

There has been some concern about possible dilution of the radioactive substrate triglyceride by plasma triglyceride added with the postheparin plasma. Especially in subjects with hypertriglyceridemia, this might lead to an incorrectly low estimate of enzyme activity (36). Attempts to delipidate postheparin plasma have not been successful (9). With the modern sensitive methods, this problem is of minor importance since very small amounts (2–10 ul) of plasma are assayed and the amount of exogenous triglyceride negligible.

Differentiation between hepatic and lipoprotein lipase activities

Since the distinction between hepatic lipase and LPL about a decade ago, several assay systems have been described for selective measurements of the two lipases. They rely upon separation of enzymes prior to assay, upon inhibition of one of the enzymes for assay of the other, or upon preparation of a substrate that is attacked only by one of the enzymes.

The separation of enzymes is most efficiently obtained by Heparin-Sepharose chromatography (37,67,73). This procedure is comparatively cumbersome and has low reproducibility, but may be useful, e.g. when it is imperative to exclude possible effects on enzymatic activity of other components in the postheparin plasma sample such as lipoproteins or apolipoproteins. This method has been reported to correlate well with an immunoinhibition method (79).

Inhibition of one of the enzymes is the most convenient way to establish specific assays. Suppression of LPL by 1 M NaCl is quantitative and does not impair hepatic lipase activity; it has been generally accepted as the most reliable way to assay hepatic lipase. Protamin, which was advocated in earlier work (36), may give variable suppression of LPL and may also affect hepatic lipase activity (6,68,76).

Selective assays for LPL are more difficult to establish by this approach since few efficient inhibitors of hepatic lipase have been described. The first methods, therefore, quantitated LPL by subtracting salt-resistant or protamin-resistant postheparin lipolytic activity from total postheparin lipolytic activity (36). This procedure is comparatively imprecise and, furthermore, each enzyme cannot be assayed under optimal conditions (25,79). Inhibition of hepatic lipase by specific antibodies is a convenient means to achieve a specific assay for LPL (31,38,71). Since such antibodies are not commercially available, they require substantial technological knowledge and resources for antibody preparation. Such immunochemical methods have been described for human (31,38,71), rat (80), pig (81), and monkey (58) postheparin plasma.

The only specific chemical inhibitor hepatic lipase activity, applicable in serial assays, is sodium dodecyl sulphate. The method described by Baginsky and Brown (30) for LPL quantitation correlates well with an immunochemical method, although the lipolytic activities were about 30% higher in the SDS procedure (2). It should be mentioned that the quantitative and selective inhibition of hepatic lipase by SDS poses certain requirements on the assay system in terms of substrate and protein concentrations which preclude the use of the convenient liquid-liquid partition systems for isolation of reaction products (2).

Another approach to establish specific assay conditions for hepatic lipase is to use a specific substrate. It was recognized early that Intralipid is not a good substrate for hepatic lipase (82), and Corey and Zilversmit (18) demonstrated that the stable emulsions prepared in glycerol provide specific substrates for LPL. Also, emulsions sonicated in buffer are specific for LPL provided that albumin and serum are added after the sonication step (35). The reason for this specificity is not clear but is probably related to the surface characteristics of the emulsion particles. In these assays, purity of the substrate triglyceride is imperative since the presence of monoglyceride affects not only accuracy but also specificity of the assay (29). If contaminated by monoglyceride, these substrates are rapidly attacked by hepatic lipase. Probably, this represents hydrolysis of monoglyceride bound to albumin and not enzyme action at the oil-water interphase.

We have recently compared two commonly used assay systems for postheparin lipases—one using gum arabic stabilized emulsions, and NaCl and anti-hepatic lipase to obtain enzyme specificity, the other employing lecithin-stabilized emulsions, NaCl inhibition to allow assay of hepatic lipase and a specific substrate for LPL (43). There was an excellent agreement for the hepatic lipase assays and a satisfactory correlation for the LPL assays. However, there was a systematic difference in the LPL assay, where the gum arabic stabilized emulsions gave significantly higher enzyme activities. This difference could be accounted for by the different emulsifiers (43).

Tissue preparations

Since the LPL activities of different organs are differently regulated, studies on enzyme regulation require direct measurements of enzyme activity in tissue samples. The two traditional techniques to extract LPL, i.e. in acetone-ether preparations (83) and in heparin eluates (84), have both been adapted for assay of enzyme activity in needle biopsy specimens from adipose tissue and skeletal muscle. This allows sequential measurements of LPL activity in patients or volunteers.

The acetone-ether preparations (11,25) are made by homogenization of tissue in acetone, further delipidation by ether, and solubilization of the precipitate in ammonium buffer or—to increase stability of the enzyme—Tris-HCl buffer containing 20% ethylene glycol (22). It is generally considered that these preparations represent the total tissue activity, i.e. both the intracellular and the extracellular pools including the physiologically active fraction at the endothelial surfaces (22,25,85).

Upon incubation of tissue samples in a heparin-containing buffer, LPL is released into the medium, providing a convenient source for assay of enzyme activity (86,87,88). In some assays, the elution of enzyme and incubation with a radiolabelled substrate are performed simultaneously, i.e. by incubating thc tissue sample in buffer containing both heparin and substrate (62,63). The elution of enzyme from the tissue is quite complex, and when performed at 37°C the enzyme activity present in the medium reflects not only elution of preformed enzyme from the tissue, but the combined effects of rates of release, activation, and inactivation of the enzyme, all of which are considerably influenced by the conditions of elution (25).

Nevertheless, in direct comparison the two enzyme preparations seem to yield largely compatible results in studies of enzyme regulation in adipose tissue (25,89,90). The effects of hormonal and dietary stimulation, however, are more pronounced when registered in heparin eluates, which is consistent with the notion that heparin eluates largely reflect extracellularly located enzyme (25,89,90).

Recently, Iverius and Brunzell (33) have tried to eliminate the undesired changes in enzyme activity which may occur during the period allowed for release of enzyme from the tissue. By performing the elution of 4°C, activation and degradation processes are minimized, thus allowing a more accurate quantitation of the physiologically relevant portion of enzyme activity.

Using only measurements of enzyme activity, it is virtually impossible to exclude losses of enzyme activity during preparation or to conclusively demonstrate which pool(s) of enzyme are recovered in acetone-ether preparations or heparin eluates under various conditions. Hopefully, future studies including measurements of enzyme protein may help to clarify this issue.

Expression of Enzyme Activity

So far there has been no general agreement on the terminology for expression of LPL activity. To facilitate comparison of data, it is recommended that the units of the SI-system, katal (*Katal*ytic activity; 1 katal = 1 mol product formed per sec) be adopted to conform to the general practice of clinical enzymology. A typical LPL activity in postheparin plasma of 200 mU per ml (200 nmol fatty acid produced per min per ml) would then correspond to the release of 12 μmol fatty acid per hour per ml and 3.33 μkat per l.

For postheparin plasma, enzyme activities are generally expressed per volume unit of enzyme source. For tissue samples, however, there are several relevant alternatives. Enzyme activity has been expressed per g wet weight, per g of tissue triglyceride, per mg protein, per mg DNA, per cell, or per organ. In theory, any difference or change in the enzymatic activity reported may be due to alterations in enzyme activity proper or to alterations in the reference variable. In some situations, e.g. where tissue wasting occurs or where cell size differs between experimental groups, the various modes of expression may convey quite different information on the outcome of the experiment. Numerous apparent discrepancies in the literature can doubtlessly be explained by such technicalities.

It is not possible to give any general recommendations as to the reference for enzyme activities in tissues. The various modes of expression emphasize different phenomena which makes them more or less helpful in the elucidation of specific problems. If possible, enough data should be provided to allow the reader to evaluate the results in alternative reference units.

Interpretation of Data

It needs to be emphasized that enzyme assays show only the enzyme activity of the particular enzyme preparation. Extrapolation from enzyme activity data may allow prediction on other variables, such as rate of lipoprotein turnover, rate of triglyceride removal from the circulation, or rate of triglyceride accumulation into tissues. It should be kept in mind, however, that several other factors may modulate these metabolic events, although LPL catalyzes the rate-limiting step. For example, substrate concentrations, proportions of stimulatory and inhibitory apoproteins, and possible circulating inhibitors may greatly affect the rate of these sequences *in vivo* although LPL activity, when measured *in vitro*, is constant (22,91).

To investigate such phenomena more directly, a number of methodologies are available. These include kinetic studies of lipoprotein turnover by tracers or by specific labelling of lipoprotein subclasses. Triglyceride removal capacity can be estimated by the intravenous fat tolerance test (92), and lipid assimilation into specific tissues can be measured directly by tracer techniques. The susceptibility to LPL activity of VLDL or chylomicrons from different individuals can be recorded by incubation of labeled lipoproteins with purified enzymes *in vitro* (93,94). Environmental factors that may affect the rate of the LPL reaction *in vivo* include circulating inhibitors, which can also be demonstrated and quantitated by separate incubations. A comprehensive system for evaluation of the quality of the reaction medium *in vivo* has been designed in assays for "LPL activating ability", which record the stimulation of a standard LPL preparation by individual sera (57,95,96).

In the near future, direct measurements of enzyme protein by immunological techniques will be available (97,98,99,100). In addition to their potential in elucidating regulation of enzyme activity, these methods will also be helpful for a better understanding of the enzymatic activity measurements presently available.

References

1. Assman, G., and H. V. Jabs. 1984. *In* Methods of Enzymatic Analysis. vol 4. 42– 50.
2. Baginsky, M. L. 1981. *In*: Methods of Enzymology. vol 72. 325–328.
3. Corey Gibson, J., J. R. Paterniti, and I.J. Goldberg. 1984. *In*: Lipid Research Methodology. Alan Liss Inc. New York. 241–286.
4. Ehnholm, C., and T. Kuusi. 1986. *Methods in Enzymology*. 129:716–738.

5. Kinnunen, P. K. J., and T. Thurén. 1984. *Methods of Enzymology.* 4:34–42.
6. Riley, S. E., and D. S. Robinson. 1974. *Biochim. Biophys. Acta.* 369:371–386.
7. Biale, Y., and E. Shafrir. 1963. *Clin. Chim. Acta.* 23:413–419.
8. Fredrickson, D. S., K. Ono, and L. L. Davis. 1963. *J. Lipid Res.* 4:24–33.
9. Greten, H., R. I. Levy, and D. S. Fredrickson. 1968. *Biochim. Biophys. Acta.* 164:185–194.
10. Kaplan, A. 1970. *Anal. Biochem.* 33:218–225.
11. Nilsson-Ehle, P., H. Tornqvist, and P. Belfrage. 1972. *Clin. Chim. Acta.* 42:383–390.
12. Schotz, M. C., A. S. Garfinkel, R. Huebotter, and J. E. Stewart. 1970. *J. Lipid Res.* 11:68–69.
13. Schotz, M. C., and A. S. Garfinkel. 1972. *J. Lipid Res.* 13:824–826.
14. Belfrage, P., and M. Vaughan. 1969. *J. Lipid Res.* 10:341–344.
15. Posner, I., and V. Bosch. 1971. *J. Lipid Res.* 12:768–772.
16. Demant, E. 1977. *Biochim. Biophys. Acta.* 489:269–287.
17. Zilversmit, D. B., N. K. Salky, M. L. Trumbull, and E. L. McCandless. 1956. *J. Lab. Clin. Med.* 48:386–391.
18. Corey, J. E., and D B. Zilversmit. 1977. *J. Lab. Clin. Med.* 89:666–674.
19. Nilsson-Ehle, P., and M. C. Schotz. 1976. *J. Lipid Res.* 17:536–541.
20. Jansen, H., and W C Hülsmann. 1973. *Biochim. Biophys. Acta.* 296:241–248.
21. Rick, W., and M. Hockeborn. 1982. *J. Clin. Chem. Clin. Biochem.* 20:627–632.
22. Nilsson-Ehle, P., A. S. Garfinkel, and M. C. Schotz. 1980. *Ann. Rev. Biochem.* 49:667–693.
23. Twu, J. S., P. Nilsson-Ehle, and M. C. Schotz. 1976. *Biochemistry.* 15:1904–1909.
24. Nilsson-Ehle, P., and P. Belfrage. 1972. *Biochim. Biophys. Acta.* 270:60–64.
25. Nilsson-Ehle, P. 1974. *Clin. Chim. Acta.* 54:283–291.
26. Nilsson-Ehle, P., P. Belfrage, and B. Borgström. 1971. *Biochim. Biophys. Acta.* 248:114–120.
27. Nilsson-Ehle, P., A. S. Garfinkel, and M. C. Schotz. 1974. *Lipids.* 9:548–553.
28. Boberg, J. 1970. *Lipids.* 5:452–456.
29. Nilsson-Ehle, P. 1984. *Clin. Chim. Acta.* 141:293–298.
30. Baginsky, M. L., and W. V. Brown. 1979. *J. Lipid Res.* 20:548–556.
31. Blache, D., D. Bouthillier, and J. Davignon. 1983. *Clin. Chem.* 29:154–158.
32. Gamlen, T R, and D. P. R. Muller. 1980. *Clin. Chim. Acta.* 106:75–83.
33. Iverius, P. H., and J. D. Brunzell. 1985. *Am. J. Physiol.* 249:E107–114.
34. Chung, J., and A. M. Scanu. 1974. *Anal. Biochem.* 62:134–148.
35. Nilsson-Ehle, P., and R. Ekman. 1977. *Artery.* 3:194–209.
36. Krauss, R. M., R. I. Levy, and D. S. Fredrickson. 1974. *J. Clin. Invest.* 54:1107–1124.
37. Boberg, J., J. Augustin, M. L. Baginsky, P. Tejada, and W. V. Brown. 1977. *J. Lipid Res.* 18:544–547.
38. Huttunen, J. K., C. Ehnholm, K. J. Kinnunen, E. A. Nikkilä. 1975. *Clin. Chim. Acta.* 63:335–347.
39. Nozaki, S., M. Kubo, Y. Matsuzawa, and S. Tarui. 1984. *Clin. Chem.* 30:748–751.
40. Blaton, V., D. Vandamme, and H. Peters. 1974. *FEBS Lett.* 44:185–188.
41. Chung, J., A. M. Scanu, and F. Reman. 1973. *Biochim. Biophys. Acta.* 296:116–123.
42. Eisenberg, S., D. Feldman, and T. Olivecrona. 1981. *Biochim. Biophys. Acta.* 665:454–462.
43. Ehnholm, C., E. A. Nikkilä, and P. Nilsson-Ehle. 1984. *Clin. Chem.* 30:568–570.
44. Datta, D. V., and H. S. Wiggins. 1963. *Proc. Soc. Exp. Biol. Med.* 115:788–792.
45. Korn, E. D. 1955. *J. Biol. Chem.* 215:1–14.
46. Fainaru, M., and R. J. Deckelbaum. 1979. *FEBS Lett.* 97:171–174.
47. Deckelbaum, R., T. Olivecrona, M. Fainaru. 1980. *J. Lipid Res.* 21:425–434.
48. Östlund-Lindqvist, A. M., and J. Boberg. 1979. *Clin. Sci. Mol. Med.* 56:99–100.
49. Hanson, R. W., and F. J. Ballard. 1968. *J. Lipid Res.* 9:667–668.
50. Whayne, T. F., and J. M. Felts. 1972. *Clin. Biochem.* 5:109–114.

51. Benson, S. M., and W. C. Love. 1982. *Clin. Chim. Acta.* 123:181–185.
52. Chen, R. F. 1967. *J. Biol. Chem.* 242:173–181.
53. Scow, R. O., and T. Olivecrona. 1977. *Biochim. Biophys. Acta.* 487:472–486.
54. Whayne, T. F., and J. F. Morelli. 1977. *Biochem. Med.* 17:247–257.
55. Fitzharris, T. J., D. M. Quinn, E. H. Goh, J. D. Johnson, M. L. Kashyap, L. S. Srinivasan, R. L. Jackson, and J. A. K. Harmony. 1981. *J. Lipid Res.* 22:921–933.
56. Matsuoka, N., K. Shirai, J. D. Johnson, M. L. Kashyap, L. S. Srinistava, T. Yamamura, A. Yamamoto, Y. Saito, A. Kumagai, and R. L. Jackson. 1981. *Metabolism.* 30:818–824.
57. Rogers, M. P., D. Barnett, and D. S. Robinson. 1976. *Atherosclerosis.* 24:551–564.
58. Goldberg, I. J., J. R. Paterniti, and W. V. Brown. 1983. *Biochim. Biophys. Acta.* 752:172–177.
59. Lukens, T. W., and J. Borensztajn. 1978. *Biochem. J.* 175:1143–1146.
60. Östlund-Lindqvist, A. M., and P. Iverius. 1975. *Biochem. Biophys. Res. Comm.* 65:1447–1455.
61. Ekman, R., and P. Nilsson-Ehle. 1975. *Clin. Chim. Acta.* 63:29–35.
62. Lithell, H., and J. Boberg. 1977. *Scand. J. Clin. Lab. Invest.* 37:551–561.
63. Lithell, H., and J. Boberg. 1978. *Biochim. Biophys. Acta.* 528:58–68.
64. LaRosa, J. L., R. I. Levy, H. G. Windmueller, and D. S. Fredrickson. 1972. *J. Lipid Res.* 13:356–363.
65. Korn, E. D., and T. W. Quigley. 1957. *J. Biol. Chem.* 226:833- 837.
66. Havel, R. J., C. J. Fielding, T. Olivecrona, V. G. Shore, P. E. Shore, and T. Egelrud. 1973. *Biochemistry.* 12:1828–1833.
67. Iverius, P. H., U. Lindahl, T. Egelrud, and T. Olivecrona. 1972. *J. Biol.Chem.* 247:6610–6616.
68. Elkeles, R. S., and J. Hambley. 1975. *Clin. Chim. Acta.* 65, 135–137.
69. Bode, G., H. U. Klör, R. Martin, R. Kulka, W. Fritz, and H. Ditschuneit. 1978. *Protides Biol. Fluids* 25:233–236.
70. Boberg, J., and L. A. Carlson. 1964. *Clin. Chim. Acta.* 10:420–427.
71. Greten, H., R. DeGrella, G. Klose, W. Rascher, J. L. deGennes, and E. Gjone. 1976. *J. Lipid Res.* 17:203–210.
72. Woolett, L. A., D. C. Beitz, R. L. Hood, and S. Aprahamian. 1984. *Anal. Biochem.* 143:25–29.
73. Wang, C. S., H. B. Bass, D. Downs, and R. K. Whitmer. 1981. *Clin. Chem.* 27:663–668.
74. Kelley, T. F. 1968. *J. Lipid Res.* 9:799–800.
75. Pittman, R. C., J. C. Khoo, and D. Steinberg. 1975. *J. Biol. Chem.* 250:4505–4511.
76. Huttunen, J. K., and E. A. Nikkilä. 1973. *Eur. J. Clin. Invest.* 3:483–490.
77. Greten, H., A. D. Sniderman, J. G. Chandler, D. Steinberg, and W. V. Brown. 1974. *FEBS Lett.* 42:157–160.
78. Persson, E., J. Nordenström, P. Nilsson-Ehle, and L. Hagenfeldt. 1985. *Eur. J. Clin. Invest.* 15:215–220.
79. Greten, H., V. Laible, G. Zipperle, and J. Augustin. 1977. *Atherosclerosis.* 26:563–572.
80. Kuusi, T., C. Ehnholm, and E. A. Nikkilä. 1980. *Atherosclerosis.* 35:363–374.
81. Kuusi, T., T. Schröder, B. Bång, M. Lempinen, and C. Ehnholm. 1979. *Biochim. Biophys. Acta.* 573:443–450.
82. Vessby, B., J. Boberg, and H. Lithell. 1978. *Clin. Sci. Mol. Med.* 54:201–209.
83. Robinson, D. S. 1963. *Adv. Lipid Res.* 1:133–181.
84. Cherkes, A., and R. S. Gordon. 1959. *J. Lipid Res.* 1:97–101.
85. Cryer, A., and H. M. Jones. 1981. *Int. J. Biochem.* 13:109–111.
86. Persson, B., P. Björntorp, and B. Hood. 1966. *Metabolism.* 15:730–741.
87. Persson, B., G. Schröder, and B. Hood. 1972. *Atherosclerosis.* 16:37–49.
88. Taskinen, M. R., E. A. Nikkilä, J. K. Huttunen, and H. Hilden. 1980. *Clin. Chim. Acta.* 104:107–117.
89. Persson, B., U. Smith, and B. Larsson. 1975. *Atherosclerosis.* 22:425–430.

90. Pykälistö, O. J., P. H. Smith, and J. D. Brunzell. 1975. *Proc. Soc. Exp. Biol. Med.* 148:297–300.
91. Robinson, D. S. 1970. *In*: Compr. Biochem. M. Florkin and E. Stoltz, editors. vol 18. Elsevier. Amsterdam. 51–116.
92. Rössner, S. 1976. *Scand. J. Clin. Lab. Invest.* 36:155–159.
93. Rosseneu, M., M. Taveirne, H. Caster, and J. P. vanBiervliet. 1985. *Eur. J. Biochem.* 152:195–198.
94. Taskinen, M. R., J. D. Johnson, M. L. Kashyap, K. Shirai, C. J. Glueck, and R. L. Jackson. 1981. *J. Lipid Res.* 22:382–386.
95. Chu, P., A. L. Miller, and G.L. Mills. 1976. *Clin. Chim. Acta.* 66:281–286.
96. Stubbe, I., A. Gustafson, and P. Nilsson-Ehle. 1982. *Scand. J. Clin. Lab. Invest.* 42:437–444.
97. Cheung, A. H., A. Bensadoun, and C. F. Cheng. 1979. *Anal. Biochem.* 94:346–357.
98. Cisar, L A, and A. Bensadoun. 1985. *J. Lipid Res.* 26:380–386.
99. Jansen, H., Garfinkel, A. S., J. S. Twu, J. Nikazy, and M. C. Schotz. 1978. *Biochim. Biophys. Acta.* 531:109–114.
100. Olivecrona, T., and G. Bengtsson. 1983. *Biochim. Biophys. Acta.* 752:38–45.

Chapter 4

ADIPOSE TISSUE LIPOPROTEIN LIPASE

Robert H. Eckel

Because of the extensive literature on lipoprotein lipase (LPL) in adipose tissue, this Chapter is arbitrarily divided in the sections outlined above. Although some overlap between sections is unavoidable, this approach should not only serve to clarify, but also to exemplify the uniqueness of LPL in adipose tissue metabolism.

Physiology and Regulation *in Vivo*

Functions of adipose tissue LPL

Triglyceride storage. There are several potential sources of acyl groups for adipose tissue triglyceride. Within adipocytes, fatty acids can either be synthesized from glucose, or provided by cyclic AMP-dependent hormone sensitive lipase-mediated lipolysis. From the extracellular compartment, both albumin-bound free fatty acids and acyl products of LPL-mediated lipoprotein triglyceride hydrolysis are potential sources. Experimental evidence suggests a predominant role of LPL in this important process in adipose tissue. However, the fact that patients with LPL deficiency maintain adipose tissue triglyceride stores indicates a compensatory role of other processes.

Although *de novo* fatty acid biosynthesis from glucose occurs in both rat (1–5) and human (6–14) adipose tissue, the relative contribution of this pathway for acyl group delivery and triglyceride storage is small. In the study by Savard et al. (14) where lipogenesis and LPL activity were compared, there was no relationship between rates of basal lipogenesis and LPL nor between lipogenesis and adipocyte size. There was, however, a direct relationship between LPL and adipocyte size. A variable and limited supply of acetyl groups (10, 11, 15, 16) and/or reduced amounts of enzymes of fatty acid biosynthesis including citrate lyase (17–19) could explain the limited role of lipogenesis in the provision of fatty acids. Despite low levels of citrate lyase in human adipose tissue, some capacity for increased fatty acid synthesis from citrate has been demonstrated following short-term hypercaloric, high carbohydrate feeding (11). Nevertheless, this is of little quantitative importance for fatty acid storage or consumption of glucose carbon. In fact, nearly all of the glucose which is incorporated into rat and human adipose tissue triglyceride stores is found in glyceride glycerol and not in acyl groups (1,5,12,17).

The reesterification of fatty acids released during intracellular lipolysis could be an alternative source of acyl groups for triglyceride replenishment, but has been less well studied. This pathway was considered less important because of the excessive energy requirements to maintain such a "futile" cycle (20). However, May (5), in a study carried out in an environment without extracellular triglyceride substrate, suggested that high rates of lipolysis and reesterification in rat adipose tissue may play an important role in regulating the rate and direction of adipose tissue triglyceride turnover. In human gluteal adipose tissue, Leibel et al. (12) using a double isotopic method demonstrated, over a wide range of lipolytic rates, a high correlation between the ratio of ^{14}C-glucose incorporated into glyceride glycerol to ^{3}H-palmitate incorporated into triglyceride and the rate of lipolysis. In addition, using the same methodology, Leibel et al. (21) estimated that reesterification in the fed state may be as high as 54% of the triglyceride fatty acid released. Reesterification however, fell to 10% in adipose tissue from fasting subjects. Nevertheless, it would appear that reesterification may be a more important mechanism than originally thought for the maintenance of adipose tissue triglyceride stores.

The ability of adipose tissue to accumulate chylomicron or very low density lipoprotein (VLDL) triglyceride fatty acids has been demonstrated following the intravenous injection of fatty acid-labeled lipoproteins into rats (22–28) and dogs (29), or following administration of ^{14}C-palmitate to human subjects (30). In the study of Bragdon and Gordon (24), carbohydrate-fed rats incorporated 32% of the label into the adipose tissue 10 minutes after chylomicron injection. In rats, with a more limited dietary carbohydrate intake, 10% of the fatty acid label was present in adipose tissue by 20 minutes (28). In fasted rats, Jones and Havel (22) found only 3.2% of the chylomicron triglyceride fatty acid in adipose tissue 3–4 minutes after injection. In the study of Bjorntorp et al. (30), uptake of label into adipose tissue related directly to fat cell size and presumably LPL. In dogs (29), 27.5% of the label was found in the adipose tissue 45 minutes following the injection of chylomicrons. A similar ability of adipose tissue to take up triglyceride fatty acids from triglyceride-rich lipoproteins has been shown in studies of perfused rat fat pads (26,31–34) and from *in vitro* incubations of rat (25,35,36) or human (37,38) adipose tissue pieces with labeled substrate. In chickens, Bensadoun and Kompiang (39) have shown total inhibition of adipose tissue and other organ removal of VLDL and chylomicron triglyceride following the injection of anti-LPL.

When the uptakes of labeled lipoprotein triglyceride glycerol and fatty acids in adipose tissue were compared, preferential uptake of the fatty acid was seen (30,31,34,40). Although free fatty acid uptake rates were similar (37) or less (36) than those measured for lipoprotein-derived fatty acids, there remains to be established an important role for free fatty acid uptake into adipose tissue from circulating fatty acid-albumin complexes. If the lateral membrane movement model of Blanchette-Mackie and Scow (41) for fatty acid transport is validated, the close proximity of lamellar structures with chylomicrons during the postprandial state, and with intracellular lipid droplets in the fasted state, would apparently function to impede the transport of non-lipoprotein or free fatty acids to or from adipocytes. However, slower mechanisms of fatty acid movement, such as molecular diffusion through aqueous media and across cell membranes (42) could allow such transport.

The established relationship between lipoprotein triglyceride fatty acid uptake and LPL activity supports a critical role for this mechanism in the maintenance of triglyceride stores in adipose tissue. Evidence comes from the experiments of Wilson et al. (37) wherein fluoride, a known inhibitor of fatty acid esterification in human adipose tissue (33), failed to diminish the incorporation of tri-palmitate fatty acid into triglyceride. Thus, the activity of LPL appeared to be rate-limiting for the deposition of fat. Relationships between lipoprotein triglyceride fatty acid uptake and LPL have been noted *in vivo* (23–25,30,43,44), *in vitro* (25,26,45–48), and in perfusion (32) studies in animals (mostly rats); in addition to *in vitro* (38,49) and *in vivo* (30) studies in humans. Such relationships have been found for both the total cellular enzyme measured in delipidated powders (23,25,26,32,43,44) and the heparin-releasable fraction eluted from tissue pieces (38,45,49). The particular importance of cell surface LPL to fatty acid uptake and incorporation into cell lipids was exemplified in the study by Verine et al. (47). Using isolated rat adipocytes, they found a very high correlation between the amount of ^{3}H-oleic acid liberated by hydrolysis and that incorporated as ^{3}H-acylglycerol, and LPL activity measured in the culture medium. The functional role of this surface fraction of LPL has also been supported by experiments in which triglyceride hydrolysis was prevented by removing this fraction with antibody (39) or heparin (50). The reduction of *in vivo* chylomicron triglyceride clearance in fed rats with larger fat cell sizes, where decreased amounts of the extracellular enzyme were found (51), also supports the role of the extracellular lipase in lipid removal from plasma.

Also relevant is the adipose tissue triglyceride loading response in rats following lipectomy (52), or refeeding after three days of fasting (53). In both studies, LPL increased before lipid loading occurred. In the study of Fried et al. (53), LPL increased to levels 60–100% above prefasting values and then returned to prefasting values after fat cell size was restored. Thus, LPL appeared not only critical for lipid loading, but may have controlled the amount of lipid entry to reach a predetermined fat cell size.

Plasma Triglyceride Removal. LPL hydrolytic activity is critical to normal lipoprotein metabolism. Patients with LPL (54) or apoliprotein CII deficiency (55,56) accumulate VLDL and chylomicrons in the plasma and have severe hypertriglyceridemia. Because all tissues which produce LPL are presumably involved in the removal of triglycerides from circulation it is not surprising that relationships between the adipose tissue enzyme activity and triglyceride levels in plasma (or in VLDL), or between adipose tissue LPL and chylomicron and VLDL triglyceride kinetics are weak or nonexistent.

In normal (57,58), streptozotocin diabetic (59,60), and pregnant (61) rats, significant inverse relationships between LPL per gram of tissue and serum triglycerides have been found. However, variations in either total or heparin-releasable LPL, induced by changing the diet and/or time of day at which the measurements were made, did not alter VLDL-triglyceride kinetics (62). In addition, the hypolipidemic effects of clofibrate in rats has been related to enhanced peripheral utilization of Intralipid, but by mechanisms independent of adipose tissue LPL (63).

Human studies have shown a more consistent, but still variable, inverse relationship between adipose tissue LPL and serum triglycerides. In studies which included normolipemic and hypertriglyceridemic subjects (64–68), variable but generally weak negative correlations between LPL activity expressed per tissue weight and serum triglycerides were reported. This, however, was not found by others (69–71). In some studies (66,72), the relationship between adipose tissue LPL and serum- or VLDL-triglycerides was not seen when the data were expressed per 10^6 cells. Persson et al. (73) found, however, an inverse relationship between serum triglycerides and LPL in normolipidemic subjects. Peltonen et al. (74) found no relationship between adipose tissue LPL and serum triglycerides in normolipidemic subjects prior to training. An inverse relationship was observed, however, following training when both trained men and controls were combined. Such a relationship was also found in athletes studied by Nikkilä et al. (75). Finally, although one study in diabetics demonstrated an inverse relationship between Intralipid clearance and adipose tissue LPL (76), such a relationship was not found by Vessby et al. (77).

In conclusion, in both rats and humans, adipose tissue LPL activity has been associated with—but is insufficient to predict—serum triglyceride levels and/or alterations in triglyceride-rich lipoprotein triglyceride kinetics. The relationship of these parameters, when existent, appears to pertain to tissue weight and not to adipocyte size.

Cholesteryl ester transport. Unlike the lipolysis of lipoprotein triglyceride which has been shown to occur with both membrane-bound and free LPL, another function of the lipase, that of chylomicron cholesteryl ester uptake (see Chapter 2) appears to occur only when the enzyme is bound to cell surfaces (78). This is true for a number of cell types, including preadipocytes and endothelial cells and for both endogenously produced and exogenously added LPL.

Physiological Changes in Adipose Tissue LPL activity

Effects of feeding and starvation. In a variety of rat strains, adipose tissue LPL activity is higher in the fed than fasted state (25,34,41,46,53,57,79–117). Increases after feeding have also been shown in cattle (118). In rat studies, this increase was seen after chow feeding, as well as after oral glucose administration (25,89,113). Although LPL has usually been measured in tissue extracts, increases in activity releasable from pieces of adipose tissue by heparin have also been found (28,34,45,56,84,86,88,90,93,94,100,103, 109,117) and have predominated over that in tissue homogenates (45,56,86, 88,90,94,103,109). Because the activity released by heparin from the tissue is believed to be extracellular, or on the adipocyte surface, the relative response of the heparin-releasable enzyme to feeding would appear adaptive for lipoprotein trigylceride hydrolysis and fatty acid delivery to adipocytes for storage. Histochemical evidence for the extracellular location of LPL was documented in the adipose tissue of fed and fasting mice (119).

LPL activity in acetone-ether homogenates of isolated adipocytes from fed rats is either similar (51,88,103,104,117,120) or higher (45,47,121) than that of fasted animals. However, when the membrane bound enzyme is eluted from adipocytes by heparin, consistently higher activities are found in adipocytes of fed animals (103,104). These data suggest the possible role of heparin on enzyme activation and/or synthesis at the adipocyte level.

Several investigations indicate that the LPL response to feeding is dependent on new enzyme synthesis. Jansen et al. (96), using immuno-titration, reported no differences in LPL specific activity between fed and fasted rats, despite increases in LPL activity of tissue extracts. The ability of cycloheximide to block the increase in LPL activity seen in adipocytes from fed rats (121), and the increased amounts of a 56,000 dalton protein on SDS/polyacrylamide gels, and incorporation of [1,3-^{3}H] diisopropyl fluorophosphate into this band (102), are also consistent with a protein synthesis-dependent effect of feeding.

The increase in rat adipose tissue LPL in response to feeding is seen as early as 3 days post-partum (80) and appears to develop over the first months of life (41,80,81,122). Although occurring simultaneously in several adipose tissue regions (53,81,83,84), the response appears to be delayed developmentally (81,83) and to be of a lesser magnitude in the subcutaneous depot (53,81,83). In one study, the total tissue LPL response to feeding was seen at forty days but not at one year of life (85). Gustafson et al. (57) reported, however, similar increases with feeding at one and fifteen months.

During progressive fasting for up to 72 hours, most of the decrease of LPL occurs within 24 hours with a maximum decrease at 48 hours (79,100,105). In one study, LPL activity remained unchanged between 48 and 72 hours (100).

In human subjects, variable increases in adipose tissue LPL activity after the ingestion of glucose (123), carbohydrate-rich meals (124–131), or four regular meals (127) have also been reported. Increases ranged from 34% (heparin-releasable LPL) in obese women six hours after three high carbohydrate meals (126), to 270% (heparin-releasable LPL) in normal weight men eight hours after four high carbohydrate meals (129). However, when LPL activity was measured in acetone-ether powders (125), or after extraction with bile salts (126), no increases were observed. Goldberg et al. (130) reported that the increase in LPL activity with feeding was inversely correlated with the levels of fasting biopsy samples. This relationship was not found in all studies (125,126) and further, Nilsson-Ehle et al. (123) reported a positive correlation between the postfeeding change in LPL and the prefeeding biopsy. An LPL response to oral glucose was not seen in massively obese women before or after 4–22 Kg weight reduction (131), or in the obese subjects studied by Dahms et al. (132).

The effects of feeding and fasting on adipose tissue LPL have also been examined in man. As in rats, the acetone-ether powder activity (133) and heparin-releasable LPL activity (69,77,134–137) decreased. Interestingly, with total fasting for up to 8 days (77,133,134,136), decreases in LPL were less marked than after hypocaloric feeding (69,135). In fact, in the study of Persson et al. (133), LPL activity actually rose after 9–13 days of fasting. There is as yet no explanation for this difference in adipose tissue responsiveness. It should be noted, however, that in two studies (69,134), the decreases in LPL were similar in different anatomical regions. Arner et al. (134), examined the abdominal wall and femoral regions and Bosello et al. (69), examined the hypogastric, gluteal and subscapular regions.

Effects of dietary composition. In general, rats fed diets high in carbohydrates had higher adipose tissue LPL activities than those fed diets high in fat (45,101,138–140). Similar data were reported from long-term (over two years) dietary manipulations in baboons (141). However, such an effect of dietary composition has not always been found in rats (44,142–145) or mice (146). In general, the shorter the time on the varied diet ($\leq$

3 weeks), the greater likelihood of differences in *LPL* response between the nutritional groups. De Gasquet et al. (140) did find, however, that the post-prandial response to meals was greater after two days of high fat intake than at 21 days.

Alterations in the degree of saturation of fatty acids in the diet have variable effects on LPL. In male Wistar rats, following a 5 week diet of 30% fat, (11% of which were polyunsaturated vs. 2.5% polyunsaturated), LPL was significantly reduced (44). In contrast, rats fed 20% fat as corn oil had higher LPL than rats fed 20% lard (147). Moreover, 4 days of a 40% fat diet rich in erucic (cis-13-docosenoic) acid resulted in increases in the enzyme (148). Similarly, long-term exposure of female guinea pigs to diets rich in corn oil resulted in increases in LPL when compared to beef tallow enriched chow (149). Finally, in seven guinea pigs, six months of cholesterol enrichment (up to 4% of dietary calories) failed to alter the heparin-releasable LPL (150).

In humans, few data on the effects of dietary composition on adipose tissue LPL have been reported. In Type I diabetics, diets with 60% of the calories from carbohydrates produced no change in fasting LPL up to 2–4 weeks when compared with diets containing 45% of calories as carbohydrates (128). However, at 4 weeks, the LPL response to a single meal was enhanced by the previously administered high carbohydrate diet. In short-term studies, Pykalisto et al. (125) found an insignificant increase in both heparin-releasable and acetone-ether LPL in normal weight subjects following 3 feedings of a fat-containing formula. As previously noted, using an identical protocol with a fat-free formula, these authors did demonstrate post-prandial increases in LPL. As expected, the fat-free formula administration was associated with greater increases in serum insulin and glucose concentrations than the fat-containing formula.

The ingestion of fat has also been shown to alter the stimulatory effect of insulin on LPL. In the studies of Sadur et al. (151), the expected increase in LPL at 6 hours following the intravenous administration of insulin and glucose was substantially blunted by corn oil ingested at the inception of the study. There was a 20% decrease in the glucose infusion rate necessary to maintain fasting euglycemia in the studies following corn oil administration when compared to infusions without oral fat. A similar effect of intravenous lipid (Intralipid) on glucose, insulin-mediated increases in LPL was not seen in patients receiving total parenteral nutrition 4 days after inception of the program (152). However, because these subjects were catabolic when total parenteral nutrition was initiated, the effect of the alteration in dietary composition on LPL in this study cannot be properly assessed.

Effects of Pregnancy Very few studies have examined adipose tissue LPL throughout pregnancy in rats. The available evidence points to a stable or slight increase in enzyme activity up to the last days of gestation (153–

156). Near parturition, a decrease (144,153,154,156,157) or no change (145) in LPL activity have been reported. In one study, LPL was not determined, but a diminished uptake of triglyceride fatty acids into adipose tissue was found (158). In guinea pigs, LPL did not decrease during the last half of pregnancy (159) whereas in sheep a terminal decline in the enzyme activity was demonstrated (160).

In humans, measurements of femoral and abdominal adipose tissue LPL at 8–11 weeks of gestation have shown no change when compared to values from non-pregnant controls (161).

Effects of Lactation. Following parturition in rats, adipose tissue LPL activity is lower than in pregnant or nonpregnant control animals (31,32,144,156,162–165). In sheep, subcutaneous adipose tissue LPL remains unchanged from levels found in the latter phases of pregnancy (160). However, omental adipose tissue LPL is lower in lactating sheep than in non-pregnant ewes (166).

The decline in LPL near parturition in rats is accompanied by increases in mammary gland LPL (31,32,144,156,162,164,165). A role of prolactin in this reciprocal regulation has been considered. First, prolactin has been shown to inhibit LPL synthesis in adipose tissue of lactating rats (165). Second, the increase in adipose tissue LPL and decrease in mammary gland LPL after hypophysectomy can be reversed by prolactin administration (165). Moreover, the fall in adipose tissue LPL and increase in mammary gland LPL induced in 20 day pregnant rats by PGF_2-α were associated with a 6-fold increase in serum prolactin (167). However, administration of the dopaminergic compound, bromocriptine, failed to alter the effect of PGF_2-α on the lipases despite the prevention of prolactin elevation. In addition, progesterone completely blocked the effect of PGF_2-α on LPL and serum prolactin. These findings suggest a primary role of progesterone, not prolactin, in controlling both adipose tissue and mammary LPL near parturition. However, Flint et al. (164) showed that treatment of lactating rats with bromocriptine increased both fatty acid synthesis and LPL activity in adipose tissue and a decrease in fatty acid synthesis and LPL in the mammary gland. The concurrent injection of prolactin prevented these effects of bromocriptine at 24 hours of litter removal, but did not at 48 hours. Such data suggest that the effect of prolactin on adipose tissue metabolism are dependent on a functioning mammary gland. Using prolactin implants, wherein the decline in milk production was prevented in lactating rats, Flint et al. (168) have further shown that prolactin prevented the expected increase in adipose tissue insulin receptors and decreased LPL. Progesterone implants, however, stimulated LPL in mammary glands and decreased insulin receptors in adipose tissue, but failed to decrease LPL. Although prolactin may prevent the decline of milk production during extended lactation through a direct effect on the mammary gland, these data are consistent with a partial effect of prolactin mediated through inhibitory effects on adipose tissue.

In humans, the higher activity of LPL in femoral vs. abdominal adipose tissue depots seen in nonpregnant women were not seen during lactation (161). In this setting, marked decreases in LPL in the femoral depot occurred. In addition, during lactation, lipolysis was significantly higher in the femoral region. These results appear to indicate that during lactation, regional metabolic patterns change to favor preferential lipid mobilization from the femoral depot. The role of prolactin in human adipose tissue LPL regulation in late pregnancy or during lactation has not been examined. However, patients with prolactin-secreting pituitary tumors have been shown to have decreases in postheparin plasma LPL (169); adipose tissue LPL was not determined in these subjects.

Effects of Alcohol Intake. In rats, a single administration of a large quantity of ethanol (6 g/kg) had very little effect on the adipose tissue LPL activity measured at 13 and 16 hours after dosing (170). However, in male rats, a 60% increase in LPL was noted after 6 hours. Ethanol (130 mM/kg) was also reported to have no effect on LPL by Giudicelli et al. (171).

In man, the effects of ethanol on adipose tissue LPL have been variable. Following the oral administration of 1 g/kg, a progressive decrease in gluteal adipose tissue LPL over 6 hours occurred that was indistinguishable from the LPL response in control subjects (172). However, when administered with glucose (30 g/m^2 orally), ethanol prevented the expected rise in gluteal heparin-releasable adipose tissue LPL. In the study of Taskinen et al. (173), when 5.5 g/kg was administered over two and a half days, a 2.3-fold increase in the lipase activity was seen. After a more long-term exposure (3 g administered 5 times/day for 5 weeks), a 3-fold increase in the gluteal enzyme occurred (174). Thus, from the limited number of studies available, the duration of ethanol exposure would appear to be the most important variable in determining the LPL response in humans.

Regulation of Adipose Tissue LPL Activity

Insulin. A working assumption for some time has been that insulin is the predominant hormonal regulator of adipose tissue LPL. Decreases in adipose tissue LPL in diabetes mellitus (insulin deficient and/or insulin resistant), and increases in LPL per adipocyte in obesity (a hyperinsulinemic state), are consistent with such a regulatory role of insulin. Although evidence from both animals, especially rats, and man support such an effect, the data are more convincing for rats. To some extent, this may relate to the *in vivo* sensitivity of the lipase response to insulin in rats. Because the effects of diabetes and obesity on adipose tissue LPL will be discussed separately, this section will focus on the effect of insulin on the *in vivo* lipase response.

A relationship between adipose tissue LPL and circulating insulin levels in rats has been reported (23,58,89,110,111,114,115,140), but in two of these reports, (89,140) this occurred only following exogenous insulin administration. In the study by Cryer et al. (23), the relationship encompassed a variety of nutritional states including *ad libitum* feeding, 24-hour starvation, and 24-hour starvation plus oral glucose, sucrose, or fructose. Following a single administration of exogenous insulin (89,108,120,175,176), or following 5–7 days of insulin administration (177–179), consistent increases in LPL have been demonstrated in experimental animals including rats (89,108,120,175,176,178,179) and mice (177). Following single administrations of insulin 1.75–6-fold increase in LPL activity occurred after three hours. Insulin administration for 5–7 days has been associated with a 2.5–8.0 fold elevation in LPL. In the study of Garfinkel et al. (120), animals injected with 0.4 units of insulin/kg intraperitoneally had a 3-fold increase in LPL four hours after injection with increments noted as early as 20 minutes following injection. This increase in LPL was only seen in adipose tissue pieces, not in isolated adipocytes. The injection of cycloheximide also eliminated the insulin-mediated effect. In all of these studies, enzyme activity was measured in extracts of whole tissue pieces.

An additional and perhaps more physiological line of experiments to examine the putative *in vivo* role of insulin on adipose tissue LPL has compared the effects of several sources of dietary carbohydrate. Insulin secretory responses to fructose are blunted in comparison to glucose (111). However, in two studies (180,181), there were no differences in the LPL response to long-term diets isocaloric for fructose and glucose. In the study by Vrana et al. (181), fructose and glucose were administered for up to 30 days and heparin-releasable LPL was measured. In the study of Kannan et al. (180), 21 days of carbohydrate administration was followed by acetone-ether powder LPL determinations. In contrast, in 24-hour fasted rats, glucose administration was associated with a 2.5 fold greater response than that seen following fructose (111). The chronic administration of fructose was also without effect on LPL in the study of Webb et al. (182). When sucrose was added to a chow diet for 7 days, hyperinsulinemia was induced and a 2.5 fold increase in LPL in postmitochondrial supernatants observed (183). However, when sucrose and starch were compared on an isocaloric basis over a two week or greater interval, dietary sucrose was associated with decreases (101) or no change in LPL (145,177,181,182). Only in the study by Shafrir et al. (177) were serum insulin levels measured and found to be equal in starch and sucrose fed mice. Overall, in short-term feeding studies in rats, the LPL response to dietary carbohydrate appeared to depend largely on the insulin secretory response to the ingested carbohydrate. In long-term studies, however, differences in the LPL response to carbohydrate sources with differing effects on insulin secretion were not apparent.

In human subjects, correlations between fasting LPL and serum insulin have been reported (69,72,125,184,185). Such a correlation however, has not always been found (150). In all but one of these studies (185), the subjects studied were both normal-weight and obese. In four studies (69,72,125,184), correlations were seen between the serum insulin concentration and the heparin-releasable enzyme expressed per 10^6 cells. Overall, the reported correlations between LPL and insulin were weak suggesting that only approximately 30% of the fasting enzyme in the respective tissue depots can be accounted for on the basis of serum insulin alone.

When normal-weight and obese subjects are combined, the response of heparin-releasable LPL to meals (125,130,132), five days of high carbohydrate feeding (69), or following caloric restriction (69) is related to the change in serum insulin. However, comparable data are not available from studies with non-obese subjects alone.

In an attempt to test the effect of insulin on LPL in non-obese humans more directly, intravenous glucose or insulin plus glucose have been administered and the LPL response monitored for 5–6 hours. Following a glucose bolus of 15 grams and a subsequent infusion rate of 30–35 g/hr, a 2.5 fold incrase in LPL occurred (186). The average blood glucose and insulin concentrations in this investigation were 134 ± 7 mg/dl and 52 ± 6 μU/ml, respectively. When obese subjects were included, both the absolute and percentage increases in LPL correlated inversely with the average insulin level achieved during the glucose infusion. In a more controlled setting utilizing the euglycemic clamp technique, Sadur and Eckel (187) showed that when insulin is infused at a rate of 40 mU/m^2/min (serum insulin concentrations of 70 μU/ml) into normal-weight subjects, a two-fold increase in LPL occurred after 6 hours of infusion. On the other hand, similar studies by Yki-Jarvinen et al. (188) failed to demonstrate any increase in LPL when insulin levels were maintained at 101 μU/ml for 5 hours. They did (188), however, report a 50% increase in the lipase response to insulin when this hormone was infused to achieve concentrations of 565 μU/ml. In a subsequent study by Sadur et al. (184), insulin concentrations were raised to 281 μU/ml and LPL responses were similar to those reported at 70 μU/ml (187).

Hyperinsulinemic clamps carried out under hyperglycemic conditions, i.e. 8.8 mM or 140 mg/dl, have demonstrated variable increases in LPL. In the study of Yki-Jarvinen et al. (188), a lesser LPL response was seen under hyperglycemic conditions than that produced at euglycemia. However, in the study of Sadur et al. (189), although the 6-hour LPL response was similar at hyperglycemia (140 mg/dl) and euglycemia (85 mg/dl), a significantly greater LPL response was seen 3 hours into the infusion at hyperglycemia than during maintenance of fasting euglycemia. In addition, over the 3-hour infusion, the LPL increase related to the glucose infusion rate (189), an effect not seen at later (5–6 hours) time points (187–189).

Adipose tissue LPL responsiveness to lower insulin infusion rates (15 mU/m^2/min) has also been demonstrated (190). In these studies (carried out only in women), a steady state insulin concentration of 27 μU/ml was achieved. Following intravenous insulin, again for 6 hours, a nearly 2-fold increase in LPL was seen. Over the range of 3 insulin infusion rates (15, 40 and 120 mU/m^2/min), the calculated steady state insulin concentration required for one-half the maximal LPL response was 15 μU/ml. On further examination, this dose response curve was markedly shifted to the right in obese women with the insulin EC_{50} for LPL at 6 hours increased to 110 μU/ml (Figure 1).

An interesting yet unexplained determinant of the LPL per gram response to insulin plus glucose is the basal (fasting) LPL activity. In several of these studies (186–188), inverse relationships between the fasting enzyme and the LPL response was seen. This was not true, however, when the data were examined per cell (R.H. Eckel, unpublished observations). Similar inverse relationships between the LPL response to high carbohydrate feedings (130,191,192), or hypocaloric feeding (135,193) and fasting LPL have been previously documented. Moreover, in some of these investigations, LPL data were expressed per 10^6 cells, not per gram weight (130,192,193).

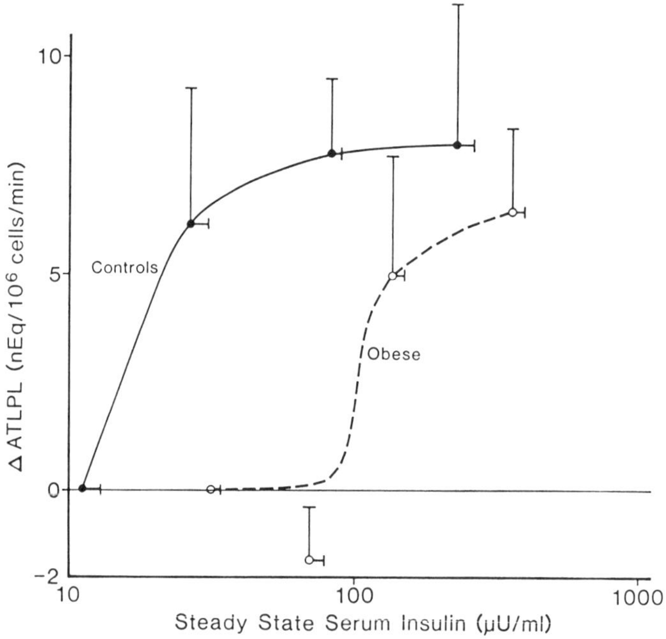

FIGURE 1 Adipose tissue LPL response to variable rate insulin infusions in control and obese women. Following two days of isocaloric formula feeding, subjects were fasted for 12 hr and underwent gluteal adipose tissue biopsies for measurements of LPL. Insulin was then administered at one of three infusion rates: 15 mU/m²/min (controls = 5, obese = 6), 40 mU/m²/min (controls = 9, obese = 9), or 120 mU/m²/min (controls = 5, obese = 14). Fasting euglycemia was maintained with a variable glucose infusion. Data for the change in LPL over 6 hrs of insulin infusion are plotted vs. log steady state serum insulin concentration. Steady state serum insulin concentrations were calculated as a mean of 9 measurements over 6 hrs. Initial data points for both groups represent the mean ±SEM for fasting serum insulin determined prior to the insulin infusion.

Thus, in humans, it appears that adipose tissue itself may play some role in determining the LPL responsiveness to changes in insulin and perhaps other regulators. A physiological role of the lipase to maintain fat cell size could, therefore, be provided by a high basal LPL which is relatively unresponsive to perturbation, or by a lower basal activity which is more responsive to potential regulators.

Glucocorticoids. In rats, conflicting data exist on the physiological *in vivo* effect of glucocorticoids on adipose tissue LPL. In one study, diurnal changes in serum corticosterone paralleled changes in LPL (115). However, 4 days following adrenalectomy, no changes were seen in LPL measured in homogenates of abdominal wall adipose tissue (194). Yet, Baggen et al. (109) demonstrated decreases in epididymal fat pad acetone-ether powder enzyme activity from rats 3 days after adrenalectomy. De Gasquet et al. (116) also demonstrated decreases in LPL after a similar period post-adrenalectomy.

Pharmacological effects of glucocorticoids have also been variable. After single injections of large doses of dexamethasone, LPL was unaltered at 3 hours (175) but increased 24 hours following dosing (116). Increases in LPL by 2 hours were, however, seen following smaller (40 mg/kg) doses of corticosterone, or 1.0 mg/kg of dexamethasone in the experiments of De Gasquet et al. (116). When 50 μg of synthetic 1–24 corticotrophin was given daily for 3 days, decreases in acetone-ether, but not heparin-releasable, LPL were seen (109). When injections were carried out for 20 days, both the acetone-ether and heparin-releasable enzyme remained unchanged from pretherapeutic values. No change in total tissue LPL was seen in uremic rats following a 5 day course of triamcinolone (0.5 ng/kg/day)(195). However, in two other investigations, doses of dexamethasone of 0.125 mg/kg intraperitoneally daily (196) and 40 μg daily (197) were associated with decreases in LPL at 2 and 4 weeks, respectively. Because this decrease occurred concomitantly with hyperinsulinemia, the effect may have been a consequence of insulin resistance produced by excessive glucocorticoids. Doses of glucocorticoids nearer the physiologic range have inconsistently decreased the enzyme activity (197).

At present, effects of glucocorticoids on adipose tissue LPL in man have not been reported.

Sex Steroids. Although sex steroids, in particular female sex steroids, play an important role in adipose tissue metabolism in the rat, sex differences in adipose tissue LPL have not been well studied in this rodent model (198,199). In humans, some studies (64,75,186,200) have demonstrated higher enzyme activities in women than men. This includes unpublished observations (R.H. Eckel et al.) wherein heparin-releasable LPL was higher in normal weight women (5.9 ± 0.6 nEq FFA/10^6 cells/min, n = 43) than men (3.0 ± 1.0, n = 13), and higher in obese women (9.4 ± 1.1, n = 46) than men (3.6 ± 1.2, n = 3). However, in most investigations, only one or predominantly one sex has been examined and, thus, comparisons were not made.

Androgens. Castration of male rats without testosterone replacement produces no alteration in adipose tissue LPL (199,201). In several studies, replacement of testosterone at lower dosages, i.e. 0.2 mg daily, for 30 days (202) or 0.5 mg three times per week for 3 weeks following castration (199) still failed to change LPL. However, when large doses, i.e. 1.0 mg/day were administered for 30 days, decreases in epididymal adipose tissue LPL were seen (202). This amount of testosterone was also associated with the depletion of cytoplasmic estrogen receptors in epididymal adipose tissue. The potential importance of the fall in estrogen receptors to the decrease in LPL was further evaluated by the daily treatment of gonadectomized male rats with a combination of testosterone propionate and the aromatase inhibitor, androsta- 1,4,6-triene-3,17-dione. Following the therapeutic manipulation, a decrease in LPL was not seen. Finally, testosterone administration (up to 0.5 μg/day for up to 6 weeks) to female rats failed to alter parametrial adipose tissue LPL (199,203).

Estrogens. Most studies in rats have demonstrated an adipose tissue LPL-lowering effect of estrogens, specifically estradiol. In both rats (198) and squirrels (204), ovariectomy alone increases parametrial adipose tissue LPL. Short-term ($\leq$1 week) administration of estradiol (2.5–25 μg/day) to ovariectomized rats was associated with an average 60% decrease in parametrial adipose tissue LPL (154,162,198,205–208). In one study, this decrease was near maximum by 1 day (162). More prolonged administration of estrogens to female rats, i.e. up to 4 weeks (58,209), caused no further decline in enzyme activity than that seen after shorter intervals. Higher doses of estradiol, i.e. $>$70 μg/day, had variable enzyme-lowering effects (198,206). In several studies, lower concentrations of estradiol either increased (206), or failed to alter LPL (210). In the only study in which isolated adipocytes were studied (211), both cell-bound and heparin-releasable LPL activities were increased by approximately 30% in rats treated with 0.6 or 6.0 μg per day of estradiol for 10 days. In male rats, estradiol administration over intervals of 3 days to 8 weeks also decreased LPL (198,199,203,205).

In humans, the administration of ethinyl estradiol, 1 μg/kg/day for 14 days failed to alter gluteal heparin-releasable or acetone-ether adipose tissue LPL (212). The observed decrease in post-heparin plasma lipolytic activity accounted for a selective decline in hepatic triglyceride lipase activity.

Progestins. Progesterone administration to female rats, in general, has been associated with increases in parametrial adipose tissue LPL (58,209,210). In one study (209) this effect of progesterone measured routinely for 3 weeks following daily injections was observed within 24 hours of the first injection. In ovariectomized rats, where LPL has been shown to be increased, progesterone had no additional stimulatory effect (198). Similarly, in estrogen-treated ovariectomized rats, 3 days of progesterone failed to prevent the expected estradiol-mediated decrease in LPL (154). However, when progesterone was administered with estrogen to non-ovariectomized rats (58,205,210), the progestin-dependent increase in LPL was observed. Unlike the results with female rats, administration of progesterone to male rats caused no increase in LPL activity (198,205). Overall, these data point to an estrogen-dependent effect of progesterone, perhaps through the progesterone receptor in adipose cells. The presence of such a receptor has been found in female (213), but not male rat (205) perigenital adipose tissue.

In humans, the role of progestins in adipose tissue metabolism has yet to be clarified. In 15 patients with endometrial carcinoma, administration of medroxyprogesterone acetate, 100 mg daily for 2 weeks, failed to alter subcutaneous adipose tissue LPL (214). However, in this study all patients were postmenopausal, the shortest interval from menopause being two years. Despite the absence of a progestin effect on LPL in these studies, positive correlations between the medroxy-progesterone acetate concentrations and LPL were seen. In younger, menstruating women, the cutaneous application of progesterone to the femoral region over a 24 hour period on the 10th day of the menstrual cycle was associated with a significant increase, albeit small (20%), in LPL when compared to the unexposed contralateral side (215). Thus, in humans, a direct effect of progesterone may be seen. Similar to the rat, estrogens may be necessary or permissive for the response. Yet, the presence of estrogen or progestin receptors in human adipose tissue has yet to be documented.

In normal weight women, the LPL activity measured during the follicular (day 10–12) and luteal (day 24–25) phases of their menstrual cycle, was unchanged (161). Preliminary cross-sectional evaluation of normal weight subjects also revealed no differences in gluteal adipose tissue LPL between menstrual cycle phases (216). However, in obese women, LPL activity during the luteal phase was 2-fold higher than during the follicular phase. In this investigation, 1.0 ng/ml of serum progesterone was used as the discriminating level of progesterone between the two phases. Using more conservative criteria, when patients with progesterone values <2.0 and >1.0 ng/ml were excluded, a nearly 3-fold difference between the two phases was seen (R.H. Eckel, unpublished data). No relationship between the serum progesterone level and LPL was found within or between groups. Overall, these data strongly suggest that the difference in LPL between normal weight and obese women are menstrual-cycle phase dependent, an effect of the cycle which could relate to the maintenance of the increased fat cell size seen in the obese state.

Thyroid Hormone. The regulation of adipose tissue LPL by thyroid hormone is one of the better examples of differences in lipid metabolism between rats and man. In rats, induction of hypothyroidism by either the inclusion of thionamides in the diet (103,114,217–220), or thyroidectomy

(221–224) for 1–6 weeks typically results in increases in the adipose tissue enzyme activity (103,114,217–220,223,224) and no change (221,222) or increases (223) in postheparin plasma LPL. Except for one study in 3–6 week old rats (220), triglyceride concentrations in serum have either fallen (103,219,224) or remained unchanged (221,225) during the hypothyroid period. In the study of Gavin et al. (224), the presence of hypothyroidism counteracted the suppressant effects of diabetes and magnified the heparin-releasable LPL response to insulin. Although increases in the total tissue and/or heparin-releasable enzyme were reported in the study of Hansson et al. (103), increases in heparin-releasable LPL predominated over that measured in acetone-ether powders. Also, in freshly prepared adipocytes, the effects of hypothyroidism on both cellular and secreted LPL were less than those found in whole tissue. Thus, a predominant effect of hypothyroidism on LPL degradation, with extracellular sites affected more than intracellular sites, could explain the increases in LPL. The synergistic effect of hypothyroidism and insulin on LPL at least provides support for independent mechanisms of response (224).

In rats made thyrotoxic with daily administrations of L-thyroxine, 50 μg intraperitoneally for 15–19 days, an age-dependent effect was seen (93). In young rats (four and a half week old), a 50% decrease in heparin-releasable LPL was observed. However, in nine and a half week old rats, increases were seen. In another study, where only the postheparin plasma LPL was determined, induction of the thyrotoxic state failed to alter the plasma enzyme activity (225). In rabbits, exogenous levothyroxine for 3 weeks was associated with a decrease in total post-heparin plasma lipolytic activity (226). Overall, these studies are insufficient for conclusions about the effects of excessive thyroid hormone on LPL.

Unlike the rat, hypothyroidism in man has been associated with variable hypertriglyceridemia (68,226–237), and in general, decreases in lipolytic enzymes. In overtly hypothyroid patients heparin-releasable LPL was reduced in both gluteal (68) and abdominal sites (234). In subclinical hypothyroidism, where serum thyroxine concentrations were normal but TSH minimally to moderately elevated, serum trigylcerides and LPL were normal (234). In hypothyroid patients, total postheparin lipolytic activities have consistently been low (168,226,231, 233), whereas postheparin plasma LPL may be normal (232,235) or decreased (236,237). Hepatic triglyceride lipase, however, has consistently been reduced (232,235–237). Yet, despite reductions of lipolytic enzymes, Abrams et al. (235) have shown that in nonobese hypothyroid patients, normal VLDL-triglyceride synthesis and clearance are maintained. Only in obese hypothyroid patients were there defects in VLDL-triglyceride metabolism. Moreover, in these patients, both increases in synthesis and decreases in fractional catabolic clearance rates were documented. Finally, when patients with primary and secondary hypothyroidism were compared, similar increases in triglyceride, decreases in adipose tissue LPL and postheparin plasma LPL, and responses to therapeutic intervention were seen (236).

In thyrotoxic human subjects, triglyceride concentrations have usually been normal (201,226,230,238) and increased after resumption of the euthyroid state (228,238). Although total postheparin lipolytic activity has been variable (226,228,230), postheparin LPL has been unchanged and hepatic triglyceride lipase increased in these subjects (201,237). This might relate to the rapid clearance of intravenous Intralipid seen in one study (230). However, an increase in triglyceride removal has not uniformly been seen (238). In this same study, heparin-releasable LPL in abdominal wall adipose tissue was unaltered.

Adrenergic system. In the mouse, Moskowitz and Moskowitz (119) have presented histochemical evidence that epinephrine administration 30 minutes before sacrifice decreased the amount of LPL reaction product on the capillary endothelium with maintenance of LPL within the adipocyte. Other agents which increase cyclic AMP and lipolysis such as ACTH (101) and cholera toxin (112) have been shown to inhibit adipose tissue LPL. This, however, was not the case for glucagon (113) when administered to starving rats. N^6-(phenyliso-propyl)adenosine, an adenosine analog which inhibits lipolysis when given intraperitoneally, also stimulated LPL (239). In experiments by Portet's group (108,175), rats acclimated to cold temperatures showed no decrease in LPL after administration of 400 μg/kg of norepinephrine 3 hours before death. In rats subjected to unilateral microsurgical denervation of epididymal adipose tissue wherein norepinephrine content was reduced to $<10\%$ of that present in the non-operated side, LPL was not altered in either the overnight fasted or fed state when compared to the contralateral pad (112). Also following administration of the beta blocker pindolol for 8 weeks, both decreases in serum free fatty acids and LPL were seen (240). Thus, the catecholaminergic regulation of LPL may depend on circulating catecholamines and not on local adrenergic mechanisms.

In man, direct effects of catecholamines on adipose tissue LPL have not been examined. However, in a study by Arner et al. (136), there was a negative correlation between the *in vitro* basal rate of lipolysis and LPL in subcutaneous adipose tissue from untreated Type II diabetics. A similar relationship was seen following one week of starvation in nondiabetic obese subjects. However, there was no relationship between lipolysis and LPL in nonobese subjects, nonstarving obese subjects and treated diabetic subjects. An inverse relationship of LPL with basal and/or norepinephrine-stimulated lipolysis was also reported in patients with lipomatous tissue (241,242), hypertriglyceridemia (243), and in the femoral region in lactating women (161). Aminophylline-induced lipolysis with concomitant falls in postheparin plasma LPL also suggest that a decline in the adipose tissue enzyme may have occurred (244).

Growth hormone. Evidence for a role of growth hormone in the modulation of adipose tissue LPL has been indirect and comes from studies of postheparin plasma only. Postheparin plasma LPL is low in acromegalics (221) and high in pituitary dwarfs who, when treated with human growth hormone, have a return of postheparin plasma LPL to levels seen in control subjects (245). Whether the insulin resistance and/or lipolysis induced by growth hormone are responsible for this alteration in postheparin plasma LPL remains untested.

Physiology and Regulation *in vitro*

Systems for the study of LPL

The interpretation of data gathered from *in vitro* experimentation on LPL depends on the system chosen for study. LPL activity is affected by the complex processing of the enzyme, its secretion from cells and relocation to extracellular sites (the extracellular matrix and/or capillary endothelium), and its biologic half-life in these different sites. In adipose tissue pieces, changes in enzyme activity could be affected by alterations of any of these parameters and could involve a multiplicity of effects at various sites. Despite such complexities, adipose tissue pieces perhaps most resemble the *in vivo* setting in that the communication networks which exist in the organism are preserved.

Isolated adipocytes are ideal for the investigation of effects of the perturbation on the lipase at the cell of origin, however, the short lifespan of such cells *in vitro* is a limitation.

Preadipocyte cultures provide for the reliable access of the perturbation to cells and, for the most part, *in vitro* longevity is not a limitation. However, these cultures contain a mixture of adipocyte-precursor cells in various stages of differentiation as well as fibroblasts and, at times, endothelial cells and may not, therefore, accurately reflect the *in vivo* adipose tissue environment. In 3T3-L1 cells, regulation of the lipase by hormones diminishes as *in vitro* lifespan increases (246). As with adipose tissue pieces, potential effects of the connective tissue matrix must be taken into consideration.

Procedures used for LPL determination are also critically important to the interpretation of LPL data. In general, measurements of enzyme activity and/or protein have been carried out 1) in the buffer or culture medium in which tissue or cells are suspended and LPL spontaneously released; 2) in the suspending buffer or medium following the addition of heparin to the incubate; and 3) after tissue or cell disruption by sonication or homogenization and extraction of protein. This last step is often preceded by delipidation with acetone and/or ether, and followed by preparation of post-mitochondrial supernatants prior to enzyme assay. Theoretically, if the rate of LPL degradation or inactivation remained constant in these arbitrary compartments, the sum of LPL in the culture medium, along with that released by heparin and extracted from cells, should be equal to that measured in the whole *in vitro* system. However, the half-life of LPL in cells and in media are affected by a number of variables. For example, at 37°, the t½ of buffer or medium-suspended LPL incubated with tissue has varied from 30 (247) to 60 (88) minutes. When measured in cycloheximide-treated 3T3-L1 cells (248), or Ob17 cells (249), a t½ of approximately 30 minutes was reported. Yet, when LPL from cycloheximide-treated fat bodies was examined at 25° rather than 37°, and in the absence of glucose to prevent the putative post-translational activation of the lipase, a markedly prolonged (t½ of five hours) was obtained. After the addition of glucose, LPL activity increased at 1 hour and then a t½ of three and a half hours was observed. At 37° in buffer removed from isolated rat adipocytes, a t½ of approximately 30 minutes was obtained (250,251). In the study of Kornhauser and Vaughn (252), a similar buffer incubated at 30° revealed an LPL t½ of 90 minutes (370). In heparin-containing medium separated from fat pads, the t½ was somewhat longer, from 1 (90) to 2 hours (253). In human adipocyte cultures, the t½ for LPL in culture medium was approximately 1 hour and for heparin-releasable enzyme approximately 2 hours (254). Although the addition of serum has generally been associated with an increase in cellular LPL activity (88,254–257), the effect of serum on the extracellular activity has been variable. In buffer-suspended rat adipocytes, a marked prolongation of the t½ occurred (252). However, in the heparin-releasable fraction from cultured isolated human adipocytes, the addition of 10% serum failed to alter the biologic half-life of approximately 2 hours (254). In cultured human adipocytes, LPL in the medium has not been measurable in the absence of serum. In summary, it appears that heparin, temperature, and serum all affect the biologic half-life of LPL, and that differences also exist between the t½ measured in the presence or absence of tissue or cells, and within versus outside cells.

The heparin-releasable compartment of LPL is worthy of additional comments. Because this enzyme fraction resides in the extra-adipocyte space or on adipocyte surfaces, its importance to the overall function of the lipase in any of the *in vitro* systems is most relevant. Whether examined in adipose tissue pieces (45,86,87,253,258–260), cultured preadipocytes (249,261–263), freshly prepared and suspended adipocytes (45,252,255,257,264,265), or cultured adipocytes (251,254), heparin increases lipolytic activity. Following heparin exposure, decreases in LPL in cellular (264) or tissue (56) homogenates, or decreases in enzyme activity released by a subsequent heparin exposure (254,259,261,262,266), have been found. Following a 24-hour exposure of preadipocytes to heparin, Rothblat and Glick (261) demonstrated a 3 day delay in replenishment of the heparin-releasable LPL pool. The dependency of the heparin release step on protein synthesis has been variable. In adipose tissue pieces (267) and cultured preadipocytes (249,262,268), time-dependent decreases in LPL activity have occurred following cycloheximide. In several studies (249,262), the effect of cycloheximide was delayed and the delay was probably in the replenishment of the heparin-releasable LPL pool. Reducing the incubation temperature to 4° also failed to alter heparin-releasable LPL (at 30 minutes) in preadipocytes (262), but did so in adipose tissue pieces from human subjects (126). In isolated adipocytes, however, decreases in heparin-releasable LPL were not seen up to 3 hours following cycloheximide (10–100μg/ml) treatment (255,265,269). Although in two of these investigations, experiments were carried out at 25° rather than 37° (255,269), it remains unclear why these data differ substantially from the marked and immediate effects of lower concentrations of cycloheximide (1 μg/ml) on heparin-releasable LPL in cultured rat adipocytes (251). Dose response curves in general have shown maximum effects of heparin over three logarithms, 0.6–130 μg/ml (254,261,265,269,270).

Adipocytes. Studies of LPL in adipocytes are usually performed in isolated cells prepared from adipose tissue pads following agitation in a collagenase-containing buffer. Generally, experiments have been carried out in buffer- or medium-suspended cells immediately after preparation. In nearly all investigations increases in LPL in the culture medium were noted at intervals of 30 minutes to 4 hours (56,129,247,252,265,271–273). In two experiments, no change was apparent 90 minutes (274) and 4 hours (129) after preparation. Only some of these experiments, however, were carried out at 37° (56,129,272); the remainder were performed at temperatures between 20° and 26°. In one experiment where 23° and 37° were compared, the increase in LPL in the culture medium at 45 minutes was greater at the higher temperature. Heparin-releasable LPL has also been shown to increase at identical intervals, as noted for culture medium LPL (56,121,252,255,265,269). Again, few studies have been performed at 37° (56,265). Changes in adipocyte or extractable enzyme activity within hours of preparation have been less predictable. Increases (247,252,255,275), decreases (56) and no change (121,250,265,271,274) have all been reported. A prior exposure to heparin has failed to predict the subsequent relative amount of cellular LPL. Here, the incubation temperature appears to be important. In only one experiment, in which LPL in adipocytes increased, were cells incubated at 37° (275). Moreover, in the only study carried out at 37° in which no change in adipocyte LPL was apparent, the experiment was concluded at 50 minutes (274).

The presence or absence of glucose (250,265,271), and changes in adipocyte protein synthesis have also been related to alterations in the lipase activity (250). Protein synthesis increased from 7 (275) to 12-fold (250) in buffer (containing glucose)-suspended adipocytes over 3 hours and 50 minutes, respectively. Thus, freshly prepared adipocytes provide a useful system in which to examine LPL regulation at the level of the adipocyte.

Recently, a system has been developed to examine the regulation of LPL in adipocytes over longer intervals. Following collagenase digestion under sterile conditions, adipocytes (both rat and human) are extensively washed, and suspended in culture medium with 10% fetal bovine serum and cephalothin in sterile polypropylene tubes (251). Adipocytes are then incubated at 37° in an atmosphere of 5% CO_2 and 95% air for up to 3 days.

Continued viability of rat adipocytes has been documented by maintenance of specific ^{125}I-insulin binding, total adipocyte number, and a linear rate of glucose utilization for up to 3 days (251). In human adipocyte cultures, cell viability was also demonstrated by constancy of specific ^{125}I-insulin binding, cell number, cell size, trypan blue exclusion, and increases in cell-associated ^{125}I-insulin following exposure to the lysosommatropic agent, chloroquine (254).

In rat adipocytes, heparin-releasable LPL fell from 7.9 ± 1.5 nEq FFA/10^6 cells/min at preparation to 1.4 ± 0.2 after overnight incubation, but remained unchanged over the subsequent 2 days (251). Nearly all the decrease in heparin-releasable LPL was seen within the first 4 hours after suspension. Cellular (extractable) activity, measured in heparin-treated cells using a modification of the bile salt detergent extraction technique of Iverius and Brunzell (126,276), fell during the first 24 hours (19.9 ± 3.3 to 7.7 ± 0.9 nEq FFA/10^6 cells/min, and remained unchanged over the subsequent 48 hours. LPL in the culture medium was stable between days 1 and 3 of culture.

Unlike cultures of rat adipocytes, heparin-releasable LPL was unmeasurable in freshly prepared cultures of human adipocytes (254), but increased progressively over the next 10 hours. This rise was enhanced by the presence of 10% fetal bovine serum in the culture medium. By 48 hours, some decline in heparin-releasable LPL was noted, with a further decrease by 72 hours. Extractable LPL was measurable after 1 hour in culture and remained unchanged over 72 hours. The presence of serum, however, failed to increase extractable LPL. Over the entire 72 hours of culture, LPL activity in the culture medium was variable, and when present, very low when serum was omitted from the culture medium. However, the addition of serum produced an activity curve very similar to that for heparin-releasable LPL. In fact, the secretory response to serum correlated strongly with heparin-releasable LPL measured 24 hours following preparation ($r_s = 0.731$, $p < 0.001$). Overall, the ability to sustain cultured adipocytes for up to 3 days *in vitro* provides a useful system for the more long-term study of LPL, as well as other aspects of adipocyte biology.

Preadipocytes. Cultured preadipocytes provide a system in which to carry out a detailed and more long-term examination of LPL *in vitro*, and an opportunity to examine the role of the enzyme in terminal differentiation and lipid filling. At the time of preparation (following collagenase digestion), the stromal vascular fraction of rat adipose tissue (including preadipocytes) fails, for the most part, to demonstrate LPL activity (34,45,88,264,277). There are several exceptions, however. Ho et al. (259), found both LPL in the culture medium and a 3-fold increase in heparin-releasable LPL immediately following preparation. In addition, after density gradient separation, two studies demonstrated the presence of LPL in rat preadipocytes (278,279). Bjorntorp et al. (278) found similar activities of LPL per 10^6 cells in the heavier (stromal) cells as well as in freshly prepared adipocytes. By immunofluorescence, the presence of LPL in connective tissue cells, including cells resembling preadipocytes (280), has been shown in human adipose tissue.

After harvesting, stromal cells are typically plated and allowed to reach confluent growth prior to spontaneous or induced differentiation. Although much of the published information on LPL and adipocyte differentiation has been gathered from studies carried out in preadipocytes exposed to agents known to induce differentation such as insulin, dexamethasone, isobutylmethylxanthine, and dibutyryl cyclic AMP (248,263,270,279,281–290), LPL has been found in cultured adipose tissue stromal cells without induction of differentiation and with minimal lipid filling (261,279,281–283,291,292). LPL has typically not been found before confluence, but in several studies including those carried out in Ob17 cells (286), 3T3-L1 cells (281) and rat preadipocytes (279,288,289), LPL was present at the time of or before confluent growth was achieved. For rodent adipocyte precursors, LPL is more assayable from 2–6 days following contact inhibition (248,263,270,282–285,291,293,294). When insulin has been added to induce differentiation, minimal (279,282) to 3-fold (281,283) increases in LPL have been noted within the first two and a half weeks of culture.

The importance of LPL to lipid filling of adipocyte precursors is related to the availability of extracellular lipoprotein substrate and to the induction of enzymes of fatty acid and triglyceride biosynthesis. The ability of 3T3-L1 (248), Ob17 (294,295) and teratogenic fibroadipogenic cells (263) to lipid-fill in the absence of serum indicates that these cells can circumvent the availability of extracellular triglyceride by inducing fatty acid biosynthesis. To a lesser extent, lipid filling also occurs in human preadipocytes where LPL activity is limited (292) or absent (290). Howver, the induction of LPL *in vitro* usually occurs before increases in neutral lipids (281,283,285,287,296,297), and in rat preadipocytes was closely related to triglyceride fatty acid uptake from the culture medium (257,288). Occasionally, triglyceride accumulation occurs prior to increases in LPL (282), or LPL has been present without lipid filling (268). These cell lines, bovine (282) and endothelial-like clones from rat stromal vascular cells (268) may not be typical and have been less well investigated than other *in vitro* models of adipocyte differentiation.

When compared to the induction of fatty acid biosynthesis, acylation of glycerophosphate, or triglyceride biosynthesis, LPL has been seen at similar postconfluent intervals (270,283,284,293) or earlier (279,285,294). The relative independence and, therefore, importance of LPL as a marker for differentiation is supported by the continued presence of the lipase when differentiation (changes in cell shape) occurs without triglyceride accumulation induced by the inclusion of extensively dialyzed serum (without biotin) in the culture medium (293). In this setting, malic enzyme and glycerophosphate acyltransferase activities rose minimally whereas LPL and glycerophosphate dehydrogenase were unaffected. The addition of biotin or serum ultrafiltrate restored these enzymes and triglyceride filling. The presence of LPL and glycerophosphate dehydrogenase, despite the limitation of triglyceride accumulation (by decreasing fatty acid synthesis or by reducting glycerophosphate acyltransferase), indicates that these two enzymes play a major role in the differentiation process.

Processing of LPL

Like many other secretory proteins, LPL is synthesized, transported, and secreted from adipocytes in a step-wise yet incompletely understood manner. Again, the systems and temperatures chosen for experiments have varied and must be taken into account before final conclusions can be reached.

Until recently when LPL antibodies became available, investigations of LPL physiology *in vitro* depended on measurements of enzyme activity in functional "compartments" and various pharmaceuticals to inhibit processes likely to be involved in LPL regulation. For the most part, this section will concentrate on LPL physiology as examined in buffer- or medium-suspended tissue or cells with glucose and/or amino acids in the absence of insulin. Mechanisms by which insulin and other hormones regulate the lipase will be subsequently covered in more detail.

Transcription. Experiments that have examined the *in vitro* effects on *LPL* of drugs which affect DNA transcription, e.g. actinomycin D and α-amanitin, did not show a decrease in cellular or tissue LPL when added for intervals up to 12 hours (88,253,275,298). In fact, in several of these experiments, increases in heparin-releasable (88) and total tissue LPL (253) were seen following actinomycin D (5 μg/ml) additions. These data suggest an effect of the inhibitor on other proteins which may be involved in intracellular activation-inactivation or degradation of the enzyme. Longer incubations in actinomycin D however, resulted in dose-dependent reductions in the cellular LPL response to insulin and glucose (275).

Protein Synthesis. Protein synthesis inhibitors, which have been more extensively studied *in vitro*, provide important information about the physiology of LPL. The addition of small concentrations of cycloheximide (298,299) or puromycin (299) to *in vitro* systems predictably and reproducibly reduce LPL or enzyme responsiveness over 24 hours. Shorter durations of exposure, however, produce a less uniform response. In adipose tissue pieces (267,273,300–302) and in freshly suspended rat adipocytes (120,121,255,265,269,271,273,275), the addition of cycloheximide in concentrations ranging from 10–100 μg/ml for up to 3 hours has, in some studies, failed to alter culture medium (120,255,265,271,273), heparin-releasable (121,255,267,269), or total cellular or tissue LPL (265,267,269,271, 273,275,300,301). These data did not appear to be influenced by incubation temperature (23–25° or 37°). Although some of these experiments were carried out in the presence of insulin in the incubate (121,255,267,269,273), the others were not, and point to protein synthesis- independent regulatory effects on the lipase or its activation. Nevertheless, a large number of investigations have not supported this position.

Whereas much of the data which support a near-complete or complete dependence of LPL activity on protein synthesis come from studies utilizing cultured preadipocytes (248,249,262,268,284,298), other systems including adipose tissue pieces (78,253,267,303,304), freshly suspended adipocytes (121,250), and cultured adipocytes (259) have also been examined. In these investigations, similar concentrations and intervals of incubation with the inhibitor were used, but nearly all experiments were carried out at 37°. The study by Spencer et al. (121) was an exception. Again, insulin was included in some (87,121,253,298,303), but not all incubations. Both decreases in extractable (87,121,248–251,253,262,284,298,303) and heparin-releasable (251,262,268,304) LPL were seen. However, as noted earlier, decreases in cellular or total tissue LPL were not always accompanied by falls in heparin-releasable LPL (121,267,284). Whether or not concominant changes in heparin-releasable LPL occur, immunotitration indicates that changes in enzyme activity parallel changes in enzyme protein (270).

Energy. The importance of cellular energy in the regulation of LPL has been shown in experiments which examined the *in vitro* effects of temperature and metabolic inhibitors on intact adipose tissue and isolated adipocytes. Stewart et al. (272) reported that the reduced release of LPL into the culture medium from freshly suspended rat adipocytes at 23° was rapidly and further reduced by sodium cyanide. In contrast, the release of malic dehydrogenase was not altered by temperature or cyanide. Subsequent studies, also carried out at room temperature, demonstrated decreases in LPL after exposure to metabolic inhibitors. In rat adipocytes, sodium cyanide reduced heparin-releasable LPL by 50% within 30 minutes of drug exposure (265). In adipose tissue pieces, the addition of dinitrophenol (1 mM) and arsenate (40 mM) resulted in a linear and time-dependent reduction in tissue LPL (273). In this experiment, insulin was included in the incubation system.

More recently, dinitrophenol has been shown to have a time- and dose-dependent effect on heparin-releasable and extractable LPL in cultured rat adipocytes (R. H. Eckel, unpublished data). In cells cultured overnight at 37°, the addition of 0.04 or 0.1 mM dinitriphenol failed to alter LPL at 30 minutes. However, by 2 hours, mean differences between controls and dinitrophenol-treated cells were statistically significant for both heparin-releasable and extractable LPL. No alteration in LPL measured in the culture medium was seen. To assure the absence of permanent cell toxicity of dinitrophenol, adipocytes were extensively washed free of drug and shown to return to basal levels of LPL production and responsiveness. The relative dependence of the decrease in heparin-releasable LPL on the decrease in extractable LPL remains untested.

Microtubules. Investigations into the role of microtubules in the regulation of LPL have used the drug colchicine, which impairs the polymerization of tubulin. Three systems have been used for such studies. In freshly prepared rat adipocytes, the addition of 0.1 mM colchicine was associated with a 75% decrease in heparin-releasable LPL over 3 hours with no alteration in culture medium or cellular enzyme (269). This effect was similar whether in the presence or absence of cycloheximide. At higher concentrations (1 mM), colchicine reduced heparin-releasable and increased cell-associated LPL over 4 hours in rat preadipocytes (262). In cultured rat adipocytes, a similar effect was seen at 0.1 mM colchicine (305). Colchicine decreased heparin-releasable LPL minimally by 2 and 4 hours and caused a 2-fold increase in extractable LPL at both timepoints. In preliminary experiments, this colchicine-mediated increase in extractable LPL was protein synthesis dependent. These data suggest that microtubules are important in regulating LPL activity as well as in its transport and synthesis within adipocytes.

Glycosylation. The role of LPL maturation, including glycosylation, in the ultimate secretion of the lipase can now be studied systematically by comparing measurements of enzyme activity with immunofluorescent microscopy. In previous studies, inhibition of glycosylation with 2-deoxyglucose produced variable results. In cultured rat adipocytes, Glick et al. (262) reported rapid decreases in both heparin-releasable and total cellular LPL following substitution of glucose with 2-deoxyglucose. In insulin and cycloheximide-exposed tissue (302) or insulin exposed glucose-deprived preadipocytes (298), the addition of 2-deoxyglucose failed to decrease cellular LPL.

More recently, Vannier et al. (249) used ionophores which affect the intra-cellular transport of membrane and secretory proteins to further examine LPL traffic and processing. After Ob17 cells were depleted of LPL with cycloheximide and heparin, the addition of monensin during the repletion phase failed to prevent the synthesis of fully active LPL. Under these conditions, however, LPL protein accumulated in the Golgi apparatus and heparin-releasable LPL was reduced. When cells were treated with carbonylcyanide m-chlorophenylhydrazone, enzyme activity was absent but immunoflourescence demonstrated LPL in the endoplasmic reticulum (*ER*). Competition for binding to anti-LPL was similar for both mature and ER-sequestered LPL. From these studies, it appears that intracellular activation of LPL takes place somewhere between the endoplasmic reticulum and the Golgi apparatus.

The importance of different stages of LPL glycosylation to LPL bioactivity and secretion has been further documented by Chajek-Shaul et al. (306). As shown by Vannier et al. (249), monensin decreased heparin-releasable and culture medium LPL in rat preadipocytes by approximately 90% at 4 hours (306). Concomitant increases in intracellular activity were seen despite reductions in ^{3}H-leucine incorporation into immunoabsorbable LPL. On the other hand, tunicamycin (5 μg/ml) caused a more limited reduction in immunoabsorbable LPL but reduced intracellular activity by 90%. Similar reductions in heparin-releasable LPL (85%) and slightly smaller decreases in extractable LPL (67%) have been observed in cultured rat adipocytes following overnight incubation in 5 μg/ml of tunicamycin (R. H. Eckel et al., unpublished data). Thus, the addition of the asparagine-linked oligosaccharide to LPL, a process inhibited by tunicamycin, appears to be necessary for the maintenance of LPL activity. Moreover, both terminal glycosylation and oligosaccharide processing may be important for the transport of LPL to the heparin-releasable compartment and subsequent secretion from the cell.

Secretion. In general, increases in LPL activity in the surrounding buffer or culture medium appear to be closely related to increases in heparin-releasable LPL. This has been most convincingly demonstrated for cultured human adipocytes (254). Increases in culture medium LPL occur more readily at 37° than 23° (272) and are enhanced by serum (252). However, both the inhibition of protein synthesis by cycloheximide (120,255,262,271) and impairment of microtubular function by colchicine (269,305) are without short-term effects (less than 4 hours). The unlikely possibility that insulin has an independent secretory effect on LPL will be subsequently addressed.

Binding and degradation. The possibility that LPL is degraded in adipose tissue has been raised by studies using ^{125}I-labeled milk LPL. The amount of binding of ^{125}I-LPL to a variety of cell types in culture at 37° is related to the enzyme concentration used (307). In cells which do not synthesize LPL (i.e. fibroblasts and endothelial cells), there is a high ratio of surface binding to degradation. However, in preadipocyte (and heart) cultures, wherein LPL is produced, this ratio is reversed. Moreover, when examined in adipose tissue pieces at 37° by a pulse-chase technique, endogenously labeled LPL is rapidly degraded (43% in 3 hours) although little degradation of the total adipose tissue protein occurs (308). Although the contribution of various cell types to this degradation process can only be inferred from the studies aforementioned with the milk lipase, these data support the concept of translocation and catabolism of LPL in the adipose tissue.

Regulation of LPL Activity

Insulin. The *in vitro* regulation of LPL by insulin has been well studied in a variety of systems. Species differences, in particular between rodent and human systems, are clearly apparent. In rat adipose tissue pads or pieces, the addition of insulin in concentrations ranging from 0.2 mU/ml (8 ng/ml) to 12.5 mU/ml (500 ng/ml) for up to 5 hours are associated with increases in total tissue (274,275,300–303,309–311) or heparin-releasable (86,304) LPL activity or both (260). In two experiments (302,311), cycloheximide was included in the suspension medium. In general, increases in LPL in the absence of cycloheximide were delayed (90 minutes to 5 hours), and of a greater magnitude (2.5-fold) than those in which the effects of insulin were protein synthesis-independent. Protein synthesis-independent effects typically occurred between 60 and 90 minutes and increases of 1.5-2-fold were noted (302,311).

In cultured preadipocytes, insulin-mediated increases in cellular LPL have also been seen over short-term incubations (< 4 hr) (246,266,298). In these experiments, similar concentrations of insulin were needed to produce responses similar to those seen in adipose tissue pads or pieces. In studies carried out over longer incubations, i.e. 24 hours, 3 (299) to 8-fold (298) increases in cellular enzyme activity were seen. Moreover, responses have been documented to occur at insulin concentrations as low as 10^{-11}M (298). In freshly suspended rat adipocytes, increases in cellular LPL have been seen by 30 minutes (252) and up to 3 hours (273) following the addition of insulin. In both of these studies, incubation temperatures were 20 and 25°, respectively. In addition, in the experiment of Ashby et al. (273), cycloheximide was included in the incubation buffer.

In cultured rat adipocytes incubated overnight at 37°, insulin-mediated increases in cellular LPL were seen as early as 30 minutes (heparin-releasable) and continued 24 hours after hormone addition (251). Dose-dependent increases in heparin-releasable LPL were noted at insulin concentrations as low as 1.0 ng/ml. Unlike experiments carried out in freshly prepared adipocytes (252,273), no increase in LPL was seen when insulin was added immediately after suspension. However, insulin did maintain enzyme activity over 4 hours (251). These data resemble those of Patten (250) in experiments also performed at 37°, and suggest that incubation temperature may be an important variable when assessing the acute effects of insulin on LPL in isolated adipocytes.

Adipocytes or cultured preadipocytes have been used to assess the effect of insulin on enzyme secretion. In all experiments (251,252,266,273,298), except one (298), insulin-mediated increases in culture medium LPL occurred simultaneously or after the increase in cellular enzyme activity. It should be noted, however, that in two of these studies (266,273), the earliest timepoints of culture medium LPL determinations were 2 and 3 hours. In the study of Spooner et al. (298), where an immediate effect of insulin on culture medium LPL was seen, no dependence on cellular metabolism or protein synthesis was required. An explanation for the differences in the data between this and other reports remains unclear.

In human adipose tissue pieces, whether studied immediately after preparation (61,312) or after 1 week of suspension (313), insulin had no stimulatory effect. When 3×10^{-7} M hydrocortisone was coincubated with 1 mU/ml (40 ng/ml) of insulin, an increase in tissue LPL (2.5-fold above hydrocortisone alone) was observed. Glucocorticoids have also been shown to enhance the effects of insulin on LPL in rat adipose tissue (311). In cultured human adipocytes incubated with insulin for 24 hours, increases in heparin-releasable (36 ± 10%) and extractable LPL (28 ± 12%) were only seen at 400 ng/ml of insulin, not at 1, 4 or 40 ng/ml (254). Because high concentrations of insulin have previously been shown to cross-react with insulin-like growth factor-1 (IGF_1) receptors (314,315), experiments were also performed over a range of IGF_1 concentrations (0.1–500 ng/ml) and compared with the responses to insulin at 400 ng/ml. IGF_1 produced a dose-dependent increase in heparin-releasable LPL that was significant at concentrations of 10, 50, and 500 ng/ml. Moreover, the magnitude of the increase in heparin-releasable LPL by IGF_1 was similar to that produced by 400 ng/ml of insulin. It should be noted that no effect of IGF_1 on LPL has been found in cultured rat adipocytes (R. H. Eckel, unpublished data). In cultured human adipocytes, concentrations of IGF_1 as low as 10 ng/ml produced increases in cellular LPL that paralleled the effects of pharmacologic concentrations of insulin. Because recent evidence suggests that microvascular endothelial cells from human adipose tissue synthesize IGF_1 (316), the effect of IGF_1 on LPL in cultured human adipocytes may have relevance *in vivo.*

In most experiments, the stimulatory effects of insulin on tissue (250,275,300,301,311) or cellular LPL (250,251,298,299,317) were reported to be blocked by cycloheximide. However, as previously discussed, the effects of insulin (and glucose) on post-synthetic events have been suggested by experiments with cycloheximide-treated cells (273) or tissue (302,311). Although a slightly greater increase has been seen in adipocytes incubated at 25° (302), increases in adipose tissue occurred at 37° (302,311). Not surprisingly, insulin-mediated effects on the lipase have also been prevented, albeit after 24 hours by actinomycin D and α-amanitin (298). The uncoupling of oxidative phophorylation with dinitrophenol, and the prevention of asparagine-linked glycosylation by tunicamycin, have also prevented insulin- mediated increases in heparin releasable and extractable LPL in cultured rat adipocytes (R. H. Eckel, unpublished data). In addition, the impairment of tubulin polymerization by colchicine has been shown to decrease insulin- stimulated heparin releasable (at 30 minutes and 2 hours), and increase insulin-stimulated extractable LPL over 4 hours in cultured rat adipocytes (305).

In summary, the insulin regulation of LPL *in vitro* appears to be species specific. In human adipocytes, the effects of insulin at physiologic concentrations have yet to be demonstrated, and the magnitude of the response after exposure to higher levels has been less than that seen *in vivo* after intravenous insulin infusions (187). In rat tissue or cells, protein synthesis-dependent effects are clearly present and a role of other cellular processes has also been established. Because in rat systems the insulin effect has not been reproduced by IGF_1 but mimicked by anti-insulin receptor antibodies (299), the ultimate mechanism(s) of the insulin-mediated increase in LPL must await further identification of the second messenger for insulin action.

Glucose. Substantial evidence supports the fact that t on LPL *in vitro* is glucose-dependent. This has been show pieces (86,260,301,302,315), cultured preadipocytes (29 rat adipocytes (250,252,273), and cultured rat (317) an (318). The only exceptions have been increases in heparin-rel in tissue pieces (260,304) incubated in insulin concentrations of 40 ng/ml for 3–4 hours. In different systems (87,298,308) including cultured rat adipocytes (R. H. Eckel, unpublished observations), near maximal responsiveness of LPL to glucose has occurred at glucose concentrations of greater than or equal to 0.25 mg/ml. In several studies, the addition of glucose to insulin-pretreated glucose-deprived cells was prevented by cycloheximide (298,302,317). In contrast, actinomycin D has failed to block this effect of glucose in 3T3-L1 cells (298). These data suggest that the glucose effect on LPL is subsequent to transcription.

In attempts to discern the role of glucose metabolism which supports the lipase response, experiments have been performed using other carbohydrates or glycolytic intermediates in place of glucose. Other than the study by Wing et al. (87), mannose has been equal to glucose in supporting the insulin-mediated LPL response (298,302, R. H. Eckel, unpublished data). Similar data have also been provided for fructose (87,298, R. H. Eckel, unpublished data), however, in the absence of insulin pretreatment, a decrease (302) and increase (304) in comparison with glucose have also been seen. Dihydroxyacetone (87,298), glucosamine (87), 2-deoxyglucose (262,298,302), ribose (302), and malate (302) have uniformly been ineffective in promoting the lipase response. However, data for both galactose and pyruvate have been conflicting. In adipose tissue (87,253,302) and preadipocytes (298), galactose and pyruvate as well as glucose failed to sustain or increase LPL, whether or not insulin-pretreatment (253,298) occurred. However, in cultured rat adipocytes, although basal and insulin-stimulated heparin-releasable LPL tended to be less with galactose (1 mg/ml) or pyruvate (2 mg/ml) than with glucose (1 mg/ml), the percentage increase with insulin-pretreatment was identical to that produced with glucose, mannose, or fructose (R. H. Eckel, unpublished data). Although the data from systems other than cultured rat adipocytes would suggest that the glucose response is only seen with hexoses that enter the glycolytic pathway, terminally differentiated fat cells may be more capable of generating ATP from galactose and pyruvate than incompletely differentiated stromal cells in culture or intact adipose tissue. At present, it remains unclear how carbohydrate assimilation affects the lipase response, but post-transcriptional protein synthesis-related events and ATP generation are almost certainly involved.

Steroids. As previously noted, glucocorticoids are permissive for the insulin-mediated increase in LPL in both rat fat pads (311) and cultured suspended human adipose tissue pieces (313). However, glucocorticoids themselves have minimal if any effect on LPL in rat adipose tissue (313)

ultured 3T3-L1 cells (298). And, an inhibitory effect in the absence of ulin has been observed in human tissue (313).

In 3T3-L1 cells, incubations with 10^{-7}M progesterone and 10^{-8}M 17-β estradiol for 4 days have been associated with modest increases in cellular LPL, 44 and 32%, respectively (298).

Pituitary Hormones. The addition of prolactin (1 μg/ml) and growth hormone (1 μg/ml) to 3T3-L1 cells over 4 days increased LPL but minimally, 35% and 25%, respectively (298). In rat adipose tissue pieces, prolactin (5 μg/ml) increased LPL in cell homogenates, but when added together with insulin (5 μg/ml), no increase was found (309). In adipose tissue pieces, Murase et al. (319) found a 20% decrease in heparin-releasable LPL more than one hour after the addition of 0.1 μg/ml of growth hormone. Higher concentrations, i.e. 1 and 10 μg/ml however, were without an inhibitory effect.

Thyroid Hormone. Again in 3T3-L1 cells, 4 days of exposure of cells to triiodothyronine (10^{-8} M) had no effect on cellular LPL (298). Recently, a role for triiodothyronine in the differentiation of adipose precursors into adipocytes in both obese and lean mice has been found (274,287). In these cell lines, low levels of triiodothyronine appear to be permissive for the insulin-stimulatory effect of LPL during differentiation.

Gastrointestinal Hormones. The original observation that gastric inhibitory polypeptide (GIP) at concentrations of 0.05–5 ng/ml enhanced culture medium and cellular LPL in cultured 3T3-L1 cells (320) has not been substantiated in experiments carried out in cultured rat preadipocytes or cultured rat adipocytes (R. H. Eckel, unpublished data). Moreover, as in the LPL response to insulin in 3T3-L1 cells, LPL responsiveness to GIP was also found to diminish with the aging of the cell *in vitro* (246). However, other gastrointestinal hormones have been shown to increase LPL *in vitro*. In adipose tissue from fasted rats, both gastrin (54 pM) and pancreozymin (12 pM) increased cellular LPL by 26 and 44%, respectively over 2 hours (301). This response was glucose-dependent for gastrin, but glucose independent and additive to that of insulin for pancreozymin. Both the gastrin and pancreozymin responses were inhibited by cycloheximide. In additional experiments performed with freshly suspended adipocytes at 26°, gastrin increased LPL in the culture medium and within cells, whereas the effect of pancreozymin was exclusively on the cellular fraction. In the adipocytes, higher concentrations of gastrin (270–540 pM) were required whereas the cellular LPL response to pancreozymin was nearly 2-fold at 12 pM. Because the concentrations of gastrin and pancreozymin were shown to simulate the fed state *in vivo*, a potential role for these hormones, in particular pancreozymin, *in vivo* remains possible.

Adrenergic System (cyclic AMP). Agents which increase cyclic AMP in adipocytes *in vitro* have been repeatedly shown to decrease LPL. In adipose tissue pads or pieces, a decrease in heparin-releasable and/or total tissue LPL occurs following exposure to epinephrine (87,253,259,273,311), norepinephrine (253,304), glucagon (218,321), ACTH (87,218,253), dibutyryl cyclic AMP (322) and theophylline (218,273,300,304). Although the mechanisms for the decrease have yet to be established, the inhibitory effects have been independent of protein synthesis (273), insulin (273,300,311), and glucose concentration (322).

In freshly suspended rat adipocytes, incubations of cells in dibutyryl cyclic AMP (250) or theophylline (247,273) have also produced decreases in culture medium (273) and cellular LPL (250,273). Again, in some studies effects have been independent of protein synthesis (273), insulin (250,273) and temperature (25° or 37°). In the study of Patten (250), a near 50% reduction of cellular LPL was seen within 60 minutes of dibutyryl cyclic AMP addition. Moreover, dibutyryl cyclic AMP also diminished protein synthesis and cellular ATP. Nevertheless, as in adipose tissue, data remain unconvincing in adipocytes to address the mechanism of the cyclic AMP-mediated diminished LPL activity. In cultured rat adipocytes, isoproterenol mediated decreases in heparin-releasable LPL have also been seen, and as early as 30 minutes following the addition of the catecholamine (R. H. Eckel, unpublished data).

Adenosine. Because adenosine has been shown to have insulin-like effects and is produced within adipose tissue, a potential regulatory role of adenosine (or its metabolite, inosine), at the tissue level have been considered. Following 2 hours of incubation at 37°, adenosine (0.1–100 μM) reduced the fall in intracellular LPL in rat adipocytes (249), but increased LPL in adipose tissue (300). Because at 25° adenosine also increased LPL in adipocytes, and the effect was also seen with adenosine deaminase or inosine but not with the adenosine analog, N^6-(phenylisopropyl)adenosine, it was concluded that the increase in cellular LPL was not due to adenosine *per se*, but rather to the intracellular metabolism of adenosine by adenosine deaminase. A similar lack of effect at 37° of the N^6 analog (0.1–1.0 μM) was found in cultured rat adipocytes, but adenosine deaminase (20–100 μg/ml) was also without effect (R. H. Eckel, unpublished data). In adipose tissue pieces (300), it has further been shown that the effects of adenosine were suppressed by cycloheximide and decreased by cyclic AMP and phosphodiesterase inhibitors. Moreover, adenosine failed to potentiate the effect of insulin. Thus, decreases in cyclic AMP could be the mechanism by which adenosine and insulin both increase LPL.

Ethanol. The addition, *in vitro*, of 20–50 mM ethanol is associated with decreases in the glucose, insulin-mediated increase in heparin-releasable LPL in rat adipose tissue pieces following 3 hours of incubation (323). Metabolites of ethanol are less effective (acetate) or ineffective (acetaldehyde, lactate) in impeding the effect of insulin and glucose.

Pathophysiology

Diabetes Mellitus

Studies *In Vivo*. Following the induction of diabetes mellitus in rats by the injection of either alloxan or streptozotocin, variable degrees of hyperglycemia and deficiencies of adipose tissue LPL have been reported (59,60,95,179,224,321,324–331). In the study of Redgrave and Sampson (225), however, differences in total tissue LPL were not seen over 10 days following streptozotocin despite severe hyperglycemia (428 ± 43 mg/dl). Decreases in both heparin-releasable (60,224,321) and total cellular LPL (59,60,95,179,324–331) have been noted. In general, the severity of the hyperglycemia has been predictive of the extent of the reduction in LPL, however, in only one study has the effect of minimal elevations in blood glucose (6.1 mM) been examined (325).

The administration of insulin to diabetic animals has been associated with increases in total tissue (179,324,327) or heparin-releasable LPL (224). In both Wistar (179) and Zucker (lean and obese)(324) models of streptozotocin-induced diabetes, dose- dependent effects of insulin on LPL have been found. In general, relatively small doses of insulin are required to normalize LPL in insulin-sensitive strains including Wistar (179), Sprague-Dawley (224) and lean Zucker (324) rats, even without substantial decreases in hyperglycemia (224,324). Intervals of insulin administration have varied from 12 hours (224) to two and a half weeks (179) in lean, and 1 month in obese (327) rats, but such variation does not appear to be an important controlling variable in the LPL response.

The impact of diabetes mellitus on human adipose tissue LPL has been examined in both Type I and Type II diabetics. In Type I patients with variable degrees of hyperglycemia (mean = 12.3 mM) and diabetic ketoacidosis (66), heparin-releasable LPL was reduced to 34% of that measured in non-diabetic control subjects. In Type II patients, similar degrees of hyperglycemia (8.3 to 16.5 mM) have been associated with LPL reductions of 40–65% (71,72,76,136,200,332). These studies have included measurements of both total tissue (71,76,125) and/or heparin-releasable LPL (71,72,76,136,200,332) activities. When compared, the effect of diabetes on the heparin releasable enzyme was greater than that on LPL measured in acetone-ether extracts (71,76). Similar efects were observed on the gluteal (72,125,200,332) and abdominal (71,76) adipose tissue enzyme.

Treatment of diabetics with either insulin (66,76,125), sulfonylureas (125) or simply weight loss (77), results in increases in LPL activity. However, this return of enzyme activity to normal values has at times been slow (66,125), and in one study LPL remained subnormal 12 weeks following therapy despite decreases in fasting plasma glucose from 248 to 140 mg/dl (125). This delay may be related to the chronicity of the insulin deficient (resistant) state. Type I diabetics, after only 12 hours of insulin withdrawal, have a significant increase in LPL (36%) following an 8-hour insulin infusion

(333). However, a six-hour insulin infusion which achieved insulin concentrations three times higher than that achieved in the study of Taskinen et al. (333), when given to Type II diabetics during maintainance of euglycemia (90 mg/dl) or fasting hyperglycemia (182–291 mg/dl), failed to increase LPL (332). Overall, the relative contributions of the duration of the hyperglycemic state, and the amount of insulin resistance to the reduced responsiveness of LPL to insulin cannot be accurately discerned from the currently available data.

Studies *In Vitro*. Few studies of LPL regulation have been carried out *in vitro* using adipose tissue or cells from animals or humans with diabetes mellitus. Murase et al. (321) have reported that adipose tissue pieces from streptozotocin-induced diabetic rats respond to 500 μU/ml (20 ng/ml) of insulin with an increase in heparin-releasable LPL after 60 minutes of incubation. Although pre-insulin heparin-releasable LPL was lower in tissue from diabetic rats than control animals, responses of LPL to insulin in tissue from non-diabetic controls were not examined.

Unpublished studies have also been carried out in overnight cultured rat adipocytes (R. H. Eckel). Following 73 ± 16 mg/kg of i.v. or i.p. streptozotocin, male Sprague-Dawley rats were sacrificed at 18 ± 1 days. At sacrifice, two groups of animals were identified. The first group (n = 4 experiments) had gained over 100 g from the time of streptozotocin administration and had a fasting serum glucose of 149 ± 8 mg/dl. The second group (n = 5 experiments) had gained only 20 g since the injection of streptozotocin and revealed a greater severity of glucose intolerance (393 ± 70 mg/dl) at sacrifice. Following overnight incubations, heparin-releasable but not extractable or culture medium LPL were reduced in cells from the second group of diabetic rats. Moreover, heparin-releasable LPL was inversely related to the extent of fasting hyperglycemia at sacrifice. Finally, the absolute (but not percentage) heparin-releasable LPL responsiveness to insulin (400 ng/ml) over 24 hours was reduced in cultured adipocytes from the more hyperglycemic rats. Thus, the diminished LPL in streptozotocin diabetic rats would appear to be, at least in part, secondary to defects within adipocytes in maintaining the heparin-releasable pool of enzyme activity. When measured in whole tissue only, this selective decrease may not be discernable.

Obesity

Studies *In Vivo*. The importance of adipose tissue LPL and its regulation in the origin and/or maintainance of the obese state remains incompletely understood. Nevertheless, experimentation in both rats and man has provided a sufficient database to strongly suggest that the enzyme functions to preserve the constancy of an increased adipocyte volume. This has been particularly true for genetic models of obesity in rodents and to some extent, in man.

Although increases in adipose tissue LPL have been noted in both genetic (82) and dietary-induced (334) forms of obesity in mice, the relevance of LPL to obesity has been most extensively investigated in the obese Zucker (fa/fa) rat. Throughout development and adult life, LPL when expressed per adipocyte or per tissue pad, measured mostly in postmitochondrial supernatants, has been found to be elevated (43,81,105,108,115,208,324,335–343). This difference between genotypes is greater within the first 10 weeks of life (81,341,343). Moreover, in several studies (335,339), both the increase in LPL per cell and the obese syndrome were not prevented when hyperphagia was eliminated by food restriction. Although some variability of LPL per cell has been shown to occur in adipose tissue from various sites differences between obese and lean Zucker rats have been, for the most part, preserved (43,81,115,324,339–342). Several additional observations in the obese Zucker rat are also noteworthy: 1) The failure of LPL per cell to fall with fasting (108,341), 2) a more sensitive response to subcutaneous insulin administration following the induction of diabetes mellitus with streptozotocin (324), 3) A further increase in enzyme activity with exercise, a response not seen in lean littermates (338).

When LPL activity is expressed per gram or per mg protein rather than per fat cell or pad, increases (43,208,337,343,344), decreases (108,343) or no changes (36,108,341,342,345) were reported compared to the LPL activities in non-obese controls. However, in the study of De Gasguet et al. (115), differences between obese and lean Zucker rats were maintained when LPL was related to surface area rather than to 10^6 cells. Moreover, when expressed per gram, food restriction was associated with a decrease in the lipase activity (105).

In obesity following ventromedial hypothalamic lesions or diet-induced obesity in rats, a somewhat different picture emerges. First, activities have not been expressed per cell, but per tissue weight or per mg protein, and an assumption must often be made that with increases in body weight, adipose tissue depot size increases as does fat cell size. Nevertheless, in cafeteria-fed Sprague-Dawley rats, increases in LPL were only seen in fed, not fasted animals (104). In high fat-fed Wistar rats, decreases in LPL per pad wre seen within the first 3 weeks of the dietary perturbation and increases were only detected at 180 days (140). Although body weight and LPL per mg protein increased following ventromedial hypothalamic knifecuts in both Wistar (179,202,326) and CD rats (178), in three of these studies the production of insulin deficiency by streptozotocin eliminated the LPL response to ventromedial hypothalamic lesions (178,179,326). In addition, prevention of hyperphagia following ventromedial hypothalamic lesions by food restriction also blunted the changes in LPL and weight gain (178). However, as in obese Zucker rats, the substitution of only small doses of insulin (2 units/rat/day) restored the differences in LPL between lesioned and control diabetic Wistar rats (179). Thus, the effects of ventromedial hypothalamic lesions on LPL in the Wistar rat may be explained only in part by the hyperinsulinemia.

In man, nearly all studies have been carried out in obese adults where genetic and environmental influences were indistinguishable. However, the marked increase in adipose tissue LPL in young adults with lifelong obesity associated with the Prader-Willi syndrome (346), has suggested that a human model of obesity resembling the obese Zucker rat may be available to gain further insight into the genetic relevance of LPL to obesity. Nevertheless, even in Prader-Willi syndrome, it remains unproven that the increased LPL precedes the marked hyperphagia which has been routinely found in these patients (347).

With one exception (348), all reports of heparin-releasable adipose tissue LPL in obese humans have demonstrated increases in enzyme activity per cell (30,38,69,72,131,136,184,346,349). When the data were expressed per gram, increases (69,70,184), decreases (males only)(186), or similar enzyme activities (38,132,136,193,348) have been found when compared to lean controls. These differences do not appear to be sex-dependent or region-specific in that samplings from gluteal (69,72,131,132,184,186,346,348,349), abdominal (38,69,70), subscapular (69) and femoral (136) depots have all been compared. Excluding the study of patients with Prader-Willi syndrome, where a 10-fold increase in LPL was found (346), the average increase of LPL per cell in obese subjects above lean controls has been 3.2 ± 0.6 (38,69,72,131,184,349). Because the extent of obesity has been variable, the emergence of a relationship between heparin-releasable LPL per cell and percent ideal body weight (125,184,346,350–352) and fat cell size (38,65,70–72,125,134,184,243,346) appears relevant. When further examined, this relationship has been inconsistent in its statistical significance when LPL was expressed per gram (38,70,71,350,353). However, in several studies, relationships between LPL and fat cell size and/or percent ideal body weight have also been shown for the acetone-ether enzyme (125,243). Relationships between the heparin-releasable LPL per cell and percent ideal body weight or fat cell size have been reported in gluteal (14,72,125,184,346,351,352), abdominal (38,65,70,71,134,243) and femoral (134) regions.

As in the animal model, the most important questions related to increased adipose tissue LPL and human obesity relate to the genesis and role of the abnormality. This question can, to some extent, be addressed by quantification of the enzyme response to alterations in body weight. For instance, following weight loss and weight stabilization, if fasting LPL or its response to stimuli decreases, one could conclude that increases in LPL per cell in obesity are largely a consequence of the obese state. However, failure of LPL or its response to decrease following weight loss (with concomitant reduction in adipocyte volume) would point to potential intrinsic defects in LPL which could serve to maintain the obese state.

The timing of the biopsy in relationship to the attainment of the reduced state is critical. In obese subjects, during or immediately after hypocaloric feeding, LPL has been repeatedly shown to be lower than that determined before the pre-reduction (69,72,77,133,135,193). However, following 2 days to 28 weeks of isocaloric feeding and weight stabilization, variable alterations of the fasting enzyme have been reported. In weight-reduced men, weight-stable for 4–28 weeks, heparin-releasable LPL was 3.6 times greater than predicted for body weight (350). In a subsequent study, Schwartz and Brunzell (351) demonstrated a 4.3-fold increase in LPL after a mean weight loss of 16% of ideal body weight and one week of isocaloric feeding. Although Sorbris et al. (131) failed to document such an increase in the lipase in 14 obese women, reductions of 13 kg and 2–3 weeks of weight maintenance was associated with a 5% increase in LPL per cell.

Other studies have not agreed with the above reports. Following a mean weight reduction of 27 kg and a subsequent 4–6 week period of weight stabilization, 8 Pima Indian men had a 50% decrease in LPL per cell (352). Similarly Rebuffe-Scrive et al. (193) demonstrated a decline in LPL from 48 to 11 mU/10^6 cells after a mean weight reduction of 8.6 kg in 6 obese women with a subsequent increase to only 26 mU/10^6 cells after 8 days of isocaloric refeeding. Although these patients had very high LPL activities before weight reduction and a threshhold weight loss may have been necessary to induce the lipase response (354), these studies suggest that the measurement of the fasting enzyme only may not resolve the questions related to the genesis and/or role of the abnormality in adipose tissue LPL in human obesity.

Although responsiveness to stimuli, e.g. oral glucose (132,191), intravenous glucose (186), or intravenous glucose and insulin (184,190) (Figure 1) may be blunted or delayed in obese subjects, this may simply be a mechanism for adipose tissue to prevent additional triglyceride loading, a function already maintained by the increase in fasting LPL. However, following weight loss, an increase in responsiveness to stimuli could be a mechanism for resumption of adipocyte volume and the obese state. In preliminary studies carried out in 8 obese women following a 12% weight reduction (11.2 $\pm$ 0.9 kg) and 3 months of weight maintenance, fasting LPL failed to change: 6.2 $\pm$ 0.6 nEq FFA/10^6 cells/min vs. 5.1 $\pm$ 0.9 before weight reduction (355). However, LPL responsiveness to both mixed meals and to 40 mU/m^2/min of intravenous insulin increased significantly. Although not statistically significant, LPL responses to 15 mU/m^2/min of insulin over 6 hours also increased in 6 of 8 subjects following weight loss.

In previous studies, five subjects achieving a near-normal or normal body weight following a weight loss of 18.9 $\pm$ 2.6 kg demonstrated falls in fasting LPL per 10^6 cells following 3 months of weight stabilization (R. H. Eckel et al., unpublished observations). Although decreases in the fasting enzyme activity were seen, all but one patient had relative increases in their LPL response to insulin over 6 hours when compared to identical studies carried out prior to weight loss. Of additional interest, the 4 patients demonstrating increases in their LPL response to insulin after weight loss regained most, if not all, of their weight within six months of the post-weight loss study. The only patient with a relative decrease in the LPL response to insulin following weight loss (3.0 vs. 16.5 nEq FFA/10^6 cells/min) has remained weight stable 25 kg under her initial weight over three years following weight loss. These data confirm the importance of examining more than the fasting enzyme to determine the relevant role of LPL in the maintenance and perhaps origin of the obese state.

Finally, the ability of fasting gluteal adipose tissue LPL to predict changes in body weight in cigarette smokers is worthy of note. Cigarette smokers usually weigh less than nonsmokers, and most experience increases in body weight following smoking cessation (356). Because Brunzell et al. (357) have demonstrated higher fasting values of gluteal adipose tissue LPL in cigarette smokers than nonsmokers, the relationship of LPL to changes in body weight has been examined in smokers and under two different conditions. In the study of Carney and Goldberg (358), fasting gluteal adipose tissue LPL was measured in 15 cigarette smokers before they stopped smoking. After 2 weeks of abstinence, the change in body weight correlated strongly with the previously measured gluteal adipose tissue LPL. ($r = 0.82$, $p < 0.0002$). In twelve of those subjects who remained abstinent for 3 weeks, this correlation remained significant ($r = 0.63$, $p < 0.05$). In a separate study, fasting gluteal adipose tissue LPL in obese smokers correlated ($r = 0.71$, $p < 0.05$) with the amount of weight loss which ensued over three weeks on hypocaloric diets (325–675 kcal/day)(359). A similar relationship was not found for 22 nonsmokers. Overall, these data suggest a regulatory role of fasting LPL in the maintenance of body weight and adipose tissue mass in smokers. In nonsmokers, the preliminary data suggests that responsiveness of the lipase may be more important.

Studies *In Vitro*. *In vitro* perturbations of LPL in adipose tissue or cells from obese animals or humans have also not been well studied. Several reports of preadipocyte cultures from the Zucker model of obesity have provided some relevant information pertinent to the genetic aspects of the syndrome. Despite similarities in proliferative capacity, heparin-releasable LPL was variably reduced over 3 days in preadipocytes from obese vs. lean rats. The variability was dependent upon which antibiotics were included in the culture medium, penicillin-streptomycin or cephalothin (360). Triglyceride accumulation was similarly affected. In a subsequent report, the response of heparin-releasable LPL over 6 days to enriched culture medium containing human serum, insulin and glucose was lower in cultures from obese vs. lean Zucker rats (361). Other responses, including ^3H_2O incorporation into total cellular lipid, fatty acid synthetase activity, and cytosolic protein content, were also lower in cells from obese rats. The substitution of lean or obese rat serum for human serum failed to alter these responses.

In overnight cultured rat adipocytes, preliminary studies suggest that alterations of LPL *in vivo* persist in the *in vitro* environment (R. H. Eckel, unpublished data). In a series of five studies, 8-week-old Zucker male rats were divided into three groups: *ad libitum* fed lean, *ad libitum* fed obese, and obese pair-fed (to equal lean) animals. After 23 ± 3 days of observation, rats were sacrificed either in the fed or 72-hour fasted condition. Following sacrifice, measurements of LPL were carried out in adipose tissue pieces and then in cultured adipocytes as previously outlined. In these experiments, only heparin-releasable LPL was determined. As expected, substantial increases were found in heparin-releasable LPL in adipose tissue pieces from obese rats. This was true in adipose tissue from both fed and fasted animals. However, unlike data previously gathered from cultured preadipocytes from lean and obese Zucker rats, heparin-releasable LPL was increased in overnight cultured adipocytes (obese and pair-fed obese). As in the tissue, these increases were seen in cells from both fed (Figure 2) and fasted animals. In addition, the heparin-releasable LPL measured in cultured adipocytes was correlated with heparin-releasable LPL meausred in the adipose tissue pieces ($r = 0.71$, $p < 0.001$). Following the addition of 400 ng/ml insulin, heparin-releasable LPL failed to increase over 4-hour cultures in cells from fed obese and pair-fed obese rats, but did so in cells from fed lean animals (Figure 2). Although overnight heparin-releasable LPL was substantially lower in fasted rats, the responses to insulin were similar in magnitude and direction as those shown in adipocytes from fed rats.

In conclusion, from these studies it would appear that the increase in heparin-releasable LPL in obese Zucker rats, at least in part, is secondary to increases in the heparin-releasable enzyme within adipocytes. Moreover, the failure of insulin to increase heparin-releasable LPL in cultured adipocytes from obese rats strongly resembles the insulin-dose response curves of the human adipose tissue enzyme in obese subjects exposed to variable insulin infusion rates (190), and again suggests that LPL regulation by insulin becomes less important for lipid filling and maintenance of fat cell size when the basal enzyme activity is high.

Hypertriglyceridemias

The role of LPL in human and animal hypertriglyceridemia, including that of the *cld* mouse (362) is discussed elsewhere in this volume (Chapters 6 and 8). The purpose of this section is to highlight the available information on the relationship between adipose tissue LPL and some forms of human and experimental hypertriglyceridemias.

In 1970 Shafrir and Biale (363) suggested the possibility that the decrease in adipose tissue LPL seen following an infusion of Intralipid or VLDL into rats was secondary to a "leaking" of the enzyme into the plasma. Although a rise in plasma lipolytic activity was detected in this investigation, subsequent support for this hypothesis has not been provided. However, the demonstration of lower activities of LPL in hypertriglyceridemic rats was not unique to this study. Similar observations were made in several rat models of hypertriglyceridemia including pregnancy (169), nephrotic syn-

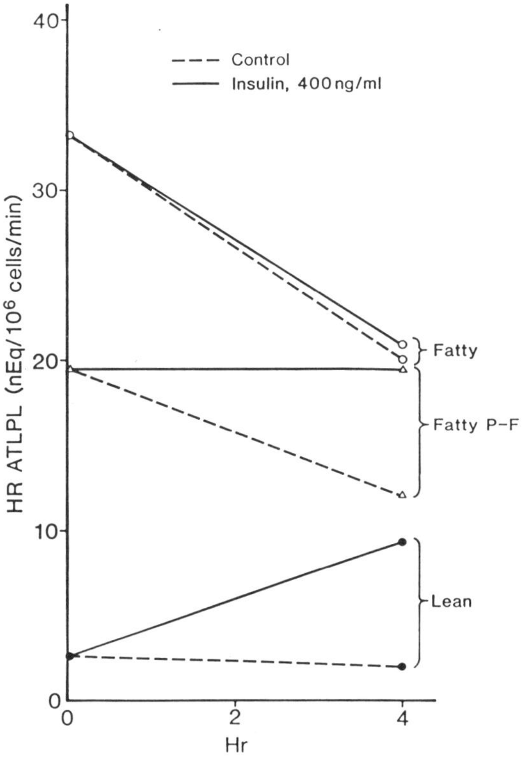

FIGURE 2 Insulin responsiveness of heparin-releasable LPL in adipocytes from fed Zucker rats. Adipocytes were prepared from epididymal fat pads of eight-week-old homozygous lean and fatty rats (two rats per group) following 23 ± 3 days of dietary control. One group of fatty rats (fatty P–F) was pair-fed to match ad libitum fed lean controls. The other fatty group had unlimited access to chow. After overnight incubation in Medium 199 ± 10% serum, heparin-releasable LPL was determined and insulin (400 ng/ml) added to one-half of the cultures for 4 hrs. Data represent the mean LPL activities for four experiments.

drome (106,364), glycerol feeding (365), endotoxemia (366,367), and during progressive growth of mammary adenocarcinoma (368). Decreases in LPL have also been produced in rat adipose tissue *in vitro* by uremic plasma (369,370). Although hypertriglyceridemia frequently occurs in uremia, in the rat this finding has been variably associated with decreased LPL (195,369,371). In the study of Ramson et al. (176), 24 hours following nephrectomy decreases in LPL and the response of LPL in isolated adipocytes to insulin was found. However, in this study, triglyceride levels were not significantly higher than levels measured in non-uremic controls. In the study of Tan (195), over 2 weeks of uremia produced a significant increase in serum triglycerides, but an insignificant decrease in LPL. In other models of hypertriglyceridemia in rats, i.e. following trauma with subsequent endotoxemia (372), sucrose feeding (373) or in the obese Zucker rat (345), adipose tissue LPL was unchanged. Clearly, alterations in triglyceride production and/or changes in LPL in other tissues such as skeletal or cardiac muscle are important additional considerations to explain the hypertriglyceridemia. The latter possibility receives support from data gathered in clofibrate-treated rats. Although repeatedly shown to decrease serum triglycerides (63,374,375), and increase intravenous fat tolerance in rats (63), increases in adipose tissue LPL were only seen in the study of Tolman et al. (375). As implicated in the study of D'Costa (63), increases in myocardial LPL were documented by Odonkor and Rogers (374). Unlike clofibrate, however the triglyceride-lowering effects of pantothene appear to be mediated in part by an increase in adipose tissue LPL (371).

In man, decreases in adipose tissue LPL in hypertriglyceridemic states have been equally unpredictable. In Type I hyperlipoproteinemia, absent or extremely reduced amounts of LPL in adipose tissue (130,376–378), in addition to postheparin plasma have been repeatedly documented. This is true both for the fasted and fed state (130,377). A similar clinical syndrome has been seen in patients with apolipoprotein CII deficiency (55,56) or circulating inhibitors to LPL (379). In both of these conditions, severe hypertriglyeridemia and absence of the adipose tissue enzyme activity have been seen when patient's serum was used as an activator (55,379). However, when pooled sera were used as an activator, increased amounts of LPL activity were seen. This suggests that a feedback mechanism of LPL regulation by tissue triglyceride-rich lipoprotein hydrolysis may exist.

Independent of the Type I abnormality, the presence of hypertriglyceridemia in humans has been associated with reductions in LPL. This has been seen in unspecified forms of hypertriglyceridemia (67,76,137,243,380) and in patients with Type III (64), Type IV (64,381,382), Type V (381,383), and Type IIb hyperlipoproteinemia (64,383), and in patients with renal failure (192,384) or infection (185). In the studies of Mirani-Oostdijk et al. (129), the postprandial increase in heparin-releasable LPL previously reported for normolipidemic controls was absent in hypertriglyceridemics (382). In hypertriglyceridemia, both decreases in the heparin-releasable enzyme (64,67,76,192,380–382,384) and/or total tissue enzyme (76,137,185,243,383) have been noted. Moreover, gluteal (64,67,192,380,384), abdominal (76,137,243,381,382), femoral (185) and omental (383) adipose tissue sites have all been utilized as sources of the lipase.

However, in a substantial number of studies, hypertriglyceridemia has not been associated with diminished adipose tissue LPL. This has included patients with genetic forms of hyperlipoproteinemia (130), obesity (72,125,186), beta adrenergic blockade (385) and unspecified etiologies of hypertriglyceridemia (70,71,386). Again, several different tissue sites and assay techniques have been employed. Moreover, fibric acid derivatives which are known to enhance triglyceride clearance, have had variable effects on adipose tissue LPL (376,384,387,388). A more consistent stimulatory effect of this class of drugs, including clofibrate and bezafibrate, has been on skeletal muscle LPL (376,388). Finally, changes in the degree of saturation of dietary fatty acids for two weeks did not alter adipose tissue LPL despite an up to 30% decrease in serum triglycerides (389). Overall, as in rats, these data imply that alternative mechanisms are the more likely explanation for many the forms of hypertriglyceridemia seen in adult humans. Because isolated defects in the production or activation of the adipose tissue enzyme have not been found, the relative contribution of adipose tissue mass to hypertriglyceridemia remains unknown.

Lipomatosis

Recent reports have provided evience for substantial increases (up to 45-fold) in LPL in lipomatous tisue when compared to LPL measured in control subjects (241,242,390,391) or non-lipomatous adjacent adipose tissue regions in lipomatous patients (390). In only one report has low levels of LPL been found (392). In addition, when examined, expected reductions in basal lipolysis have been found (241,242,393). In most of the reports, heparin-releasable LPL was measured (241,242,390). However, the regions from which lipomatous tissue was obtained were variable including the abdomen, deltoid region, and back. Whether patients with single lipomas have an alternative pathophysiologic explanation for lipomatous tissue development than patients with multiple symmetric lipomatosis (241) has yet to determined.

Brown Adipose Tissue

Especially in hibernating animals, brown adipose tissue has an important role in non-shivering thermogenesis through its ability to generate heat by the oxidation of fatty acids. Fatty acids can be provided either from the hydrolysis of triglyceride stores within brown adipose tissue, *de novo* fatty acid synthesis, or LPL-mediated uptake from circulating triglyceride-rich lipoproteins. LPL activity has also been demonstrated in brown adipose tissue of man (394), rat (395) and mice (396). As in white adipose tissue, LPL is releasable by heparin (342,397,398), but in one experiment the heparin-releasable LPL/total tissue LPL ratio in brown fat was less than that measured in white adipose tissue (342). Although the time course of development of the lipase in brown adipose tissue does not differ substantially from that in white adipose tissue (80,342,397,399), the functional differences between the two adipose tissues indicate differences in regulation.

Nutritional influences on brown adipose tissue LPL have been variable. In mice, brown adipose tissue LPL did not differ postprandially in lean and obese (ob/ob) mice (82). In Wistar rats during development (80), moderate increases were noted in fed rats at birth and on days 7 and 60 of life. In Zucker rats, total cellular brown adipose tissue LPL was higher in 6-hour fasted lean and obese rats than fed rats (108). However, 3 days of fasting decreased brown adipose tissue LPL in Wistar rats (400). Upon refeeding, increases in the brown adipose tissue lipase were greater when only 50–75% of the average *ad libitum* caloric intake was given (400). This adaptation could have served to sustain the delivery of lipoprotein fatty acids for maintenance of thermogenesis during undernutrition. Diets high in fat, however, did not increase brown adipose tissue LPL at 28° but increases were seen at 4° (108). Finally, whereas 8 weeks of overfeeding with sucrose supplements increased body weight, white adipose tissue LPL, and lipogenesis in brown adipose tissue in rats, brown adipose tissue LPL actually fell (183).

Perhaps most reproducible has been the brown adipose tissue LPL response to cold. Following cold exposures for intervals as short as 3 hours (401) to 70 days (402), brown adipose tissue LPL was repeatedly shown to be elevated (108,175,207,395,398,402–404). In the study of Bertin et al. (108), cold induced changes were only seen in fed, not fasted rats. Because this response was inhibited by propranolol (402), beta adrenergic receptors appear important for the effect. Additional support comes from studies demonstrating norepinephrine stimulation of the brown adipose tissue lipase (108,175,402), with inhibition of this response by propranolol and no inhibitory effect of the alpha adrenergic agent phenylephrine (402). Isoprenaline, a beta adrenergic agonist, also reproduced the norepinephrine effect (402).

Few experiments have been performed to examine the effects of specific hormones on brown adipose tissue LPL. As in white adipose tissue, hypothyroidism is associated with increases in brown adipose tissue LPL (397) and decreases occur after excessive triiodothyronine administration (398). In cold-acclimated rats, a single injection of dexamethasone increased brown adipose tissue LPL but not when animals were kept in warmer environments (28°) (175). Opposite effects at these two temperatures were produced after a single injection of insulin (175). No effect of insulin or glucose injections, however, were seen in the cold or at room temperatures in the experiments by Carneheim et al. (108,403). In rodent models of obesity, brown adipose tissue LPL was either diminished (108,342) or unchanged (82,337). However, as in white adipose tissue, decreases in the brown adipose tissue lipase were observed in streptozotocin-diabetic rats (329). Finally, estradiol benzoate administration to ovariectomized hamsters (but not rats,) was associated with increases in brown adipose tissue LPL (207). Opposite effects were seen in the white adipose tissue depot. The overall effect of estradiol in the setting of weight loss appears to be to shift fatty acids away from white adipose tissue storage depots to brown adipose tissue where oxidation can ensue.

Summary and Conclusions

Further insights into adipose tissue LPL and its regulation will come from the consolidation of emerging observations in the basic science arena, including at the level of the LPL gene, with forthcoming *in vivo* data from studies of adipose tissue LPL physiology and pathophysiology in animals and man. If either basic scientists ignore the ongoing developments in the clinical environment, or clinical investigators overlook new information about adipose tissue LPL processing and regulation at the cellular and tissue level, a comprehensive report will not ensue. With the recent advent of the molecular age, undoubtedly questions related to adipose tissue LPL will soon be addressed at the level of the LPL gene. Only then will tissue-dependent differences in the physicochemical properties and regulation of LPL be effectively evaluated. Isolation of the LPL gene will also permit new approaches to the origin of interspecies differences in adipose tissue LPL regulation. Examples of such areas of pursuit will be the differences between rats and man in the adipose tissue LPL response to thyroid hormone, and IGF_1.

Many areas of ongoing basic investigation will have obvious extensions into the clinical arena. Studies related to *in vitro* differentiation of adipocyte precursors, with further pursuits of the regulation of terminal differentiation at the LPL gene level, will provide important information about the role of LPL in adipose tissue development. This may have important relevance in the area of adipose tissue hyperplasia, wherein the onset of obesity occurs early in life. Further insights into the coordinate regulation of LPL with other processes that control adipocyte triglyceride loading and maintenance of fat cell size such as lipolysis, reesterification, and lipogenesis may lead to interventions which could regulate adipocyte fatty acid flux *in vivo*. The use of patients with LPL deficiency will be useful here.

Additional studies of transcription, translation, and secretion of LPL from cultured adipocytes should lead to more detailed studies of regulation of LPL in adipose tissue. Such studies might proceed by the utilization of co-cultures of adipocytes and microvascular endothelium in a medium of connective tissue matrix proteins. In co-cultures, the relative roles of LPL transport between cells, binding and degradation to enzyme physiology and pathophysiology can be systematically approached. Insights into the relationship between the basal (fasting) enzyme activity and the lipase response to perturbations may be provided by such investigations. In addition, there remains a limited knowledge of the heparin-releasable pool of enzyme activity and its important relationship to the *in vivo* function of the enzyme. This is relevant to metabolic disease states such as diabetes mellitus, wherein selective alterations in the heparin-releasable pool of adipose tissue LPL occur. By the use of anti-LPL antibodies, further insights into the anatomic location of this pool should occur. Additional information about the physiology and pathophysiology of the functional heparin-releasable adipose tissue LPL pool will require indepth studies at every level of LPL synthesis and processing.

Finally, the contributory role of adipose tissue LPL to the origin and maintenance of the expanded adipocyte size in obesity must be approached at both levels. It will be important to discover if some of the genetic syndromes of obesity are associated with primary abnormalities in the expression and/or function of adipose tissue LPL. It is also possible that the increased LPL per fat cell present in obese rodents and humans is simply a response on the part of adipose tissue to the *in vivo* environment. Alternatively, with increases in body weight and fat cell size, augmented LPL gene expression could result in sustained increases in basal adipose tissue LPL. Subsequent to weight loss, LPL responsiveness to perturbations such as food and/or hormones would then occur and resumption of the obese state follow. Although these questions may all be dissectable with molecular tools, the necessity of a continued pursuit of the *in vivo* regulation of adipose tissue LPL activity in obese animals and patients should not be minimized. Particularly intriguing in man would be studies of adipose tissue LPL regulation prior to the development of the obese state. Identification of such subjects might be only randomly achieved, however, and could be in part aided by the selection of subjects with a high prevalence of obesity in the family.

References

1. Hollenberg, C. H. 1966. *J. Clin. Invest.* 45:205–216.
2. Patkin, J. K., and E. J. Masoro. 1964. *Canad. J. Physiol. Pharmacol.* 42:101–107.
3. De Freitas, A. S. W., and F. Depocas. 1965. *Canad. J. Biochem.* 43:437–450.
4. Himms-Hagen, J. 1965. *Canad. J. Physiol. Pharmacol.* 43:379–403.
5. May, J. M. 1982. *J. Lipid. Res.* 23:428–436.
6. Bray, G. A. 1972. *J. Clin. Invest.* 51:537–548.
7. Hirsch, J., and R. B. Goldrick. 1964. *J. Clin. Invest.* 43:1776–1792.
8. Kuo, P. T., L. Feng, N. N. Cohen, W. T. Fitts, Jr., and L. D. Miller. 1967. *Amer. J. Clin. Nutr.* 26:116–125.
9. Bray, G. A., S. Mothon, and A.Cohen. 1969. *J. Clin. Invest.* 48:1413–1422.
10. Galton, D. J. 1968. *J. Lipid Res.* 9:19–26.
11. Sjostrom, L. 1973. *Scand. J. Clin. Lab. Invest.* 32:339–349.
12. Leibel, R. L., J. Hirsch, E. M. Berry, and R. K. Gruen. 1984. *J. Lipid. Res.* 25:49–57.
13. Patel, M. S., O. E. Owen, L. I. Goldman, and R. W. Hanson. 1975. *Metabolism* 24:161–173.
14. Savard, R., Y. Deshaies, J. -P. Despres, M. Marcotte, L. Bukowiecki, C. Allard, and C. Bouchard. 1984. *Canad. J. Physiol. Pharmacol.* 62:1448–1452.
15. Winegrad, A. I., and A. E. Renold. 1958. *J. Biol.Chem.* 233:267–270.
16. Bray, G. A. 1968. *J. Lipid. Res.* 9:681–686.
17. Shrago, E., T. Spennetta, and E. Gordon. 1969. *J. Biol. Chem.* 244:2761–2766.
18. Shrago, E., J. A. Glennon, and E. S. Gordon. 1967. *J. Clin. Endocrinol.* 27:679–685.
19. Shrago, E., J. A. Glennon, and E. S. Gordon. 1971. *Metabolism* 20:54–62.
20. Katz, J., and R. Rognstad. 1978. *Trends in Biochem. Sci.* 3:171–174.
21. Leibel, R. L., J. Hirsch, E. M. Berry, and R. K. Gruen. 1985. *Am. J. Clin. Nutr.* 42:198–206.
22. Jones, N. L., and R. J. Havel. 1967. *Am. J. Physiol.* 213:824–828.
23. Cryer, A., S. E. Riley, E. R. Williams, and D. S. Robinson. 1976. *Clin. Sci. Molec. Med.* 50:213–221.
24. Bragdon, J. H., and R. S. Gordon, Jr. 1958. *J. Clin. Invest.* 37:574–578.
25. Garfinkel, A. S., N. Baker, and M. C.Schotz. 1967. *J. Lipid Res.* 8:274–280.

26. Linder, C., S. S.Chernick, T. R. Fleck, and R. O. Scow. 1976. *Am. J. Physiol.* 231:860–864.
27. Olivercrona, T., and P. Belfrage. 1965. *Biochim. Biophys. Acta.* 98:81–93.
28. Olivecrona, T. 1962. *J. Lipid. Res.* 3:439–444.
29. Nestel, P. J., R. J. Havel, and A. Bezman. 1962. *J. Clin. Invest.* 41:1915–1921.
30. Bjorntorp, P., G. Enzi, R. Ohlson, B. Persson, P. Sponbergs, and U. Smith. 1975. *Horm. Metab. Res.* 7:230–237.
31. Scow, R. O., E. J. Blanchette-Mackie, and L. C. Smith. 1976. *Circ. Res.* 39:149–162.
32. Scow, R. O., S. S. Chernick, and T. R. Fleck. 1977. *Biochim. Biophys. Acta.* 487:297–306.
33. Fielding, C. J., J. P. Renston, and P. E. Fielding. 1978. *J. Lipid Res.* 19:705–711.
34. Rodbell, M., and R. O. Scow. 1965. In: *Handbook of Physiology,* Sect. 5, Adipose Tissue. Renold, A. E., and G. F. Cahill, editors. 491–498.
35. Nestel, P. J., W. Austin, and C. Foxman. 1969. *J. Lipid Res.* 10:383–387.
36. McNamara, J. P., M. Azain, T. R. Kasser, and R. J. Martin. 1982. *Am. J. Physiol.* 243:R258–R264.
37. Wilson, J. P. D., R. Gutman, and D. J. Galton. 1973. *Metabolism* 22:913–921.
38. Taskinen, M. -R. and E. A. Nikkila. 1977. *Acta. Med. Scand.* 202:399–408.
39. Bensadoun, A. and I. P. Kompiang. 1979. *Fed. Proc.* 38:2622–2626.
40. Robinson, D. S. 1970. In: *Comprehensive Biochemistry.* M. Florkin, and E. H. Stotz, editors. Elsevier Publishing Co., New York. Vol. 18:51–116.
41. Blanchette-Mackie, E. J., and R. O. Scow. 1981. *J. Ultrastruct. Res.* 77:295–318.
42. Dietschy, J. M. 1978. In: *Distrubances in lipid and lipoprotein metabolism.* Dietschy, J. M., A. M. Gotto, Jr., and J. A. Ontko, editors. American Physiology Society, Bethesda. 1–28.
43. Maggio, C. A., and M. R. C. Greenwood. 1982. *Physiol. Behav.* 29:1147–1152.
44. Paik, H. S., and E. S. Yearick. 1978. *J. Nutr.* 108:1798–1805.
45. Pokrajac, N., and W. J. Lossow. 1967. *Biochim. Biophys. Acta.* 137:291–295.
46. Bezman, A., J. M. Felts, and R. J. Havel. 1962. *J. Lipid. Res.* 3:427–431.
47. Verine, A., P. Salers, and J. Boyer. 1982. *Am. J. Physiol.* 243:E175–E181.
48. Lasuncion, M. A., and E. Herrera. 1983. *Biochem. J.* 210:639–643.
49. Walldius, G. 1976. *Acta. Med. Scand.* (Suppl.) 591:1–47.
50. Borensztajn, J. A., and D. S. Robinson. 1970. *J. Lipid. Res.* 11:111–117.
51. Hartman, A. D. 1977. *Am. J. Physiol.* 232:E316–E323.
52. Roth, J., M. R. C. Greenwood, and P. R. Johnson. 1981. *Int. J. Obesity* 5:131–143.
53. Fried, S. K., J. O.Hill, M. Nickel, and M. DiGirolamo. 1983. *J. Nutr.* 113:1861–1869.
54. Nikkila, E. A. 1983. In: *The Metabolic Basis of Inherited Disease.* Stanbury, J. B., J. B. Wyngaarden, D. S. Fredrickson, J. L. Goldstein, and M. S. Brown, editors. McGraw-Hill, Inc. 5th Edition. 622–642.
5. Breckenridge, W. C., J. A. Little, G. Steiner, A. Chow, and M. Poapst. 1978. *N. Engl. J. Med.* 298:1265–1273.
56. Yamamura, T., H. Sudo, K. Ishikawa, and A. Yamamoto. 1979. *Atherosclerosis* 34:53–65.
57. Gustafsson, K., H. Kiessling, and J. Boberg. 1981. *Artery* 9:394–404.
58. Kim, H. -J., and R. K. Kalkhoff. 1975. *J. Clin. Invest.* 56:888–896.
59. Chen, Y. -D. I., T. R. Risser, M. Cully, and G. M. Reaven. 1979. *Diabetes* 28:893–898.
60. Chen, Y. -D. I., J. Howard, V. Huang, F. B. Kraemer, and G. M. Reaven. 1980. *Diabetes* 29:643–647.
61. Hamosh, M., T. R. Clary, S. S. Chernick, and R. O. Scow. 1970. *Biochim. Biophys. Acta.* 210:473–482.
62. Verschoor, L., Y. -D. I. Chen, and G. M. Reaven. 1982. *Metabolism* 31:499–503.
63. D'Costa, M. A, F. C. Smigura, K. Kulhay, and A. Angel. 1977. *J. Lab. Clin. Med.* 90:823–836.
64. Persson, B. 1973. *Acta. Med. Scand.* 193:447–456.
65. Lithell, H., and J. Boberg. 1978. *Int. J. Obesity* 2:47–52.
66. Taskinen, M. -R. and E. A. Nikkila. 1979. *Diabetologia* 17:351–356.

67. Persson, B., P. Bjorntorp, and B. Hood. 1966. *Metabolism* 15:730–741.
68. Pykalisto, O., A. P. Goldberg, and J. D. Brunzell. 1976. *J. Clin. Endocrinol. Metab.* 43:591–600.
69. Bosello, O., M. Cigolini, A. Battaggia, F. Ferrari, R. Micciolo, R. Olivetti, and M. Corsato. 1984. *Int. J. Obesity* 8:213–220.
70. Gunther, W., W. Leonhardt, M. Hanefeld, and H. Haller. 1977. *Endokrinol.* 70:176–181.
71. Lithell, H., J. Boberg, K. Hellsing, and U. Waern. 1978. *Upsala J. Med. Sci.* 83:45–52.
72. Guy-Grand, B., and B. Bigorie. 1975. *Horm. Metab. Res.* 7:471–475.
73. Persson, B., G.Schroder, and B. Hood. 1972. *Atherosclerosis* 16:37–49.
74. Peltonen, P., J. Marniemi, E. Hietanen, I. Vuori, and C. Ehnholm. 1981. *Metabolism* 30:518–526.
75. Nikkila, E. A., M. -R. Taskinen, S. Rehunen, and M. Harkonen. 1978. *Metabolism* 27:1661–1670.
76. Taylor, K. G., D. J. Galton, and G. Holdsworth. 1979. *Diabetologia* 16:313–317.
77. Vessby, B., I. Selinus, and H. Lithell. 1985. *Arteriosclerosis* 5:93–100.
78. Chajek-Shaul, T., G. Friedman, O.Stein, T. Olivecrona, and Y. Stein. 1982. *Biochim. Biophys. Acta.* 712:200–210.
79. Hietanen, E., and M. R. C. Greenwood. 1977. *J. Lipid Res.* 18:480–490.
80. Planche, E., A. Boulange, P. De Gasquet, and N. T. Tonnu. 1980. *Am. J. Physiol.* 238:E511–E517.
81. Gruen, R. K., and M. R. C. Greenwood. 1981. *Am. J. Physiol.* 241:E76– E83.
82. Rath, E. A., D. A. Hems, and A. Beloff-Chain. 1974. *Diabetologia* 10:261–265.
83. Tan, M. H., T. Sata, and R. J. Havel. 1977. *J. Lipid Res.* 18:363–370.
84. Cherkes, A., and R. S.Gordon, Jr. 1959. *J. Lipid Res.* 1:97–101.
85. Chen, Y. -D. I., and G. M. Reaven. 1979. *J. Gerontol.* 36:3–6.
86. Hollenberg, C. H. 1959. *Am. J. Physiol.* 197:667–670.
87. Wing, D. R., M. R. Salaman, and D. S. Robinson. 1966. *Biochem. J.* 99:648–656.
88. Cunningham, V. J., and D. S. Robinson. 1969. *Biochem. J.* 112:203–209.
89. Borensztajn, J., D. R. Samols, and A. H. Rubenstein. 1972. *Am. J. Physiol.* 223:1271–1275.
90. Pykalisto, O. J., W. C. Vogel, and E. L. Bierman. 1974. *Biochim. Biophys. Acta.* 369:254–263.
91. Riley, S. E., and D. S. Robinson. 1974. *Biochim. Biophys. Acta.* 369:371–386.
92. Etienne, J., M. Breton, A. Vanhove, and J. Polonovski. 1976. *Biochim. Biophys. Acta.* 429:198–204.
93. Wilson, D. E., W. Jubiz, C. M. Flowers, S. I. Carlile, and A. M. Adolf. 1977. *Atherosclerosis* 26:253–262.
94. Benson, J. D., and A. Bensadoun. 1977. *J. Nutr.* 107:990–997.
95. Elkeles, R. S., and J. Hambley. 1977. *Diabetes* 26:58–60.
96. Jansen, H., A. S. Garfinkel, J. -S. Twu, J. Nikazy, and M. C. Schotz. 1978. *Biochim. Biophys. Acta.* 541:109–114.
97. Kruszynska, Y. T., P. D. Home, and K. G. M. M. Alberti. 1985. *Diabetes* 34:611–616.
98. Ashby, P., A. M. Tolson, and D. S. Robinson. 1978. *Biochem. J.* 171:305–311.
99. Vanhove, A., C. Wolf, M. Breton, and M. -C. Glangeaud. 1978. *Biochem. J.* 172:239–245.
100. Sedlakova, A., I. Ahlers, and N. Praslicka. 1979. *Folia Biol.* 25:254–265.
101. Lawson, N., A. D. Pollard, R. J. Jennings, M. I. Gurr, and D. N. Brindley. 1981. *Biochem. J.* 200:285–294.
102. Parkin, S. M., B. K. Speake, and D. S. Robinson. 1982. *Biochem. J.* 207:485–495.
103. Hansson, P., G. Nordin, and P. Nilsson-Ehle, 1983. *Biochim. Biophys. Acta.* 753:364–371.
104. Walks, D., M. Lavau, E. Presta, M. -U. Yang, and P. Bjorntorp. 1983. *Amer. J. Clin. Nutr.* 37:387–395.

105. Quig, D. W., D. K. Layman, P. J. Bechtel, and L. R. Hackler. 1983. *J. Nutr.* 113:1150–1156.
106. Kikuchi, H., S. Tamura, S. Nagase, and S. Tsuiki. 1983. *Biochim. Biophys. Acta.* 744:165–170.
107. Knobler, H. J., T. Chajek-Shaul, O. Stein, J. Etienne, and Y. Stein. 1984. *Biochim. Biophys. Acta.* 795:363–371.
108. Bertin, R., M. Triconnet, and R. Portet. 1985. *Comp. Biochem. Physiol.* 81:797–801.
109. Baggen, M. G., R. Lammers, H. Jansen, and J. C. Birkenhager. 1985. *Metabolism* 34:1053–1056.
110. Reichl, D. 1972. *Biochem. J.* 128:79–87.
111. Cryer, A., S. E. Riley, E. R. Williams, and D. S. Robinson. 1974. *Biochem. J.* 140:561–563.
112. Hansson, P., T. Holmin, and P. Nilsson-Ehle. 1981. *Biochem. Biophys. Res. Comm.* 103:1254–1257.
113. Borensztajn, J., P. Keig, and A. H. Rubenstein. 1973. *Biochem. Biophys. Res. Comm.* 53:603–608.
114. Nikkila, E. A., and O. Pykalisto. 1968. *Biochim. Biophys. Acta.* 152:421–423.
115. De Gasquet, P., and E. Pequignot. 1973. *Horm. Metab. Res.* 5:440–443.
116. De Gasquet, P., E. Pequignot-Planche, N. T. Tonnu, and F. A. Diaby. 1974. *Horm. Metab. Res.* 7:152–157.
117. Nilsson-Ehle, P., A. S. Garfinkel, and M. C. Schotz. 1976. *Biochim. Biophys. Acta.* 431:147–156.
118. DiMarco, N. M., D. C. Beitz, and G. B. Whitehurst. 1981. *J. Anim. Sci.* 52:75–82.
119. Moskowitz, M. S., and A. A. Moskowitz. 1965. *Science* 149:72–73.
120. Garfinkel, A. S., P. Nilsson-Ehle, and M. C. Schotz. 1976. *Biochim. Biophys. Acta.* 424:264–273.
121. Spencer, I. M., A. Hutchinson, and D. S. Robinson. 1978. *Biochim. Biophys. Acta.* 530:375–384.
122. Cryer, A., and H. M. Jones. 1979. *J. Dev. Physiol.* 1:261–265.
123. Nilsson-Ehle, P., S. Carlstrom, and P. Belfrage. 1975. *Scand. J. Clin. Lab. Invest.* 3:373–378.
124. Nilsson-Ehle, P., H. Tornqvist, and P. Belfrage. 1972. *Clin. Chim. Acta.* 42:383–390.
125. Pykalisto, O. J., P. H. Smith, and J. D. Brunzell. 1975. *J. Clin. Invest.* 56:1108–1117.
126. Iverius, P. -H. and J. D. Brunzell. 1985. *Am. J. Physiol.* 249:E107–E114.
127. Lithell, H., J. Boberg, K. Hellsing, G. Lundqvist, and B. Vessby. 1977. *Atherosclerosis* 30:89–94.
128. Taskinen, M. -R. E. A. Nikkila, and A. Ollus. 1983. *Diabetes Care* 6:224–230.
129. Pagano Mirani-Oostdijk, C., L. Havekes, J. Terpstra, M. Frolich, C. M. Van Gent, and H. Jansen. 1982. *Eur. J. Clin. Invest.* 13:301–309.
130. Goldberg, A. P., A. Chait, and J. D. Brunzell. 1980. *Metabolism* 29:223–229.
131. Sorbis, R., B. -G. Petersson, and P. Nilsson-Ehle. 1981. *Eur. J. Clin. Invest.* 11:491–498.
132. Dahms, W. T., P. Nilsson-Ehle, A. S. Garfinkel, R. L. Atkinson, G. A. Bray and M. Schotz. 1981. *Int. J. Obesity* 5:81–84.
133. Persson, B., B. Hood, and G. Angervall. 1970. *Acta. Med. Scand.* 188:225–229.
134. Arner, P., P. Engfeldt, and H. Lithell. 1981. *J. Clin. Endocrinol. Metab.* 53:948–952.
135. Taskinen, M. -R., and E. A. Nikkila. 1978. *Atherosclerosis* 32:289–299.
136. Arner, P., J. Bolinder, P. Engfeldt, and H. Lithell. 1982. *Int. J. Obesity* 7:167–172.
137. Taylor, K. G., G. Holdsworth, and D. J. Galton. 1980. *Eur. J. Clin. Invest.* 10:133–138.
138. Weisenburg Delorme, C. L., and K. L. Harris. 1975. *J. Nutr.* 105:447–451.
139. De Gasquet, P., S. Griglio, E. Pequignot-Planche, and M. I. Malewiak. 1977. *J. Nutr.* 107:199–212.
140. De Gasquet, P., E. Planche, and A. Boulange. 1981. *Int. J. Obesity* 5:701–705.
141. Kotze, J. P., and I. V. Menne. 1977. *So. African J. Sci.* 73:91–92.

142. Summerfield, J. A., D. Applebaum-Bowden, and W. R. Hazzard. 1984. *Proc. Soc. Exp. Biol. Med.* 175:158–163.
143. Kimball, T. J., M. T. Childs, D. Applebaum-Bowden, and W. L. Sembrowich. 1983. *Metabolism* 32:497–503.
144. Steingrimsdottir, L., J. Brasel, and M. R. C. Greenwood. 1980. *Metabolism* 29:837–841.
145. Childs, M. T., J. Tollefson, R. H. Knopp, and D. Applebaum-Bowden. 1981. *Metabolism* 30:27–34.
146. Robeson, B. L., E. J. Eisen, and J. M. Leatherwood. 1981. *Growth* 45:198–215.
147. Pawar, S. S., and H. C. Tidwell. 1968. *J. Lipid Res.* 9:334–336.
148. Hulsmann, W. C., M. M. Geelhoed-Mieras, H. Jansen, and U. M. T. Houtsmuller. 1978. *Biochim. Biophys. Acta.* 572:183–187.
149. Cryer, A., J. Kirtland, H. M. Jones, and M. I. Gurr. 1978. *Biochem. J.* 170:169–172.
150. Heller, E. R. 1983. *Biochim. Biophys. Acta.* 752:357–360.
151. Sadur, C. N., T. J. Yost, and R. H. Eckel. 1984. *Metabolism* 3:1043–1047.
152. Taskinen, M. -R. and E. A. Nikkila. 1981. *Clin. Chim. Acta* 112:325–332.
153. Flint, D. J., P. A. Sinnett-Smith, R. A. Clegg, and R. E. Vernon. 1979. *Biochem. J.* 182:421–427.
154. Gray, J. N., and M. R. C. Greenwood. 1983. *Am. J. Physiol.* 245:E132–E137.
155. Vernon, R. G., R. A. Clegg, and D.J. Flint. 1979. *Biochem. Soc. Trans.* 7:992–993.
156. Hamosh, M., T. R. Clary, S. S. Chernick, and R. O. Scow. 1970. *Biochim. Biophys. Acta.* 210:473–482.
157. Llobera, M., A. Montes, and E. Herrera. 1979. *Biochem. Biophys. Res. Comm.* 91:272–277.
158. Lasuncion, M. A., and E. Herrera. 1981. *Biochem. Biophys. Res. Comm.* 98:227–233.
159. Jones, C. T. 1976. *Biochem. J.* 156:357–365.
160. Vernon, R. G., R. A. Clegg, and D. J. Flint. 1981. *Biochem. J.* 200:307–314.
161. Rebuffe-Scrive, M., L. Enk, N. Crona, P. Lonnroth, L. Abrahamsson, U. Smith, and P. Bjorntorp. 1985. *J. Clin. Invest.* 75:1973–1976.
162. Ramirez, I. 1981. *Am. J. Physiol.* 240:E533–E538.
163. Otway, S., and D. S. Robinson. 1968. *Biochem. J.* 106:677–682.
164. Flint, D. J., R. A. Clegg, and R. G. Vernon. 1981. *Molec. Cell. Endocrinol.* 22:265–275.
165. Zinder, O., M. Hamosh, T. R. Clary Fleck, and R. O. Scow. 1974. *Am. J. Physiol.* 226:744–748.
166. Smith, R. W., and A. Walsh. 1984. *Res. Veterin. Sci.* 37:320–323.
167. Spooner, P. M., M. M. Garrison, and R. O. Scow. 1977. *J. Clin. Invest.* 60:702–708.
168. Flint, D. J., R. A. Clegg, and C. H. Knight. 1984. *J. Endocrinol.* 102:231–236.
169. Pelkonen, R., E. A. Nikkila, and B. Grahne. 1982. *Clin. Endocrinol.* 16:383 390.
170. Johnson, O., and O. Hernell. 1975. *Nutr. Metabl.* 19:41–44.
171. Giudicelli, Y., R. Nordmann, and J. Nordmann. 1975. *Clin. Sci. Molec. Med.* 48:153–156.
172. Nilsson-Ehle, P., S. Carlstrom, and P. Belfrage. 1978. *Lipids* 13:433–437.
173. Taskinen, M. -R., N. Valimaki, E. A. Nikkila, T. Kuusi, and R. Ylikahri. 1985. *Metabolism* 34:112–119.
174. Belfrage, P., B. Berg, I. Hagerstrand, P. Nilsson-Ehle, H. Tornqvist, and T. Wiebe. 1977. *Eur. J. Clin. Invest.* 7:127–131.
175. Goubern, M., and R. Portet. 1981. *Horm. Metab. Res.* 13:73–77.
176. Ransom, J., A. S. Garfinkel, J. Nakazy, M. C. Schotz, and K. Kurokawa. 1981. *Metabolism* 30:1165–1169.
177. Shafrir, E., A. Benchimol, and M. Orevi. 1975. *Isr. J. Med. Sci.* 11:738–752.
178. Lowell, B. B., G. N. Wade, J. M. Gray, R. M. Gold and J. Petrulavage. 1980. *Physiol. Behav.* 25:113–116.
179. Hansen, F. M., P. Nilsson, B. E. Hustvedt, P. Nilsson-Ehle, and A. Lovo. 1983. *Am. J. Physiol.* 244:E203–E208.
180. Kannan, R., N. Baker, and K. R. Bruckdorfer. 1981. *J. Nutr.* 111:1216–1223.

181. Vrana, A., P. Fabry, and L. Kazdova. 1974. *Nutr. Metab.* 17:282–288.
182. Webb, W., P. J. Nestel, C. Foxman, and A. Lynch. 1970. *Nutr. Rep. Int.* 1:189–195.
183. Granneman, J. G., and G. N. Wade. 1983. *Metabolism* 32:202–207.
184. Sadur, C. N., T. J. Yost, and R. H. Eckel. 1984. *J. Clin. Endocrinol. Metab.* 59:1176–1182.
185. Robin, A. P., J. Askanazi, M. R. C. Greenwood, Y. A. Carpentier, F. E. Gump, and J. M. Kinney. 1981. *Surgery* 90:401–408.
186. Taskinen, M. -R., and E. A. Nikkila. 1981. *Metabolism* 30:810–817.
187. Sadur, C. N., and R. H. Eckel. 1982. *J. Clin. Invest.* 69:1119–1125.
188. Yki-Jarvinen, H., M. -R. Taskinen, V. A. Koivisto, and E. A. Nikkila. 1984. *Diabetologia* 27:364–369.
189. Sadur, C. N., T. J. Yost, and R. H. Eckel. 1984. (Abst.). *Clin. Res.* 32:86A.
190. Eckel, R. H., C. N. Sadur, and T. J. Yost. 1986. (Abst.). *Clin. Res.* 34:58A.
191. Brunzell, J. D., R. S. Schwartz, R. H. Eckel, and A. P. Goldberg. 1981. *Int. J. Obesity* 5:685–694.
192. Goldberg, A., D. J. Sherrard, and J. D. Brunzell. 1978. *J. Clin. Endocrinol. Metab.* 47:1173–1182.
193. Rebuffe-Scrive, M., A. Basdevant, and B. Guy-Grand. 1983. *Am. J. Clin. Nutr.* 37:974–980.
194. Plucinski, T., and R. L. Baldwin. 1975. *J. Dairy Sci.* 59:157–160.
195. Tan, M. H. 1985. *Horm. Metab. Res.* 17:580–582.
196. Bagdade, J. D., E. Yee, J. Albers, and O. J. Pykalisto. 1976. *Metabolism* 25:533–542.
197. Krotkiewski, M., P. Bjorntorp, and U. Smith. 1976. *Horm. Metab. Res.* 8:245–246.
198. Hamosh, M., and P. Hamosh. 1975. *J. Clin. Invest.* 5:1132–1135.
199. Wilson, D. E., C. M. Flowers, S. I. Carlile, and K. S. Udall. 1976. *Atherosclerosis* 24:491–499.
200. Taskinen, M. -R., E. A. Nikkila, T. Kuusi, and K. Harno. 1982. *Diabetologia* 22:46–50.
201. Hansson, P., S. Valdemarsson, and P. Nilsson-Ehle. 1983. *Horm. Metab. Res.* 15:449–452.
202. Gray, J. M., A. A. Nunez, L. I. Siegel, and G. N. Wade. 1979. *Physiol. Behav.* 23:465–469.
203. Tomita, T., I. Yonekura, T. Okada, and E. Hayashi. 1984. *Horm. Metab. Res.* 16:525–528.
204. Dark, J., G. N. Wade, and I. Zucker. 1984. *Physiol. Behav.* 32:75–78.
205. Gray, J. M., and G. N. Wade. 1980. *Am. J. Physiol.* 239:E237–241.
206. Benoit, V., A. Vallette, L. Mercier, J. M. Meignen, and J. Boyer. 1982. *Biochem. Biophys. Res. Comm.* 109:1186–1191.
207. Edens, N. K., and G. N. Wade. 1983. *Physiol. Behav.* 31:703–709.
208. Gray, J. M., and M. R. C. Greenwood. 1984. *Proc. Soc. Exp. Biol. Med.* 175:374–379.
209. Steingrimsdottir, L., J. Brasel, and M. R. C. Greenwood. 1980. *Am. J. Phys.* 239:E162–E167.
210. Kim, H. -J. and R. K. Kalkhoff. 1978. *Metabolism.* 27:571–587.
211. Valette, A., L. Mercier, A. Verine, J. M. Meignen, and J. Boyer. 1983. *Molec. Cell Endocrinol* 29:243–254.
212. Applebaum, D. M., A. P. Goldberg, O. J. Pykalisto, J. D. Brunzell, and W. R. Hazzard. 1977. *J. Clin. Invest.* 59:601–608.
213. Gray, J. M., and G. N. Wade. 1979. *Endocrinology* 104:1377–1382.
214. Lehtonen, A., M. Gronroos, J. Marniemi, P. Peltonen, M. Mantyla, J. Niskanen, A. Rautio, and E. Hietanen. 1985. *Horm. Metab. Res.* 17:32–34.
215. Rebuffe-Scrive, M., A. Basdevant, and B. Guy-Grand. 1983. *Horm. Metab. Res.* 15:566.
216. Eckel, R. H., C. N. Sadur, and T. J. Yost. 1985. (Abst.) *Int. J. Obesity* 9:A27.
217. Mjos, O. D., O. Faergeman, R. L. Hamilton, and R. J. Havel. 1975. *J. Clin. Invest.* 56:603–615.
218. Nestel, P. J., and W. Austin. 1969. *Life Sci.* 8:157–164.

219. Rosenqvist, U., R. Mahler, and L. A. Carlson. 1981. *J. Endocrinol. Invest.* 4:75–80.
220. Levacher, C., C. Sztalryd, M. -F. Kinebanyan, and L. Picon. 1984. *Am. J. Physiol.* 246:C50–C56.
221. Murase, T., and H. Uchimura. 1980. *Metabolsim* 29:797–801.
222. Murase, T., N. Yamada, and H. Uchimura. 1983. *Metabolism* 32:146–150.
223. Skottova, N., L. Wallinder, and G. Bengtsoon. 1983. *Biochim. Biophys. Acta.* 750:533–538.
224. Gavin, L. A., F. McMahon, and M. Moeller. 1985. *Diabetes* 34:1266–1271.
225. Redgrave, T. G., and D. A. Snibson. 1977. *Metabolism* 26:493–503.
226. Kirkeby, K. 1968. *Acta Endocrinol.* 59:555–563.
227. Porte, D., Jr., D. D. O'Hara, and R. H. Williams. 1966. *Metabolism* 15:107–113.
228. Nikkila, E. A. and M. Kekki. 1972. *J. Clin. Invest.* 51:2103–2114.
229. Hazzard, W. R., and E. L. Bierman. 1972. *Arch. Int. Med.* 130:822–828.
230. Tulloch, B. R., B. Lewis, and T. R. Fraser. 1973. *Lancet* 1:391–394.
231. Baum, D., R. Guthrie, J. D. Brunzell, W. C. Vogel, and E. L. Bierman. 1973. *Am. J. Dis. Child.* 125:612–613.
232. Krauss, R. M., R. I. Levy, and D. S. Frederickson. 1974. *J. Clin. Invest.* 54:1107–1124.
233. Arons, D., P. H. Schreibman, and P. Downs. 1972. *N. Engl. J. Med.* 286:233–237.
234. Lithell, H., J. Boberg, K. Hellsing, S. Ljunghall, G. Lundqvist, B. Vessby, and L. Wide. 1981. *Eur. J. Clin. Invest.* 11:3–10.
235. Abrams, J. J., S. M. Grundy, and H. Ginsberg. 1981. *J. Lipid. Res* 22:307–322.
236. Valdemarsson, S., P. Hedner, and P. Nilsson-Ehle. 1983. *Acta. Endocrinol.* 103:192–197.
237. Valdemarsson, S., P. Hansson, P. Hedner, and P. Nilsson-Ehle. 1983. *Acta. Endocrinol.* 104:50–56.
238. Lithell, H., B. Vessby, I. Selinus, and P. A. Dahlberg. 1985. *Acta. Endocrinol.* 109:227–231.
239. Ohisalo, J. J., H. Strandberg, E. Kostianinen, T. Kuusi, and C. Ehnholm. 1981. *Febs. Lett.* 132:121–123.
240. Maebashi, M., K. Yoshinaga, and M. Suzuki. 1984. *Tohuku J. Exp. Med.* 143:71–77.
241. Enzi, G., N. Favaretto, S. Martini, R. Fellin, A. Baritussio, G. Baggio, and G. Crepaldi. 1983. *J. Lipid Res.* 24:566–574.
242. Giudicelli, Y., R. Pecquery, B. Agli, C. Jamin, and J. Quevauvilliers. 1976. *Clin. Sci. Molec. Med.* 50:315–318.
243. Larsson, B., P. Bjorntorp, J. Holm, T. Schersten, L. Sjostrom, and U. Smith. 1975. *Metabolism* 24:1375–1389.
244. Zanaboni, L., D. Bonfiglioli, D. Sommariva, D. D'Adda, and A. Fasoli. 1981. *Eur. J. Clin. Pharmacol.* 19:349–351.
245. Asayama, K., S. Amemiya, S. Kusano, and K. Kato. 1984. *Metabolism* 33:129–131.
246. Eckel, R. H., W. Y. Fujimoto, and J. D. Brunzell. 1981. *Int. J. Obesity* 5:571–577.
247. Bordeaux, A. -M., M. -C. Rebourcet, J. Nordmann, R. Nordmann, and Y. Giudicelli. 1982. *Biochem. Biophys. Res. Comm.* 107:59–67.
248. Wise, L. S., and H. Green. 1978. *Cell* 13:233–242.
249. Vannier, C., E. -Z. Amri, J. Etienne, R. Negrel, and G. Ailhaud. 1985. *J. Biol. Chem.* 260:4424–4431.
250. Patten, R. L. 1970. *J. Biol. Chem.* 245:5577–5584.
251. Eckel, R. H., J. E. Prasad, P. A. Kern, and S. Marshall. 1984. *Endocrinology* 114:1665–1671.
252. Kornhauser, D. M., and M. Vaughan. 1975. *Biochim. Biophys. Acta* 380:97–105.
253. Wing, D. R., and D. S. Robinson. 1968. *Biochem. J.* 106:667–676.
254. Kern, P. A., S. Marshall, and R. H. Eckel. 1985. *J. Clin. Invest.* 75:199–208.
255. Cryer, A., P. Davies, E. R. Williams, and D. S. Robinson. 1975. *Biochem. J.* 146:481–488.
256. Stewart, J. E., and M. C. Schotz. 1973. *Nature* (London) *New Biol.* 244:250–251.
257. De la Llera, M., J. M. Glick, and G. Rothblat. 1981. *J. Lipid Res.* 22:245–253.

258. Korn, E. D., and T. W. Quigley, Jr. 1955. *Biochim. Biophys. Acta.* 18:143–145.
259. Ho, S. J., R. J. Ho, and H. C. Meng. 1967. *Am. J. Physiol.* 212:284–290.
260. Salaman, M. R., and D. S. Robinson. 1966. *Biochem. J.* 99:640–647.
261. Rothblat, G. H., and F. D. DeMartinis. 1977. *Biochem. Biophys. Res.* Comm. 78:45–50.
262. Glick, J. M., and G. H. Rothblat. 1980. *Biochim. Biophys. Acta.* 618:163–172.
263. Serrero, G., and J. C. Khoo. 1982. *Anal. Biochem.* 120:351–359.
264. Patten, R. L, and C. H. Hollenberg. 1969. *J. Lipid Res.* 10:374–382.
265. Stewart, J. E., andM. C. Schotz. 1974. *J. Biol. Chem.* 249:904–907.
266. Eckel, R. H., W. Y. Fujimoto, and J. D. Brunzell. 1978. *Biochem. Biophys. Res. Comm.* 84:1069–1075.
267. Cryer, A., B. Foster, D. R. Wing, and D. S. Robinson. 1973. *Biochem. J.* 142:833–836.
268. Glick, J. M., and S. J. Adelman. 1983. *In Vitro* 19:421–428.
269. Cryer, A., A. A. McDonald, E. R. Williams, and D. S. Robinson. 1975. *Biochem. J.* 152:717–720.
270. Vannier, C., H. Jansen, R. Negrel, and G. Ailhaud. 1982. *J. Biol. Chem.* 257:12387–12393.
271. Stewart, J. E., and M. C. Schotz. 1971. *J. Biol. Chem.* 246:5749–5753.
272. Stewart, J. E., C. F. Whelan, and M. C. Schotz. 1969. *Biochem. Biophys. Res. Comm.* 34:376–381.
273. Ashby, P., D. P. Bennett, I. M. Spencer, and D. S. Robinson. 1978. *Biochem. J.* 176:865–872.
274. Bordeaux, A. -M., Y. Giudicelli, M. -C Rebourcet, J. Nordmann, and R. Nordmann. 1980. *Biochem. Biophys. Res. Comm.* 95:212–219.
275. Vydelingum, N., R. L. Drake, J. Etienne, and A. H. Kissebah. 1983. *Am. J. Physiol.* 245:E121–E131.
276. Chait, A., P. -H Iverius, and J. D. Brunzell. 1982. *J. Clin. Invest.* 69:490–493.
277. Rodbell, M. 1964. *J. Biol. Chem.* 239:753–755.
278. Bjorntorp, P., M. Karlsson, H. Pertoft, P. Pettersson, L. Sjostrom, and U. Smith. 1978. *J. Lipid Res.* 19:316–324.
279. Gaben-Cogneville, A. -M., A. Quignard-Boulange, Y. Aron, L. Brigant, T. Jahchan, J.-Y. Pello, and E. Swierczewski. 1984. *Biochim. Biophys. Acta* 805:252–260.
280. Jonasson, L., G. K. Hansson, G. Bondjers, G. Bengtsson, and T. Olivecrona. 1984. *Atherosclerosis* 51:313–326.
281. Spooner, P. M., S. S. Chernick, M. M. Garrison, and R. O. Scow. 1979. *J. Biol. Chem.* 254:1305–1311.
282. Plaas, H. A. K., and A. Cryer. 1980. *J. Devel. Physiol.* 2:275–289.
283. Negrel, R., P. Grimaldi, and G. Ailhaud. 1978. *Proc. Natl. Acad. Sci.* U.S.A. 75:6054–6058.
284. Murphy, M. G., R. Negrel, and G. Ailhaud. 1981. *Biochim. Biophys. Acta.* 664:240–248.
285. Amri, E. -Z., P. Grimaldi, R. Negrel, and G. Ailhaud. 1984. *Exp. Cell Res.* 152:368–377.
286. Gaillard, D., P. Poli, and R. Negrel. 1985. *Exp. Cell Res.* 156:513–527.
287. Forest, C., P. Grimaldi, D. Czerucka, R. Negrel, and G. Ailhaud. 1983. *In Vitro* 19:344–354.
288. Bjorntorp, P., M. Karlsson, P. Pettersson, and G. Sypniewska. 1980. *J. Lipid Res.* 21:714–723.
289. Friedman, G., T. Chajek-Shaul, O. Stein, and Y. Stein. 1983. *Biochim. Biophys. Acta.* 752:106–117.
290. Kern, P. A., and R. H. Eckel. 1984. *Arteriosclerosis* 4:232–237.
291. Eckel, R. H., W. Y. Fujimoto, and J. D. Brunzell. 1977. *Biochem. Biophys. Res. Comm.* 78:288–293.
292. Van, R. L. R., C. E. Bayliss, and D. A. K. Roncari. 1976. *J. Clin. Invest.* 58:699–704.
293. Kuri-Harcuch, W., L. S. Wise, and H. Green. 1978. *Cell* 14:53–59.
294. Gaillard, D., G. Ailhaud, and R. Negrel. 1985. *Biochim. Biophys. Acta.* 846:185–191.

295. Grimaldi, P., D. Czerucka, N. Rassoulzadegan, F. Cuzin, and G. Ailhaud. 1984. *Proc. Natl. Acad. Sci.* U.S.A. 81:5440–5444.
296. Hausman, G. J., J. E. Novakofski, T. Ramsay, and R. J. Martin. 1985. *J. Anim. Sci.* 60:1553–1561.
297. Gaben-Cogneville, A. -M., Y. Aron, G. Idriss, T. Jahchan, J. -Y. Pello, and N. E. Swierczewski. 1983. *Biochim. Biophys. Acta.* 762:437–444.
298. Spooner, P. M., S. S. Chernick, M. M. Garrison, and R. O. Scow. 1979. *J. Biol. Chem.* 254:10021–10029.
299. Van Obberghen, E., P. M. Spooner, C. R. Kahn, S. S. Chernick, M. M.Garrison, F. A. Karlsson, and C. Grunfeld. 1979. *Nature* 280:500–502.
300. Bourdeaux, A. -M., R. Nordmann, and Y. Giudicelli. 1984. *Febs. Lett.* 178:132–136.
301. Bourdeaux, A. -M., Y. Giudicelli, M. -C. Rebourcet, J. Nordmann, and R. Nordmann. 1979. *Experientia.* 36:913–914.
302. Parkin, S. M., K. Walker, P. Ashby, and D. S. Robinson. 1980. *Biochem. J.* 188:193–199.
303. Vydelingum, N., A. H. Kissebah, and V. Wynn. 1978. *Horm. Metab. Res.* 10:38–46.
304. Nikkila, E. A., and O. Pykalisto. 1968. *Life Sci.* 7:1303–1309.
305. Eckel, R. H. and Prasad, J. M. (1985). (Abst.). *Int. J. Obesity* 9:A28.
306. Chajek-Shaul, T., G. Friedman, H. Knobler, O. Stein, J. Etienne, and Y. Stein. 1985. *Biochim. Biophys. Acta.* 837:123–134.
307. Friedman, G., T. Chajek-Shaul, T. Olivecrona, O. Stein, and Y. Stein. 1982. *Biochim. Biophys. Acta.* 71:114–122.
308. Speake, B. K., S. M. Parkin, and D. S. Robinson. 1985. *Biochim. Biophys. Acta.* 840:419–422.
309. Emery, R. S. 1979. *J. Anim. Sci.* 48:1530–1537.
310. Austin, W., and P. J. Nestel. 1968. *Biochim. Biophys. Acta.* 164:59–63.
311. Ashby, P., and D. S. Robinson. 1980. *Biochem. J.* 188:185–192.
312. Ekleles, R. S. 1974. *Clin.Sci., Mol. Med.* 46:753–762.
313. Cigolini, M., and U. Smith. 1978. *Metabolism* 28:502–510.
314. Czech, M. P. 1982. *Cell* 31:8–10.
315. Nissley, S. P., and M. M. Rechler. 1984. *Clin. Endocrinol. Metab.* 13:43–67.
316. Kern, P. A., D. Graves, J. Baskin, R. H. Eckel, and J. J. Van Wyk. 1985. (Abst.). *Clin. Res.* 33:434A.
317. Eckel, R. H. 1985. (Abst.). *Clin. Res.* 33:429A.
318. Kern, A. P., and R. H. Eckel. 1986. (Abst.). *Clin. Res.* 34:547A.
319. Murase, T., N. Yamada, and F. Matsuzaki. 1980. *Life Sci.* 28:199–201.
320. Eckel, R. H., W. Y. Fujimoto, and J. D. Brunzell. 1979. *Diabetes* 28:1141–1142.
321. Murase, T., K. Tanaka, Y. Iwamoto, Y. Akanuma, and K. Kosaka. 1981. *Horm. Metab. Res.* 13:212–213.
322. Wing, D. R., and D. S. Robinson. 1968. *Biochem. J.* 109:841–849.
323. Hansson, P., and P. Nilsson-Ehle. 1983. *Ann. Nutr. Metab.* 27:328–337.
324. Chan, C. P., and J. S. Stern. 1982. *Am. J. Physiol.* 242:E445–E450.
325. Rauramaa, R. 1982. *Med. Biol.* 60:139–143.
326. Hansen, F. M., P. Nilsson, O. Sonne, B. -E. Hustvedt, P. Nilsson-Ehle, J. H. Nielsen, and A. Lovo. 1983. *Diabetologia* 24:131–135.
327. Brown, D. F., K. Daudiss, and J. Durrant. 1967. *Diabetes* 16:90–95.
328. Schnatz, J. D., and R. H. Williams. 1963. *Diabetes* 12:174–178.
329. Rauramaa, R., P. Kuusela, and E. Hietanen. 1980. *Horm. Metab. Res.* 12:591–595.
330. Ishikawa, A., T. Murase, N. Yamada, K. Tanaka, and Y. Iwamoto. 1982. *Endocrinol. Jpn.* 29:379–381.
331. Dall'Aglio, E., F. Chang, H. Chang, J. Stern and G. Reaven. 1983. *Diabetes* 32:46–50.
332. Sadur, C. N., T. J. Yost, and R. H. Eckel. 1984. (Abst.). *Diabetes* 33 (Suppl 1):623.
333. Taskinen, M. -R., E. A. Nikkila, R. Nousianen, and A. Gordin. 1981. *Scand. J. Clin. Lab. Invest.* 41:263–268.

334. Lemonnier, E., J. -P. Suquet, R. Auberi, P. De Gasquet, and E. Pequignot. 1975. *Diabet. Metab.* 1:77–85.
335. Vasselli, J. R., M. P. Cleary, K. -L. C. Jen, and M. R. C. Greenwood. 1980. *Physiol. Behav.* 25:565–573.
336. Shepherd, A., and M. P. Cleary. 1984. *Am. J. Physiol.* 246:E123–E128.
337. Horwitz, B. A., T. Inokuchi, S. J. Wickler, and J. S. Stern. 1984. *Metabolism* 33:354–357.
338. Walberg, J. L., M. R. C. Greenwood, and J. S. Stern. 1983. *Am. J. Physiol.* 245:R706–R712.
339. Cleary, M. P., J. R. Vasselli, and M. R. C. Greenwood. 1980. *Am. J. Physiol.* 238:E284–E292.
340. Greenwood, M. R. C., C. A. Maggio, H. S. Koopmans, and A. Sclafani. 1982. *Int. J. Obesity* 6:513–525.
341. Hartman, A. D. 1981. *Am. J. Physiol.* 241:E108–E115.
342. Boulange, A., E. Planche, and P. De Gasquet. 1981. *Metabolism* 30:1045–1052.
343. Gruen, R., E. Hietanen, and M. R. C. Greenwood. 1978. *Metabolism* 27:1955–1966.
344. Schonfeld, G., C. Felski, and M. A. Howald. 1974. *J. Lipid Res.* 15:457–464.
345. Wang, C. -S., N. Fukuda, and J. A. Ontko. 1984. *J. Lipid Res.* 25:571–579.
346. Schwartz, R. S., J. D. Brunzell, and E. L. Bierman. 1979. *Trans. Assn. Am. Phys.* 92:89–95.
347. Holm, V. A., and P. L. Pipes. 1976. *Am. J. Dis. Child.* 130:1063–1067.
348. Olsson, S. -A., B. G. Petersson, R. Sorbris, and P. Nilsson-Ehle. 1984. *Am. J. Clin. Nutr.* 40:1273–1280.
349. Taskinen, M. -R., I. Tulikoura, E. A. Nikkila, and C. Ehnholm. 1981. *Eur. J. Clin. Invest.* 11:317–323.
350. Schwartz, R. S., and J. D. Brunzell. 1978. *Lancet* 1:1230–1231.
351. Schwartz, R. S., and J. D. Brunzell. 1981. *J. Clin. Invest.* 67:1425–1430.
352. Reitman, J. S., F.C. Kosmakos, B. V. Howard, M. -R. Taskinen, T. Kuusi, and E. A. Nikkila. 1982. *J. Clin. Invest.* 70:791–797.
353. Jaillard, J., G. Sezille, J. C. Fruchart, R. Dewailly and M. Romon. 1976. *Diabete Metab.* 2:5–9.
354. Schwartz, R. S., and J. D. Brunzell. 1984. (Correspondence). *Am. J. Clin. Nutr.* 39:641.
355. Eckel, R. H., and T. J. Yost. 1986. (Abst.). *Diabetes* 35:10A.
356. Comstock, G. W., and R. W. Stone. 1972. *Arch. Environ. Health* 24:271–276.
357. Brunzell, J. D., A. P. Goldberg, and R. S. Schwartz. 1980. *Int. J. Obesity* 4:101–103.
358. Carney, R. M., and A. P. Goldberg. 1984. *N. Engl. J. Med.* 310:614–616.
359. Eckel, R. H., C. N. Sadur, and T. J. Yost. 1984. *N. Engl. J. Med.* 311:259–260.
360. Goldstein, A. L., and P. R. Johnson. 1982. *Metabolism* 31:601–607.
361. Bourgeois, F., A. L. Goldstein, and P. R. Johnson. 1983. *Metabolism* 32:673–680.
362. Paterniti, J. R., Jr., W. V. Brown, H. N. Ginsberg, and K. Artzt. 1983. *Science* 221:167–169.
363. Shafrir, E., and Y. Biale. 1970. *Eur. J. Clin. Invest.* 1:19–24.
364. Gutman, A., and E. Shafrir. 1963. *Am. J. Physiol.* 205:702–706.
365. Abe, R., I. MacDonald, Y. Maruhama, and Y. Goto. 1979. *Metabolism* 28:97– 99.
366. Bagby, G. J., and J. A. Spitzer. 1980. *Am. J. Physiol.* 238:H325–H330.
367. Lanza-Jacoby, S., S. C. Lansey, M. P. Cleary, and F. E. Rosato. 1982. *Arch. Surg.* 117:144–147.
368. Lanza-Jacoby, S., S. C. Lansey, E. E. Miller, and M. P. Cleary. 1984. *Cancer Res.* 44:5062–5067.
369. Murase, T., D. C. Cattran, B. Rubenstein, and G. Steiner. 1975. *Metabolism* 24:1279–1286.
370. Bagdade, J. D., E. Yee, D. E. Wilson, and E. Shafrir. 1978. *J. Lab. Clin. Med.* 91:176–186.
371. Noma, A., M. Kita, and T. Okamiya. 1984. *Horm. Metab. Res.* 16:233–236.
372. Bagby, G. J., and J. A. Spitzer. 1980. *J. Surg. Res.* 29:110–115.

373. Suzuki, M., Y. Satoh, and N. Hashiba. 1983. *J. Nutr. Sci. Vitaminol.* 29:663–670.
374. Odonkor, J. N., and M. P. Rogers. 1984. *Biochem. Pharmacol.* 33:1337–1341.
375. Tolman, E. L., H. M. Tepperman, and J. Tepperman. 1970. *Am. J. Physiol.* 218:1313–1318.
376. Lithell, H., J. Boberg, K. Hellsing, G. Lundqvist, and B. Vessby. 1978. *Eur. J. Clin. Invest.* 8:67–74.
377. Brunzell, J. D., A. Chait, E. A. Nikkila, C. Ehnholm, J. K. Huttunen, and G. Steiner. 1980. *Metabolism* 29:624–629.
378. Harlan, W. R., Jr., P. S. Winesett, and A. J. Wasserman. 1967. *J. Clin. Invest.* 46:239–247.
379. Brunzell, J. D., N. E. Miller, P. Alaupovic, R. J. St. Hilaire, C. S. Wang, D. L. Sarson, S. R. Bloom, and B. Lewis. 1983. *J. Lipid Res.* 24:12–19.
380. Persson, B. 1974. *Clin. Sci. Molec. Med.* 47:631–634.
381. Taskinen, M. -R., E. A. Nikkila, and T. Kuusi. 1982. *Eur. J. Clin. Invest.* 12:433–438.
382. Pagano Mirani-Oostdijk, C., L. Havekes, C. M. Van Gent, M. Frolich, H. Jansen, and J. Terpstra. 1985. *Atherosclerosis* 57:129–137.
383. Lisch, H. -J., W. Patsch, L. Riedler, S. Sailer, and H. Braunsteiner. 1978. *Klin. Wochenschr.* 56:1067–1069.
384. Goldberg, A. P., E. M. Applebaum-Bowden, E. L. Bierman, W. R. Hazzard, L. B. Haas, D. J. Sherrard, J. D. Brunzell, J. K. Huttunen, C. Ehnholm, and E. A. Nikkila. 1979. *N. Engl. J. Med.* 301:1073–1076.
385. Fager, G., G. Berglund, G. Bondjers, D. Elmfeldt, I. Lager, S. -O. Olfsson, U. Smith, and O. Wiklund. 1983. *Artery* 11:283–296.
386. Holdsworth, G., K. G. Taylor, and D. J. Galton. 1979. *Atherosclerosis* 33:253–258.
387. Taylor, K. G., G. Holdsworth, and D. J. Galton. 1977. *Lancet* 2:1106–1107.
388. Vessby, B., H. Lithell, and H. Ledermann. 1982. *Atherosclerosis* 44:113–118.
389. Boberg, J., I. -B., Gustafsson, B. Karlstrom, H. Lithell, B. Vessby, and I. Werner. 1981. *Ann. Nutr. Metab.* 25:320–333.
390. Solvonuk, P. F., G. P. Taylor, R. Hancock, W. S. Wood, and J. Frohlich. 1984. *Lab. Invest.* 51:469–474.
391. Etienne, J., M. Van Den Akker, Y. Mafart, R. Pieron, J. Debray, and J. Polonovski. 1974. *Pathologie Biol.* 22:611–615.
392. Marshall, F. N. 1965. *Experientia* 21:130–131.
393. Enzi, G., E. M. Inelmen, A. Baritussio, P. Dorigo, M. Prosdocimi, and F. Mazzoleni. 1977. *J. Clin. Invest.* 60:1221–1229.
394. Chakrabarty, K., B. Chaudhuri, and H. Jeffay. 1983. *J. Lipid Res.* 24:381–390.
395. Guerrier, D., and H. Pellet. 1979. *Febs. Lett.* 106:115–120.
396. Olivecrona, T., S. S. Chernick, G. Bengtsson-Olivecrona, J. R. Paterniti, Jr., W. V. Brown, and R. O. Scow. 1985. *J. Biol. Chem.* 260:2552–2557.
397. Hemon, P., D. Ricquier, and G. Mory. 1975. *Horm. Metab. Res.* 7:481–484.
398. Radomski, M. M., and T. Orme. 1971. *Am. J. Physiol.* 220:1852–1856.
399. Cryer, A., and H. M. Jones. 1978. *Biochem. J.* 174:447–451.
400. Fried, S. K., J. O. Hill, M. Nickel, and M. DiGirolamo. 1983. *J. Nutr.* 113:1870–1874.
401. Pequignot-Planche, E., P. DeGasquet, A. Boulange, and N. T. Tonnu. 1977. *Biochem. J.* 162:461–463.
402. Carneheim, C., J. Nedergaard, and B. Cannon. 1984. *Am. J. Physiol.* 246:E327–E333.
403. Goubern, M., N. C. Laury, L. B. Zizine, and R. Portet. 1985. *Horm. Metab. Res.* 17:176–180.
404. Bertin, R., M. Goubern, and R. Portet. 1978. In: *Effectors of Thermogenesis.* Girardier, L., and J. Seydoux, editors. Birkhauser Verlag, Basel. 185–189.

Chapter 5

HEART AND SKELETAL MUSCLE LIPOPROTEIN LIPASE

Jayme Borensztajn

The presence of lipoprotein lipase (LPL) activity in skeletal muscle was first reported in 1959 (1). In subsequent years, this observation was confirmed in studies showing LPL activity in single muscles [e.g. diaphragm (2), soleus (3)] and in groups of muscles [e.g. thigh muscles (4)]. In all these studies, the enzyme activity per unit weight was shown to be considerably lower than that found in adipose tissue, heart, and lactating mammary gland. Further, the reported range of enzyme activity of various muscles was quite broad. In one study (5), for example, the LPL activity in the rat soleus muscle was reported to be about four times that in the tibial muscle. The reason for this variation among individual muscles became apparent with the observation that LPL activity is significantly higher in fast-twitch red and slow-twitch red fibers than in fast-twitch white fibers (6–9). Since muscles are made up of a mixture of fiber types, the LPL activity depends on whether the muscle has predominantly red fibers or white fibers (8). In the rat, skeletal muscle forms about 45% of the body weight (10), and based on the conservative estimate that one third of the muscle mass is made up of red fibers, the total LPL activity in this tissue is substantial. For example, in fed rats, the LPL activity in the muscle mass could be two thirds (8) or more (7,11) that present in the total adipose tissue mass, and several-fold greater (7) than that in the adipose tissue mass of starved rats.

The presence of substantial LPL activity in muscle suggests that it has a major role in the uptake of plasma triglyceride fatty acids by that tissue. The uptake of plasma triglycerides by skeletal muscle was assessed in early studies (12–15) by measuring the amount of radioactive fatty acids in a single muscle (e.g. psoas, gluteal) or a group of muscles (e.g. abdominal, leg, and back muscles) at different times after the intravenous injection of chylomicrons containing radioactive triglycerides. The results of these studies, which assumed that the small muscle sample examined was representative of the total muscle mass, indicated that only 3–18% of the injected chylomicron triglyceride fatty acids was taken up by the skeletal muscle. However, most of the muscles sampled in these studies contain a large proportion of white fibers which have very low LPL activity. Thus, the amount of triglyceride fatty acids taken up by the total muscle mass may have been underestimated. This interpretation is supported by the observations that the recovery of injected labelled triglyceride fatty acids in muscles containing mainly red fibers, with high LPL activity, is substantially greater than those containing mainly white fibers (7–9). Linder et al. (7) for example, reported that ten minutes after the injection of chylomicrons containing labelled triglyceride fatty acids into starved rats, when most of the radioactivity had been cleared from the plasma, about 1% of the injected label was recovered per gram of slow-twitch red soleus muscle. Based on the previously noted assumption that red muscle fibers account for only one third of the muscle mass, it can be calculated that in their experiments, about 30% of the injected label was taken up by the muscle. This estimate corresponds, in all probability, to minimal values since some of the fatty acids taken up by the high oxidative red fibers may have been oxidized. Muscle has only a limited lipid storage capacity, and not all fatty acids formed by LPL action on lipoprotein triglycerides are taken up by the tissue. Consequently, the contribution that muscle LPL makes to the clearance of triglyceride-rich lipoproteins from circulation cannot be accurately estimated from the recovery of label in the muscle. However, these studies together with the results of studies on the clearance of triglyceride-rich lipoproteins from circulation of the supra-diaphragmatic portion of the rat (16), intact rat (17), dog (18), and man (19), as well as the measurement in humans of arterio-venous differences of exogenous triglycerides infused into the deep veins of the forearm (20, 21), which drain mainly muscle tissue (22–24), provide compelling evidence that muscle LPL makes a quantitatively major contribution to the clearance from circulation of triglyceride-rich lipoproteins, particularly in conditions when the metabolic requirements of muscle are met by the oxidation of fatty acids (e.g. starvation).

In contrast to skeletal muscle, heart LPL accounts for only a small fraction of the total enzyme activity present in extra-hepatic tissues and makes, therefore, a quantitatively minor contribution to the catabolism of plasma triglyceride-rich lipoproteins. Nevertheless, since the presence of LPL in heart was first reported by Korn (25), interest in the myocardial enzyme has been much greater than that in skeletal muscle and second only to that in the adipose tissue enzyme. This interest in heart LPL can be accounted for by the following: a) The heart, unlike most other extra-hepatic tissues, can be isolated intact and its vascular bed perfused with relative ease. Since the hydrolysis of lipoprotein triglycerides occurs on the surface of the capillaries, the isolated perfused heart preparation has been extensively used for the study of the interaction of LPL with its substrate at its normal site of action. b) In general, the isolated perfused heart is held to be a valid model system for the study of many characteristics of LPL. The results of extensive studies on the localization, transport, and synthesis of LPL using this system, are considered generally applicable to skeletal muscle as well as other extra-hepatic tissues. c) Myocardial cells can be isolated and maintained metabolically active in culture. d) Finally, LPL activity in the heart, per unit weight, is higher than that of skeletal muscle, and because of the greater homogeneity of the heart tissue, measurements of the heart enzyme are easier to make and less variable. As a result, studies on the regulation of muscle LPL activity have been carried out mainly using heart muscle. Evidence has become available, however, showing that not all results obtained with heart LPL can be extrapolated to the skeletal muscle. This has become apparent from studies showing that the enzyme in the heart and skeletal muscle may respond differently to the same stimuli (see below). In spite of these reported differences, heart and skeletal muscle LPL appear to share many properties and will, therefore, be discussed together in this Chapter.

Localization

Muscle LPL activity has been found in cells and in extracellular locations. Cellular LPL activity has been conclusively demonstrated a) in neonatal rat heart cells (both myocytes and cells of mesenchymal origin) (26–34), b) in subcellular fractions of isolated rat heart cells (35), and c) in isolated adult rat heart myocytes (35–41). In the latter case, only a fraction of the total heart LPL activity can be recovered. Homogenates of intact cells isolated from hearts by collagenase perfusion yield only about 30% of the total heart LPL activity of fed rats. When rats are starved, the total heart activity is greatly increased, while the cell-associated activity remains unchanged and thus accounts for only 15% of the total (37). These results suggest that the balance of the total heart LPL activity is extracellular and is lost or destroyed during cell isolation with collagenase. But the possibility has not yet been ruled out that at least part of the adult rat heart LPL activity is present in cells other than myocytes (42), that are destroyed by collagenase during the cell isolation procedure.

An extracellular location for heart LPL was first inferred from studies which suggested the presence of activity on the surface of capillary endothelial cells. Perfusion of isolated rat hearts with heparin caused an immediate release of LPL activity into the perfusate, with peak activity appearing within seconds (43–49). The rapid appearance of this activity suggested that the released enzyme had been located at an extracellular site easily accessible to heparin, such as the surface, or a site close to the surface, of the capillary endothelium (43,50). Corroborating evidence of this hypothesis was subsequently provided by studies in which triglyceride-rich lipoproteins were perfused through the isolated heart. Although these particles are too large to penetrate the endothelial cells or their junctions, their triglycerides were nevertheless hydrolyzed (see below). More direct evidence of the presence of LPL on the endothelial surface of heart capillaries has been provided by an immunocytochemical reaction of the enzyme at that site, followed by visualization by electron microscopy (51).

The proportion of the total heart LPL activity that can be rapidly released by heparin, depends not only on the concentration of heparin used (52), but also on a variety of physiological and pathological stimuli. Under all conditions, however, the rapidly releasable activity accounts for not more than half of the total activity present in the tissue (52–55). In isolated hearts, the initial rapid heparin-mediated release of LPL activity is followed by a continuous, although slower, release which persists for the duration of the perfusion (53,54), lasting over 1 hour in some studies (43,44,53). The rapid and slow phases of LPL release have also been observed in skeletal muscle (22,24). In the heart, depending on the duration of perfusion, the total activity released in the slow phase can be considerable, accounting in some studies for 30–50% of the total enzyme present in the muscle (43,44,53). It is noteworthy, however, that even after prolonged perfusion with heparin, not all of the heart initial enzyme activity is released from the tissue. What remains is presumed to be primarily the cell-associated enzyme. The location of the slowly releasable LPL activity has not yet been determined. It has been suggested to be present in the interstitial space in transit from its site of synthesis or storage in the cells to its binding sites on the surface of the capillary endothelium (44). This suggestion of an interstitial rather than an intracellular location is supported by the results of experiments (56) in which the heart is perfused with a calcium-free medium, which presumably disrupts cellular junctions, and allows rapid access of the perfusate to the interstitial spaces. The addition of heparin to this calcium-free perfusate has been shown to cause the rapid release of the otherwise slowly releasable LPL activity (56). The addition of collagenase to a calcium-free perfusing medium also causes the release or destruction of the interstitial LPL, depending on the protease concentration used (57).

Functions of Muscle Liproprotein Lipase

As described above, muscle LPL is distributed throughout the tissue in several compartments. Studies on the function of the enzyme in the heart have demonstrated that the fraction that can be rapidly released by heparin is involved in the hydrolysis of circulating lipoprotein triglycerides. The function of the remaining activity has not yet been definitely established.

There is considerable evidence that links the rapidly releasable LPL activity to hydrolysis of circulating triglycerides. Removal or inactivation of this LPL fraction by pre-perfusion with heparin (53,58) or anti-LPL antibodies (59), respectively, virtually abolishes the ability of the heart to hydrolyze lipoprotein triglycerides during subsequent perfusion. Also, when a variety of stimuli (e.g. starvation, cold exposure) are employed which alter heart LPL activity, changes in the ability of the heart to hydrolyze lipoprotein triglycerides parallel the changes which occur in the rapidly releasable fraction, but not those in the remaining fraction (53,60,61). It is noteworthy that not all of the rapidly releasable fraction appears to be involved in the hydrolysis of circulating triglycerides. Inhibition of only 60% of the rapidly releasable LPL activity by Triton WR-1339 almost completely abolishes the ability of isolated perfused hearts to hydrolyze chylomicron triglycerides (61). These findings suggest that the remaining 40% of the rapidly releasable fraction is sequestered in such a way that it is inaccessible to the non-ionic detergent and to the large circulating chylomicrons.

The function of the LPL fraction that is not readily releasable from the organ by heparin, like its location in the tissue (see above), has not yet been clearly established. To distinguish it from the rapidly releasable LPL activity, this fraction has been variously referred to as "residual" (54,62,63); "tissue-bound" (64); "non-releasable" (45,53,60), even though most of it can be released by heparin, albeit at a slow rate; "non-functional" (55), indicating its non-involvement in the hydrolysis of circulating lipoprotein triglycerides; and "intra-cellular" (47,65) even though its exact distribution between intra and extracellular spaces remains to be determined. It has been postulated (66–70) that this fraction functions in the hydrolysis of endogenous triglycerides. In support of this hypothesis, these authors reported that in conditions where the LPL activity remaining in heart and skeletal muscle after a brief perfusion with heparin is increased (e.g. following exposure of the heart to epinephrine), the concentration of endogenous triglycerides is decreased. Further, these authors reported an inverse correlation between the LPL activity of isolated cardiac myocytes and intracellular triglyceride levels (41). This postulated function assumes the enzyme to be localized primarily in intracellular sites in proximity to the endogenous triglycerides (71). Yet, as described above, much of the LPL activity remaining in the heart after brief heparin perfusion cannot be recovered in the myocytes. Furthermore, such a function for intracellular LPL presupposes its activity in the absence of apoprotein CII, the required LPL co-factor, which is not present in heart cells. Hulsmann et al. (56) have reported that at neutral pH, LPL which remains in the heart after a prolonged (twenty-five minutes) perfusion with heparin, is active even in the absence of apoprotein CII. But these authors concluded that this enzyme is extracellular and is not involved in the hydrolysis of endogenous triglycerides. The role of LPL in the hydrolysis of endogenous myocardial triglycerides has also been questioned by Goldberg and Khoo (72). These authors reported the existence of a neutral triglyceride hydrolase in rat heart with properties similar to those of the triglyceride hydrolyzing hormone-sensitive lipase of adipose tissue. They suggested that it is this neutral lipase, rather than LPL, that is involved in the hydrolysis of myocardial triglycerides.

Synthesis and Transport

In muscle, as well as in other tissues, the site of action of LPL is the endothelial surface, to which the enzyme is bound. It appears, however, that endothelial cells are incapable of synthesizing LPL (73). Current evidence indicates instead that the LPL is synthesized in other cell types and is transported to the endothelial surface. In muscle, support for this hypothesis is derived primarily from studies of the heart which show that interference with cellular synthesis and transport of protein affects endothelial LPL activity. LPL has been found to be synthesized in both myoctyes and non-muscle cells. In cultures of neonatal (two day old) rat heart cells, LPL activity is found to be associated primarily with mesenchymal cells, which are presumably derived from the vascular and interstitial elements of the heart (27–29). In contrast to these studies, other work with isolated adult rat heart cells has shown LPL activity to be present predominantly in myocytes (36,37,40) and absent from non-muscle cells (39). Thus, in neonatal and adult rat hearts, mesenchymal cells and myocytes, respectively, could serve as the source of endothelial LPL. Not only are both cell types capable of synthesizing the enzyme, but in culture both are able to release it into the medium, albeit under the influence of heparin (26–41) or steroid hormones (38). The heparin-mediated LPL release into the medium is not accompanied by an appreciable decrease in the cell-associated enzyme activity (39), suggesting that the enzyme may be stored in an inactive form which is activated upon release. However, evidence in support of this hypothesis is lacking. An alternative hypothesis is that synthesis of LPL is linked to its release (74). The heparin-mediated release of LPL from neonatal cells in culture ocurs, as in the intact heart, in a rapid and a slow phase (29), suggesting that some of the enzyme activity (i.e. the rapidly releasable) is present on the cell surface. This hypothesis is supported by the finding that mesenchymal cells in culture are able to hydrolyze lipoprotein triglycerides in the medium, even though there is no soluble LPL activity present (30). In contrast, adult heart myocytes release LPL only slowly (39) in response to heparin and do not hydrolyze lipoprotein triglycerides in the medium, suggesting that their LPL is predominantly intracellular (75). The slow phase release of LPL from both myocytes and mesenchymal cells is dependent on continued protein synthesis as is shown by the absence of this release when the cells are treated with cycloheximide (29,38). The heparin-mediated releasable activity from isolated cells is greatly decreased by the addition of colchicine in concentrations which are insufficient to inhibit protein synthesis (29,38). The mechanism of action of colchicine is considered to be the disruption of the microtubular-mediated system of intracellular protein transport. Thus, its inhibitory effect on heparin-releasable activity indicates that this fraction represents intracellular LPL transported to the cell surface. In addition, it appears that glycosylaton of the enzyme is also required for its cellular secretion. Incubation of cardiomyocytes (38) and mesenchymal cells (34) with tunicamycin, which inhibits protein glycosylation, decreases heparin-releasable activity.

The synthesis, transport, and secretion of LPL have also been examined in the intact rat heart *in vivo* and in the isolated perfused preparation. In the intact heart, the LPL that is transported to the surface of the synthesizing cell must be transported further to the surface of the capillary endothelial cells. The integrity of this latter phase of the transport process can be assessed by measuring the enzyme activity that can be readily released by heparin from the capillary bed. Inhibition of the transport of LPL to the endothelium would result in a marked decrease in the LPL activity that is rapidly released by heparin and by a corresponding accumulation of LPL activity at sites that are not readily accessible to heparin. Such an inhibition of LPL transport has, in fact, been shown to occur in hearts of rats treated with colchicine at doses that do not inhibit protein synthesis (54,55,64,70). The site within the heart, where the non-transported LPL activity accumulates as a result of the colchicine treatment, has not yet been determined. It is noteworthy that the effect of colchicine on the intact heart differs somewhat from its effects on isolated heart cells. While there is a reduction of heparin releasable activity in both preparations, isolated cells show no accumulation of enzyme activity (29,38). As described above, cellular secretion of LPL requires glycosylation which is prevented by tunicamycin. The inhibitory effect of this drug is also seen in intact hearts. When isolated perfused hearts are treated with tunicamycin, LPL activity is decreased in the rapidly releasable and the remaining fractions (64). Total LPL activity of intact hearts is also decreased by cycloheximide treatment (55,64). Again, the rapidly releasable and remaining fractions are affected. The rates of decrease of activity of these fractions after cycloheximide treatment differ, however. The half-life of the rapidly releasable fraction is about half that of the enzyme which remains associated with the tissue (55). The more rapid decline in the activity of the former enzyme fraction might be due to its continuous elution from the endothelial surface by circulating lipoproteins (47,52,76–79). In summary, the results of the studies described above suggest that in the intact heart, LPL is being continuously synthesized and glycosylated in either myocytes or mesenchymal cells and transported first to the external surface of these cells and then to the external surface of the capillary endothelial cells. The pathway followed by the enzyme to reach its site of action on the endothelium is not known.

Physiological Changes in Lipoprotein Lipase Activity

Muscle LPL activity is responsive to various physiological changes. In this section, only the effects of starvation, feeding, and cold exposure are considered. Changes in LPL activity in pathological conditions are described in other Chapters.

Effect of starvation

The first reported alteration of muscle LPL activity in response to a physiological challenge was that showing that heart LPL activity increases during starvation (80). This finding was confirmed and extended to skeletal muscle by Hollenberg (2) who showed that its LPL activity was also increased in response to food deprivation. Since it was known that adipose tissue LPL activity decreases during starvation, Hollenberg suggested that these opposite changes in adipose tissue and muscle LPL might serve as a mechanism to divert more of the circulating triglycerides from adipose tissue to muscle where they could be utilized. Subsequent studies have shown this phenomenon to be generally true. In various physiological and pathological situations, muscle LPL activity parallels the use by this tissue of exogenous fatty acids for oxidation. In the rat, starvation causes an increase in the LPL activity of all types of muscle fibers (53,81–84), with the maximum activity being reached about twelve hours after the fed animal is deprived of food (81). This effect of starvation on rat muscle LPL activity occurs only in animals that are at least fourteen days old (11). In man, skeletal muscle LPL activity is also increased after an overnight fasting period (85). In the rat heart, the increase in LPL activity with starvation (2,53,60,80,81,86–88) occurs in the fraction that can be readily released from the vascular bed by heparin as well as in the fraction that remains associated with the tissue (53,60,62). It is noteworthy, however, that when fed rats are deprived of food, the progressive increase in the activity of the heparin-releasable fraction levels off after about seven hours whereas the activity of the enzyme which is not readily accessible to the heparin continues to increase, reaching its maximum at about twelve hours of starvation (J. Borensztajn, unpublished observations). In contrast to many well-documented studies showing increases in skeletal muscle and heart LPL activity with starvation, several studies have failed to show such changes (1,8,43). These exceptions are not readily explained, although a possible explanation may reside in the timing of the experiments. In the course of a day, heart and skeletal muscle LPL activities of rats with free access to food undergo oscillatory changes which follow closely the cyclic feeding habits of the animal (81,89–91). Oscillations also occur, and are more pronounced, in animals deprived of food (81). Thus, differences in heart and skeletal muscle enzyme activities between fed and starved animals may vary considerably depending on the length of starvation, the eating schedule of the "fed" animals, and the time of day at which the animals are sacrificed.

Effect of carbohydrate and fat feeding

In man and experimental animals, the consumption of carbohydrate causes muscle LPL activity to be maintained at low levels (81,83,92–95). In animals and humans deprived of food, in whom muscle LPL activity is elevated, carbohydrate feeding, but apparently not its parenteral administration (96,97), causes the rapid decline in the high LPL activity of muscle (38,46,49,53,82,84,98). This phenomenon occurs when the animals are given glucose but not fructose (46,84). Sucrose feeding has been reported to have either no effect (84) or to cause the decline in heart LPL activity (46). The effect of glucose feeding is most pronounced on the heart LPL activity fraction that can be readily released by heparin. Within eighty minutes of glucose feeding to twelve-hour starved rats, the activity of this fraction was reported to decline by 85% (46,98). No significant changes were observed in enzyme activity that remained associated with the tissue. The mechanism for this rapid decline only in the fraction that is directly involved in the hydrolysis of circulating lipoprotein triglycerides is not known.

In rats fed fat-rich diets for at least ten days, the heart LPL activity has been reported to be significantly higher (83) or not different (94,99) from that of control rats fed a carbohydrate-rich diet. Feeding rats fat-rich diets for shorter periods was also reported to result in either no change (94) or an increase (68,99) in heart LPL activity compared to control animals eating a regular chow diet. In the latter two studies, the increase in enzyme activity was observed in the fraction that is readily releasable by heparin (99) as well as in the fraction that remains associated with the tissue (68,99). The acute feeding of fat to starved (86) or fed (94) rats has been reported to result in no change in heart LPL activity. But in contrast, Pedersen et al. (49,98) reported that one hour after the acute feeding of fat to starved rats, the heart LPL fraction that is readily releasable by heparin was significantly increased. When carbohydrate-fed rats were given fat, the activity of this LPL fraction was increase ten fold within three hours. The reasons for the differences among these various studies are not clear.

Effect of exposure to cold temperatures

When starved or freely eating rats are exposed to 2–4 C for a few hours or up to several weeks, there is a signficant increase in the LPL activities of their heart and skeletal muscles (60,68,88,91,100–103). In the heart, this increase has been shown in the LPL fraction that can be readily released from the vascular bed by heparin (60), as well as in the fraction that remains associated with the tissue (60,68). It is noteworthy, however, that the increase in the heparin-releasable enzyme activity, although insignificant, was small compared to that of the tissue-associated enzyme which accounted for most of the increased LPL activity of the heart. The reasons for the smaller increase in the enzyme activity on the endothelium are not apparent. A possible explanation is that the number of LPL binding sites on the endothelium surface is limited and that once these sites become saturated, any further increase in LPL synthesis or activation results in the accumulation of enzyme at sites not accessible to heparin. During non-shivering thermogenesis, the caloric demands of muscle are met by the increased utilization of fatty acids. The observed increase in LPL activity could satisfy this metabolic requirement. The decrease in the concentration of plasma triglycerides during cold exposure (104) lends support to this hypothesis.

Regulation

Many studies, involving primarily the heart, have sought to establish that changes in muscle LPL activity are regulated by hormones. There are two reasons for this emphasis on hormones; first, it is well documented that the LPL of adipose tissue and mammary gland is under hormonal control; second, many physiological and pathological stresses which alter muscle LPL activity are accompanied by changes in specific hormone levels. However, despite the numerous studies described below, the identification of the hormone(s) primarily involved in this regulatory process remains to be determined.

Insulin

The possible involvement of insulin in regulating muscle LPL activity has been investigated in studies *in vivo* that have sought to establish a correlation between the plasma levels of this hormone and the activity of the enzyme. The rationale for these studies is based on observations that in adipose tissue and muscle, LPL activity often change in opposite directions (e.g. feeding after a period of starvation). Since a positive correlation can be demonstrated between plasma insulin levels and adipose tissue LPL activity, it was considered likely that an inverse correlation between the hormone level and the muscle LPL activity could also be demonstrated. Cryer et al. (84) using rats maintained under different nutritional conditions, did report such an inverse correlation involving both heart and skeletal muscle. In contrast, studies in which rat heart LPL activity and plasma insulin levels were monitored over twenty hours (105), and also in rats with mammary gland tumors (106) in which insulin levels were significantly depressed, such a relationship could not be demonstrated. In starved rats, an increased plasma insulin level produced by injection of the hormone was not accompanied by a decrease in heart or skeletal muscle LPL activity (91,102,107). In rats made insulin deficient by the administration of alloxan (44,108), streptozotocin (63,81,109), mannoheptulose (107), or by pancreatectomy (7), heart and skeletal muscle LPL activities were reported to be decreased or unchanged; although in one study (110) the heart activity of alloxan diabetic rats was reported elevated. In man, normal or insulin deficient, no correlation has been found between elevated skeletal muscle activity and low plasma insulin levels (111–115).

The possibility that insulin has a direct effect on muscle LPL activity was investigated by O'Looney et al. (63) using the isolated perfused rat heart. They reported that perfusion with insulin of hearts from rats with steptozotocin-induced diabetes restores to normal levels the organ's depressed LPL activity. The increase in LPL activity occurred in both the fraction rapidly releasable by heparin and the fraction which remained associated with the tissue. In contrast to these findings, insulin perfusion had no effect on normal hearts (63,64) or on hearts from alloxan diabetic rats (44).

Glucagon

A role for glucagon in the regulation of muscle LPL activity has been suggested by studies showing that administration of this hormone to rats resulted in significant increases in heart LPL activity (66,82,116). Glucagon has also been shown to have a direct effect on the LPL activity of isolated perfused rat heart (24,117). In contrast, other studies *in vivo* have failed to show either a response of heart and skeletal muscle activity to the administration of glucagon (88,118) or a correlation between plasma levels of this hormone and muscle LPL activity (81,103). The addition of glucagon to the incubation medium of isolated cardiomyocytes (38) or cultured mesenchymal rat heart cells (31) also failed to cause an increase in LPL activity. In man, plasma glucagon/insulin ratios, rather than insulin or glucagon levels alone, have been suggested to be involved in the regulation of muscle LPL activity (111–113).

Glucocorticoids

Unlike the conflicting results of the studies with insulin and glucagon, administration of glucocorticoids to normal fed rats or adrenalectomized rats, has consistently resulted in increases in heart LPL activity (49,91,116,118). The oscillatory changes in heart LPL activity that occur during a twenty-four hour period also appear to parallel changes in plasma corticosterone levels (105). The LPL activity of neonatal rat heart mesenchymal cells in culture is also significantly increased following the addition of glucocorticoids to the incubation medium (31).

Thyroid hormones

The role of these hormones in regulating muscle LPL activity has been inferred mainly from studies with hypo- or hyperthyroid animal models. Hypothyroidism produced by thyroidectomy (102) or the administration of propylthiouracyl has been reported to result in an increase (119), compared to control animals matched for age, weight and food consumption; a decrease (120) or no change (121) in heart LPL activity. In the latter study, however, the enzyme activity in the soleus and vastus lateralis muscles was increased. In hypothyroid man, skeletal muscle LPL activity was reported decreased (122). Hyperthyroidism in the rat is accompanied by an increase in heart LPL activity (121–123) whereas in skeletal muscle the enzyme activity is either decreased (121) or increased (123). The administration of triiodothyronine to normal (100) or hypothyroid rats (124) caused an increase in heart LPL activity.

Catecholamines

The acute and chronic administration of epinephrine and norepinephrine to rats results in an increase in the LPL activity of heart (91,94,100) and red skeletal muscle fibers (118). A direct effect of these hormones on heart LPL activity has also been shown. Thus, in the isolated rat heart preparation perfused with norepinephrine, the activity of the fraction readily releasable by heparin is increased (64). The activity of the fraction that remains associated with the tissue is also increased following the perfusion of hearts with epinephrine (67,69). Addition of epinephrine to heart slices or homogenates, however, has no effect (34).

Cyclic AMP

The possibility that the regulation of muscle LPL activity by hormones might be mediated by cyclic AMP was investigated by Palmer et al. (67,69). They reported that in rat hearts perfused with dibutyryl cyclic AMP or with 3-isobutyl-1-methylxanthine, a phosphodiesterase inhibitor, there was a marked increase in the LPL fraction that remains associated with the tissue after heparin perfusion. Also, exposure of cardiomyocytes, isolated from adult rat hearts, to epinephrine (41) resulted in increases in the intracellular concentration of cyclic AMP and in the LPL activity. Support for a role of cyclic AMP in regulating muscle LPL activity has also been provided by the observtions that the administration of cholera toxin to fed or starved rats (62) results in a marked rise in skeletal muscle LPL activity as well as in the heart LPL fractions that a) are readily releasable by heparin and b) remain associated with the tissue. This effect has been ascribed to a rise in the intracellular cyclic AMP as a result of the increase in tissue adenylate cyclase activity. In contrast to these observations, however, intracellular increases in cyclic AMP resulting from the incubation of isolated adult rat cardiomyocytes or cultured neonatal mesenchymal heart cells with dibutyryl cyclic AMP (33,38), cholera toxin or 3-isobutyl-1-methylxanthine (33), had either no effect (38) or actually caused a decrease (33) in the LPL activity of the cells.

Summary and Conclusions

Skeletal muscle is composed of distinct fiber types which, according to their metabolic and mechanical characteristics, can be classified as fast-twitch red, slow-twitch red and fast-twitch white fibers. Although the presence of LPL in skeletal muscle has long been known, it was only established relatively recently that most of the activity is associated with the red-fibers, which have high oxidative capacity and are, therefore, capable of utilizing fatty acids. Per unit weight, the LPL activity in the skeletal muscle is low when compared to that of other tissues, e.g. adipose tissue and heart of fed and starved animals, respectively. However, because a large portion of the body mass is made up of red-fiber type muscle, the contribution that this tissue makes to the removal of triglyceride-rich lipoproteins from circulation can be equal to- or greater than- that of adipose tissue.

Compared to skeletal muscle, heart muscle, because of its relatively small mass, has only a limited role in the removal of triglyceride-rich lipoproteins from circulation. Nevertheless, because heart and skeletal muscle LPL share common properties and because of convenience of experimentation, most studies on muscle LPL have been carried out using the heart rather than skeletal muscle. These studies have greatly contributed to our present understanding of the function of the enzyme, its actions and its properties. However, several basic questions regarding muscle LPL remain unanswered:

1. What is the distribution of the enzyme between intra-and extracellular spaces of muscle?
2. What portion of the skeletal muscle LPL activity is responsible for the hydrolysis of circulating triglycerides and how can it be quantitated?
3. What is the function of the substantial LPL activity which is not directly involved in the hydrolysis of circulating triglycerides? Does it, as has been suggested, function in the hydrolysis of endogenous triglycerides?
4. What pathway is followed by LPL from its site of synthesis to the surface of endothelial cells?
5. Which hormones, or other factors, have a direct effect in the regulation of muscle LPL *in vivo* and what is the mechanism of this regulation.

Although many investigations aimed at answering these questions have been carried out in the past two decades, they have relied mainly on the measurement of enzyme activity and only incomplete—often contradictory—results have been obtained. New experimental approaches are clearly needed to examine these basic questions if definitive answers are to be forthcoming.

References

1. Cherkes, A., and R. S. Gordon, Jr. 1959. *J. Lipid Res.* 1:97–101.
2. Hollenberg, C. H. 1960. *J. Clin. Invest.* 39:1282–1287.
3. Parizkova, J., Z. Koutecky, and L. Stankova. 1966. *Physiol. Behemoslav.* 15:237–243.
4. Nikkilä, E. A., P. Torsti, and O. Penttila. 1963. *Metabolism* 12:863–865.
5. Parizkova, J., and Z. Koutecky. 1968. *Physiol. Behemoslav.* 17:179–189.
6. Borensztajn, J., M. S. Rone, S. P. Babirak, J. A. McGarr, and L. B. Oscai. 1975. *Am. J. Physiol.* 229:394–397.
7. Linder, C., S. S. Chernick, T. R. Fleck, and R. O. Scow. 1976. *Am. J. Physiol.* 231:860–864.
8. Tan, M. H., T. Sata, and R. J. Havel. 1977. *J. Lipid Res.* 18:363–370.
9. Mackie, B. G., G. A. Dudley, H. Kaciuba-Uscilko, and R. L. Terjung. 1980. *J. Appl. Physiol.* 49:851–855.
10. Caster, W. O., J. Poncelet, A. B. Simon, and W. D. Armstrong. 1956. *Proc. Soc. Exp. Biol. Med.* 91:122–126.
11. Planche, E., A. Boulange, P. de Gasquet, and N. T. Tonu. 1980. *Am. J. Physiol.* 238:511–517.
12. Bragdon, J. H., and R. S. Gordon, Jr. 1958. *J. Clin. Invest.* 37:574–578.
13. Havel, R. J., J. M. Felts, and C. M. Van Duyne. 1962. *J. Lipid Res.* 3:297–308.
14. Olivecrona, T., and B. Belfrage. 1965. *Biochim. Biophys. Acta* 98:81–93.
15. Jones, N., and R. J. Havel. 1967. *Am. J. Physiol.* 213:824–828.

16. Bezman-Tarcher, A., S. Otway, and D. S. Robinson. 1965. *Proc. Roy. Soc. B.* 162:411–426.
17. Harris, K. L., and J. M. Felts. 1973. *Biochim. Biophys. Acta* 316:288–295.
18. Terjung, R. L., L. Budohoski, K. Nazar, A. Kobryn, and H. Kaciuba-Uscilko. 1982. *J. Appl. Physiol.* 52:815–820.
19. Rossner, S. 1974. *Acta med. scand.* (Suppl. 564): 3–24.
20. Kaijser, L., and S. Rossner. 1975. *Acta med. scand.* 197:289–294.
21. Rossner, S., B. Eklund, L. Kaijser, A. G. Olsson, and G. Walldius. 1976. *Europ. J. Clin. Invest.* 6:299–305.
22. Nestel, P. 1970. *Proc. Soc. Expt. Biol. Med.* 134:896–899.
23. Heaf, D. J., L. Kaijser, B. Eklund, and L. A. Carlson. 1977. *Europ. J. Clin. Invest.* 7:195–199.
24. Ehnholm, C., D. J. Heaf, L. Kaijser, P. K. J. Kinnunen, and L. A. Carlson. 1977. *Atherosclerosis* 27:35–39.
25. Korn, E. D. 1955. *J. Biol. Chem.* 215:1–14.
26. Pinson, A., C. Frelin, and P. Padieu. 1973. *Biochimie* 55:1261–1264.
27. Henson, L. C., M. C. Schotz, and I. Harary. 1977. *Biochim. Biophys. Acta* 487:212–221.
28. Chajek, T., O. Stein, and Y. Stein. 1977. *Biochim. Biophys. Acta* 488:140–144.
29. Chajek, T., O. Stein, and Y. Stein. 1978. *Biochim. Biophys. Acta* 528:456–465.
30. Chajek, T., O. Stein, and Y. Stein. 1978. *Biochim. Biophys. Acta* 528:466–474.
31. Friedman, G., O. Stein, and Y. Stein. 1978. *Biochim. Biophys. Acta* 531:222–232.
32. Friedman, G., O. Stein, and Y. Stein. 1979. *Biochim. Biophys. Acta* 573:521–534.
33. Friedman, G., T. Chajek-Shaul, O. Stein, and Y. Stein. 1983. *Biochim. Biophys. Acta* 752:106–117.
34. Friedman, G., O. Stein, and Y. Stein. 1980. *Atherosclerosis* 36:289–298.
35. Choan, P., and A. Cryer. 1979. *Biochem. J.* 181:83–93.
36. Bagby, G. J., M. S. Liu, and J. A. Spitzer. 1977. *Life Sci.* 21:467–474.
37. Choan, P., and A. Cryer. 1978. *Biochem. J.* 174:663–666.
38. Cryer, A., P. Choan, and J. J. Smith. 1981. *Life Sci.* 29:923–929.
39. Choan, P., and A. Cryer. 1980. *Biochem. J.* 186:873–879.
40. Vahouny, G. V., A. Tamboli, M. V. Maten, H. Jansen, J. S. Twu and M. C. Schotz. 1980. *Biochim. Biophys. Acta* 620:63–69.
41. Palmer, W. K., and T. A. Kane. 1983. *Biochem. J.* 216:241–243.
42. Jansen, H., H. Stam, C. Kalkman, and W. C. Hulsmann. 1980. *Biochem. Bipophys. Res. Comm.* 92:411–416.
43. Robinson, D. S., and M. A. Jennings. 1965. *J. Lipid Res.* 6:222–227.
44. Atkin, E., and H. C. Meng. 1972. *Diabetes* 21:149–156.
45. Ben-Zeev, O., H. Schwalb, and M. C. Schotz. 1981. *J. Biol. Chem.* 256:10550–10554.
46. Pedersen, M. E., and M. C. Schotz. 1980. *J. Nutr.* 110:481–487.
47. Bagby, G. J. 1983. *Biochim. Bipophys. Acta* 753:47–52.
48. Ho, R. J., E. Atkin, and H. C. Meng. 1966. *Am. J. Physiol.* 210:299–304.
49. Pedersen, M. E., L. E. Wolf, and M. C. Schotz. 1981. *Biochim. Biophys. Acta* 666:191–197.
50. Robinson, D. S. 1963. *Adv. Lipid Res.* 1:133–182.
51. Pederson, M. E., M. Cohen, and M. C. Schotz. 1983. *J. Lipid Res.* 24:512–521.
52. Crass, M. F., and H. C. Meng. 1964. *Am. J. Physiol.* 206:610–614.
53. Borensztajn, J., and D. S. Robinson. 1970. *J. Lipid Res.* 11:111–117.
54. Chajek, T., O. Stein, and Y. Stein. 1975. *Biochim. Biophys. Acta* 388:260–267.
55. Borensztajn, J., M. S. Rone, and T. Sandros. 1975. *Biochim. Biophys. Acta* 398:394–400.
56. Hulsmann, W. C., H. Stam, and W. A. P. Breeman. 1982. *Biochem. Biophys. Res. Comm.* 108:371–378.
57. Rajaram, O. V., M. G. Clark, and P. J. Barter. 1980. *Biochem. J.* 186:431–438.
58. Fielding, C. J., and J. M. Higgins. 1974. *Biochemistry* 13:4324–4330.

59. Schotz, M. C., J. S. Twu, M. E. Pedersen, C. H. Chen, A. S. Garfinkel, and J. Borensztajn. 1977. *Biochim. Biophys. Acta* 489:214–224.
60. Rogers, M. P., and D. S. Robinson. 1974. *J. Lipid Res.* 15:263–272.
61. Borensztajn, J., M. S. Rone, and T. J. Kotlar. 1976. *Biochem. J.* 156:539–543.
62. Knobler, H., T. Chajek-Shaul, O. Stein, and Y. Stein. 1984. *Biochim. Biophys. Acta* 795:363–371.
63. O'Looney, P., M. V. Maten, and G. V. Vahouny. 1983. *J. Biol. Chem.* 258:12994–13001.
64. Stam, H., and W. C. Hulsmann. 1984. *Biochim. Biophys. Acta* 794:72–82.
65. Bagby, G. J., and J. A. Spitzer. 1981. *Proc. Soc. Expt. Biol. Med.* 168:395–398.
66. Oscai, L. B. 1979. *Biochem. Biophys. Res. Comm.* 91:227–232.
67. Palmer, W. K., R. A. Caruso, and L. B. Oscai. 1981. *Biochem. J.* 198:159–166.
68. Miller, W. C., and L. B. Oscai. 1984. *Am. J. Physiol.* 247:621–625.
69. Palmer, W. K., and T. A. Kane. 1983. *Biochem. J.* 212:379–383.
70. Miller, W. C., W. K. Palmer, and L. B. Oscai. 1984. *Biochem. J.* 224:793–798.
71. Wetzel, M. G., and R. O. Scow. 1984. *Am. J. Physiol.* 246:467–485.
72. Goldberg, D. I., and J. C. Khoo. 1985. *J. Biol. Chem.* 260:5879–5882.
73. Howard, B. V. 1977. *J. Lipid Res.* 18:561–571.
74. Cryer, A. 1981. *Int. J. Biochem.* 13:525–541.
75. Tamboli, A., P. O'Looney, M. V. Maten, and G. V. Vahouni. 1983. *Biochim. Biophys. Acta* 750:404–410.
76. Nakatani, M., M. Nakamura, and S. Torii. 1961. *Proc. Soc. Exp. Biol. Med.* 107:853–856.
77. Enser, M. B., F. Kunz, J. Borensztajn, L. H. Opie, and D. S. Robinson. 1967. *Biochem. J.* 104: 306–316.
78. Felts, J. M., H. Itakura, and R. T. Crane. 1975. *Biochem. Biophys. Res. Comm.* 66:1467–1475.
79. Friedman, G., O. Stein, and Y. Stein. 1979. *FEBS Lett.* 100:371–373.
80. Zemplenyi, T., and D. Grafnetter. 1959. *Arch. Intern. Pharmacodyn.* 122:57–66.
81. Kotlar, T. J., and J. Borensztajn. 1977. *Am. J. Physiol.* 233:316–319.
82. Borensztajn, J., P. Keig, and A. H. Rubenstein. 1973. *Biochem. Biophys. Res. Comm.* 53:603–608.
83. Delorme, C. L. W., and K. L. Harris. 1975. *J. Nutr.* 105:447–451.
84. Cryer, A., S. E. Riley, E. R. Williams, and D. S. Robinson. 1976. *Clin. Sci. Mol. Med.* 50:213–221.
85. Lithell, H., J. Boberg, K. Hellsing, G. Lundqvist, and B. Vessby. 1978. *Atherosclerosis.* 30:89–94.
86. Borensztajn, J., S. Otway, and D. S. Robinson. 1970. *J. Lipid Res.* 11:102–110.
87. Schotz, M. C., and A. S. Garfinkel. 1972. *Biochim. Biophys. Acta* 270:472–478.
88. Rault, C., J. C. Fruchart, P. Dewailly, J. Jaillard, and G. Seizille. 1974. *Biochem. Biophys. Res. Comm.* 59:160–166.
89. De Gasquet, P., S. Griglio, E. Pequinot-Planche, and M. I. Malewiak. 1977. *J. Nutr.* 107:199–212.
90. Goldberg, D. I., W. L. Rumsey, and Z. V. Kendrick. 1984. *Metabolism* 33:964–969.
91. Goubern, A., and R. Portet. 1981. *Horm. Metab. Res.* 13:73–77.
92. Lithell, H., I. Jacobs, B. Vessby, K. Hellsing, and J. Karlsson. 1982. *Metabolism* 31:994–998.
93. Jacobs, I., H. Lithell, and J. Karlsson. 1982. *Acta Physiol. Scand.* 115:85–90.
94. Alousi, A. A., and S. Mallov. 1964. *Am. J. Physiol.* 206:603–609.
95. Vrana, A., P. Fabry, and L. Kazdova. 1974. *Nutr. Metabol.* 17:282–288.
96. Taskinen, M. R., I. Tulikoura, E. A. Nikkilä, and C. Ehnholm. 1981. *Europ. J. Clin. Invest.* 11:317–323.
97. Taskinen, M. R., and E. A. Nikkilä. 1981. *Metabolism* 30:810–817.
98. Kronquist, K. E., M. E. Pedersen, and M. C. Schotz. 1980. *Life Sci.* 27:1153–1158.

99. Jansen, H., W. C. Hulsmann, A. van Zuylen-van Wiggen, C. B. Struijk, and U. M. T. Houtsmuller. 1975. *Biochem. Biophys. Res. Comm.* 64:747–751.
100. Radomski, M. W., and T. Orme. 1971. *Am. J. Physiol.* 220:1852–1856.
101. Begin-Heick, N., and H. M. C. Heick. 1977. *Can. J. Biochem.* 55:1241–1243.
102. Keig, P., and J. Borensztajn. 1974. *Proc. Soc. Exp. Biol. Med.* 146:890–893.
103. Grafnetter, D. J., J. Grafnetterova, E. Grossi, and P. Morganti. 1965. *Med. Pharmacol. Exp.* 12:266–273.
104. Himms-Hagen, J. 1972. *Lipids* 7:310–323.
105. De Gasquet, P., and E. Pequinot. 1973. *Horm. Metab. Res.* 5:440–443.
106. Lanza-Jacoby, S., S. C. Lansey, E. E. Miller, and M. P. Cleary. 1984. *Cancer Res.* 44:5062–5067.
107. Borensztajn, J., D. R. Samols, and A. H. Rubenstein. 1972. *Am. J. Physiol.* 223:1271–1275.
108. Elkeles, R. S., and E. Williams. 1974. *Clin. Sci. Mol. Med.* 46:661–664.
109. Rauramaa, R. 1982. *Med. Biol.* 60:139–143.
110. Kessler, J. I. 1963. *J. Clin. Invest.* 42:362–367.
111. Robin, A. P., M. R. C. Greenwood, J. Askanazi, D. H. Elwyn and J. M. Kinney. 1981. *Ann. Surg.* 194:681–686.
112. Taskinen, M. R., E. A. Nikkilä, S. Rehunen, and A. Gordin. 1980. *Artery* 6:471–483.
113. Lithell, H., J. Boberg, K. Hellsing, and G. Lundqvist. 1978. *Eur. J. Clin. Invest.* 8:67–74.
114. Taskinen, M. R., and E. A. Nikkilä. 1979. *Diabetologia* 17:351–356.
115. Taskinen, M. R., E. A. Nikkilä, R. Nousiainen, and A. Gordin. 1981. *Scand. J. Clin. Lab. Invest.* 41:263–268.
116. De Gasquet, P., E. Pequinot-Planche, N. T. Tonnu, and F. A. Diaby. 1974. *Horm. Metab. Res.* 7:152–157.
117. Simpson, J. 1979. *Biochem. J.* 182:253–255.
118. Gorski, J., and B. Stankiewicz-Choroszucha. 1982. *Horm. Metab. Res.* 14:189–191.
119. Hansson, P., G. Nordin, and P. Nilsson-Ehle. 1983. *Biochim. Biophys. Acta* 753:364–371.
120. Mallov, S., and A. A. Alousi. 1967. *Am. J. Physiol.* 212:1158–1164.
121. Kaciuba-Uscilko, H., G. A. Dudley, and R. L. Terjung. 1980. *Am. J. Physiol.* 238:518–523.
122. Lithell, H., J. Boberg, K. Hellsing, S. Ljunghall, G. Lundqvist, B. Vessby, and L. Wide. 1981. *Eur. J. Clin. Invest.* 11:3–10.
123. Wilson, D. E., W. Jubiz, C. M. Flowers, S. I. Carlile, and A. M. Adolf. 1977. *Atherosclerosis* 26:353–362.
124. Silverman, L. H., M. Beznak, and K. J. Kako. 1972. *Arch. Int. Pharmacodyn.* 199:368–375.

Chapter 6

ROLE OF LIPOPROTEIN LIPASE DURING LACTATION

Robert O. Scow and Sidney S. Chernick

Fat is an important constituent of milk from many species (1,2). Its content is 4% in human and bovine milk, 11% in rodent milk, and 53% in seal's milk, but zero in rhinoceros's milk. Fat provides half of the calories in human and bovine milk, three-fourths in rodent milk, and nearly all in seal's milk (1–3).

Fat is present in milk as oil droplets, 1–7 μm in diameter, enclosed by a monolayer of amphipathic lipids and possibly protein, and a bilayered structure, located outside the monolayer, derived from plasma membrane of mammary epithelial cells (4,5). Milk fat consists of triglycerides composed mostly of long chain (C_{14}-C_{18}) fatty acids (1,2,6). Triglyceride of milk may also contain, depending on both species and dietary fatty acid composition (1,7,8), medium chain (C_8-C_{12}) and, sometimes, short chain (C_4-C_6) fatty acids (1–3). Long chain fatty acids in milk fat are either unsaturated or saturated, whereas the medium and short chain fatty acids are only saturated. The membranous structures surrounding the fat droplet consist of proteins, phospholipids, cholesterol, and other lipids (9,10). Cholesteryl esters are present in milk, but they account for less than 14% of the cholesteryl moiety in milk (3,11).

Long chain fatty acids in milk are derived primarily from diet (7,8,12–14) and fatty acid synthesis in mammary gland and liver (7,15), and to a lesser extent from fat stores in adipose tissue (7). Fatty acids are transported from intestines and liver in the blood stream as triglyceride in chylomicrons and VLDL, respectively (16,17). Most of the fatty acids mobilized from fat stores for milk production are probably first taken up and incorporated by liver into VLDL-triglyceride and then transported as such to mammary gland (12).

Uptake of fatty acids from triglyceride of chylomicrons and VLDL requires the action of lipoprotein lipase (LPL) at the luminal surface of capillaries (16–19). LPL activity is greatly increased in mammary gland (20–23) and markedly decreased in adipose tissue during late-pregnancy and lactation (22,23), resulting in the diversion of plasma triglyceride from storage in adipose tissue to milk production in mammary gland (24). This chapter describes the effects and regulation of LPL activity in these tissues during pregnancy and lactation, the action of LPL in capillaries, and the mode of transport of fatty acids, monoglyceride, cholesterol, and other substances from chylomicrons and VLDL in blood to mammary secretory cells.

Lethal hypertriglyceridemia with levels as high as 20,000 mg/dl, develops within 3 days in newborn mice with combined lipase deficiency (*cld/cld*) if allowed to suckle (25). This condition, which involves both LPL and hepatic lipase (25–27), is caused by a recessive mutation (*cld*) within the T/t complex of chromosome 17 of the mouse (25). This chapter reviews recent studies concerning the nature and consequence of lack of LPL activity in combined lipase deficient (*cld/cld*) mice.

Relationship Between Hyperlipemia of Pregnancy and Lipoprotein Lipase Activity

Hypertriglyceridemia develops in several species during pregnancy and disappears at or near parturition (21, 28–32). We found that hypertriglyceridemia developed in pregnant rats fed a diet containing 4.5% fat, but not in rats fed a fat-free diet, demonstrating the dietary origin of hyperlipemia in pregnant rats (31). Studies by others (32) showed that as little as 0.3% fat in the diet was sufficient for development of hypertriglyceridemia in pregnant rats. Hypertriglyceridemia in fed pregnant rats is very different from that in fasted pregnant rats (31). The latter results from glucose lack and increased fat mobilization, and is characterized by severe ketosis (31,33).

The relationship between hyperlipemia of pregnancy and LPL activity has been studied in the rat (22,32). Earlier studies showed that LPL activities in heart, diaphragm muscle and lung of rat were unaffected by pregnancy, and that LPL activity in adipose tissue began to decrease several days before parturition (22,32). Development of hyperlipemia occurred before the fall in LPL activity of adipose tissue and may be attributed to greater food intake (22,32). The rise in LPL activity in mammary gland observed in pregnant guinea pigs (20,21) and rats (22) 1–2 days before parturition occurred at the same time hyperlipemia disappeared in rats (22,30,31). Increased uptake of plasma triglyceride by mammary gland accounted for the decrease in plasma triglyceride concentration (22).

Liproprotein Lipase Activity During Lactation

Lipoprotein Lipase Activity in Mammary Gland

LPL activity in mammary gland is greatly increased during lactation in guinea pig (20,21), rat (22,32), goat (34), and cow (35,36). The high level of LPL activity in breast milk (37) suggests that human mammary gland also has high lipase activity during lactation. LPL activity in mammary gland of rats increased very slowly during the first 20 days of pregnancy, from 0.9 to 7 U/g (Fig. 1). It increased two fold the next day to 21 U/g, decreased sharply during parturition (on the 22nd–23rd day) to 6 U/g, and then increased within 2 days after parturition to more than 40 U/g (Fig. 1). The drop in activity at parturition was due to transient engorgement of the glands with milk (see below). LPL activity in mammary gland of pregnant guinea pigs also began to increase 2 days before parturition and reached a maximum several days after parturition (20). LPL activity remained high in lactating mammary gland of both rats and guinea pigs as long as the dams suckled (20,22,23). When the sucklings were taken from the dams, LPL activity in mammary gland decreased within 18 hours to the very low level in nulliparous animals (Fig. 2).

Lipoprotein Lipase Activity in Adipose Tissue

LPL activity in adipose tissue is markedly decreased during lactation in rat (22,23,32), goat (38) and cow (36). The activity in adipose tissue of rats increased two fold during the second week of pregnancy, remained at that high level for 8 days, and then decreased, during the 19th day to a level 20% of that in nulliparous animals (Fig. 1). LPL activity in adipose tissue remained at this low level as long as the dams suckled (22,23). When the sucklings were taken from the dams, LPL activity in adipose tissue returned within 48 hours to the high level in nulliparous animals (Fig. 2)(22,23).

Effect of Lipoprotein Lipase Activity on Plasma Triglyceride Concentration

We studied in detail the relationship during pregnancy and lactation of the concentration of triglyceride in plasma to LPL activity in adipose tissue and mammary gland (22). We found that plasma triglyceride concentration in pregnant rats increased two fold during the third week of gestation and

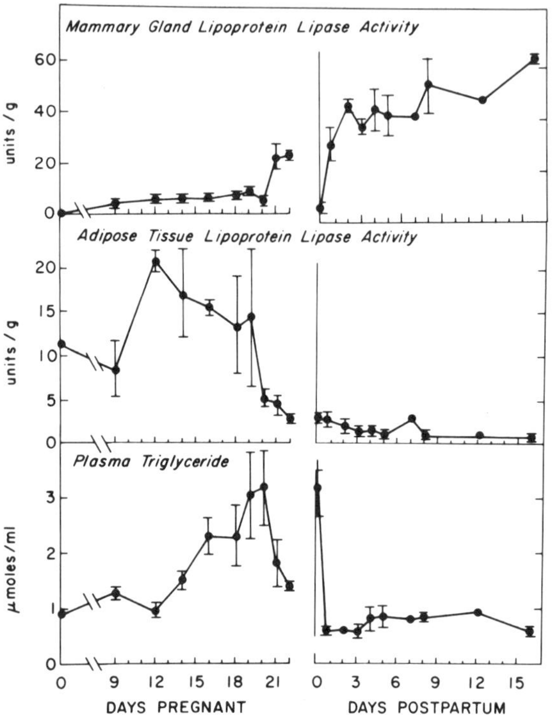

FIGURE 1 Lipoprotein lipase activity in inguinal-abdominal mammary glands and parametrial adipose tissue and plasma triglyceride concentration in pregnant and lactating rats. Parturition occurred on the 22nd day of gestation in half of the animals and on the 23rd day in the other half. The vertical line through each point represents ± 1 SE. One unit of activity = 1 μmol of glycerol released per h. [From Hamosh et al. (22), with permission.]

reached a maximum of 3.3 mM on the 20th day of gestation (Fig. 1). This increase occurred with very little change in the concentration of phospholipids or total cholesterol in blood (31), as also observed in humans (28). Plasma triglyceride concentration decreased 50% on the 21st day, increased to 3.0 mM at parturition, and decreased again, to below 1.0 mM, on the day after parturition. It remained at that low level as long as the dams suckled. The brief hyperlipemia at parturition occurred simultaneously with a transient loss of LPL activity in mammary gland. Between the 20th day of gestation and the 16th day of lactation, the latest time studied, the mean values for plasma triglyceride concentration ranged from 0.6 to 3.3 mM and the values for LPL activity in mammary gland ranged from 6 to 61 U/g, while the values for adipose tissue LPL activity remained low, below 5.3 U/g (Fig. 1). The changes in mammary tissue LPL activity were always accompanied by opposite changes in plasma triglyceride concentration

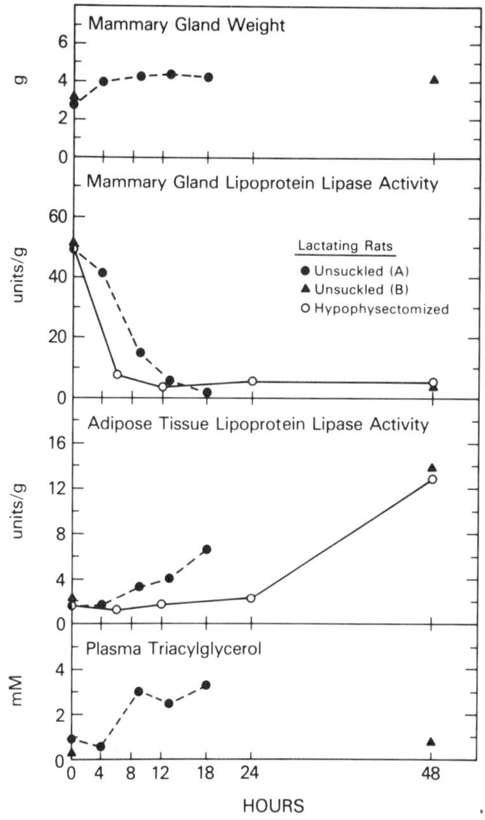

FIGURE 2 Effect of hypophysectomy and nonsuckling on lipoprotein lipase activity in mammary gland and adipose tissue in lactating rats. Hypophysectomized rats were injected with oxytocin every 6 h and allowed to suckle. One unit of activity = 1 μmol of glycerol released per h. Data on hypophysectomized rats are from Zinder et al. (43), that on unsuckled rats group A are from Hamosh et al. (22), and that on unsuckled rats group B are from Scow et al. (24).

(Fig. 3). The findings suggest that hpertriglyceridemia would develop in late-pregnant or lactating rats whenever LPL activity in mammary gland was less than 15 U/g. This was confirmed in lactating rats unsuckled for 9–18 hours (Fig. 2).

Regulation of Lipoprotein Lipase Activity

Role of Suckling. Suckling is essential for the continuation of high LPL activity in mammary gland of lactating animals (20,22,23). Nonsuckling for 4 hours in rats caused engorgement of mammary gland, and a small decrease in LPL activity of mammary gland, but had no effect on LPL activity in adipose tissue or plasma triglyceride (Fig. 2). Nonsuckling for 9 hours caused a 70% reduction in LPL activity in mammary gland, a doubling of LPL

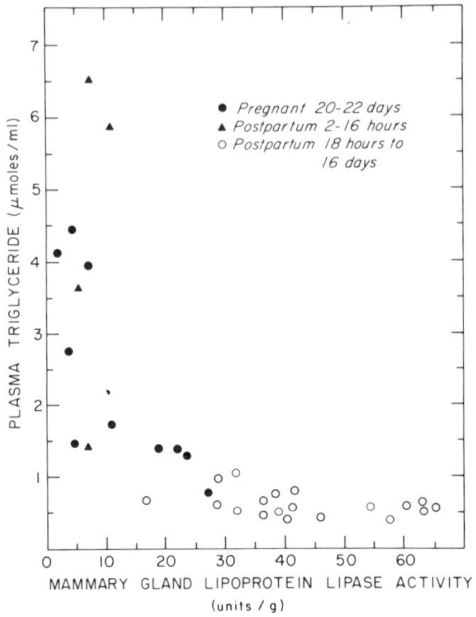

FIGURE 3 Relationship in individual rats between lipoprotein lipase activity in mammary gland and plasma triglyceride concentration in late pregnant and lactating rats. Lipoprotein lipase activity in the parametrial adipose tissue of these rats was less than 5 units/g. One unit of activity = 1 μmol of glycerol released per h. [From Hamosh et al. (22), with permission].

activity in adipose tissue, and development of hyperlipemia. Nonsuckling for 18 hours reduced LPL activity in mammary gland by 95% in both rats (22,23) and guinea pigs (20), increased LPL activity in adipose tissue in rats to a level about 50% of that in nulliparous animals, and maintained the hyperlipemia that developed earlier. Nonsuckling for 44 hours in rats reduced LPL activity in mammary gland to the very low level in nulliparous animals, increased LPL activity in adipose tissue by six fold, and decreased plasma triglyceride concentration to 0.9 mM (24).

Nonsuckling caused engorgement and loss of LPL activity in mammary gland, return of LPL activity in adipose tissue, and development of hypertriglyceridemia (Fig. 2). These effects on LPL and plasma triglyceride are mediated, as described below, through the anterior pituitary gland. In order to determine the local effect of engorgement on LPL activity in mammary gland of lactating rats, the lactiferous ducts draining the inguinal-abdominal glands on one side were ligated while those on the opposite side and the pectoral glands on both sides were left intact, and the dams were allowed to suckle. LPL activity in the duct-ligated glands was reduced 90% in 18 hours and the weight of the glands was doubled, while lipase activity and weight in the intact glands were unaffected. Duct-ligation of one-fourth of the glands also had no effect on LPL activity in adipose tissue or on plasma triglyceride concentration. Others (39,40) observed that many hormone-dependent enzymes involved in carbohydrate metabolism and in synthesis of lipid and lactose in lactating mammary gland were also depressed in duct-ligated glands as well as in unsuckled glands. The localized suppression of enzyme activities in duct-ligated glands with normal levels of activities in the other glands indicates that the effects of duct-ligation are independent of hormone concentrations in plasma. The effects of duct-ligation probably result from mechanical compression of capillaries (22), impairing delivery of nutrients and hormones to mammary cells.

Hormonal Control During Lactation. The abrupt changes in LPL activity in mammary gland and adipose tissue that occur at the onset and the termination of lactation (Figs. 1 and 2) suggested that one or more of the anterior pituitary hormones responsible for milk secretion (prolactin, growth hormone or ACTH) (41,42) might regulate LPL activity during lactation. The effects of these and other hormones on LPL activity in lactating rats were studied in rats that were hypophysectomized on the 5th–6th day of lactation and allowed to suckle (43). Since the posterior pituitary gland was also removed, all operated rats were given oxytocin to ensure milk ejection and prevent engorgement of the mammary glands (44). Hypophysectomy caused in lactating rats severe but transient diabetes insipidus and loss of body weight during the first 24 hours after surgery (43). Some of the rats continued to lose weight, whereas others gained body weight during the second 24 hours after surgery. Since failure to gain weight affected the response of adipose tissue to hypophysectomy (see below), only rats that gained body weight during the second 24 hours are presented at 48 hours in Fig. 2 and used as controls for rats given hormone replacement (Table I and II). All hormones were injected every 6 hours for 2 days, starting 2 hours after surgery unless indicated otherwise.

Hypophysectomy in lactating rats lowered LPL activity in mammary gland from 50 U/g to 8 U/g in 6 hours, and increased LPL activity in adipose tissue from 2 U/g to 13 U/g in 48 hours, restoring these activities to the same levels as those in nulliparous animals. Prolactin injection begun 2 hours after hypophysectomy increased LPL activity in mammary gland to 18 U/g at 24 hours and to 50 U/g at 48 hours (Table I). It also blocked return of LPL activity in adipose tissue. Prolactin treatment begun 24 hours after hypophysectomy increased LPL activity of mammary gland from 6 U/g to 12 U/g in 24 hours and blocked completely the return of LPL activity in adipose tissue.

The effects of prolactin on LPL activity in mammary gland and adipose tissue were not altered by simultaneous administration of growth hormone and thyroxine (Table II). Dexamethesone, however, administered with or without growth hormone and thyroxine, increased the effect of prolactin on LPL activity in mammary gland and milk secretion. Dexamethasone injected alone also increased LPL activity in mammary gland, but only to 50% of that in prolactin-treated animals, and it had no effect on milk se-

TABLE I Effect of prolactin on lipoprotein lipase activity in mammary gland and adipose tissue in hypophysectomized lactating rats[a].

Treament	Onset of treatment	Time after hypophysectomy	Lipoprotein Lipase Activity[b]	
			Mammary gland	Adipose tissue
	h	h	units/g	units/g
None	—	0	50 ± 4 (7)	2.4 ± 0.6
None	—	48	5 ± 2 (4)	13.0 ± 2
Prolactin	2	12	6 (1)	2.6
Prolactin	2	24	18 ± 6 (7)	0.6 ± 0.2
Prolactin	2	48	50 ± 4 (4)	4.4 ± 1.5[c]
Prolactin	24	48	12 ± 2 (7)	1.2 ± 0.6

Hypophysectomy was performed on 5th–6th day of lactation and prolactin injections, 0.5 mg every 6 h, were begun 2 or 24 h later. All rats were injected with oxytocin every 6 h and allowed to suckle. [From Zinder et al. (43).]

[a]Data for untreated hypophysectomized lactating rats are presented in Fig. 2.

[b]One unit of activity = 1 μmol of glycerol released per h. Values are means ± SE with number of animals per groups indicated by figure in parentheses.

[c]This value is not significantly different from that in lactating rats prior to hypophysectomy ($P > 0.1$).

TABLE II Effect of various hormones on milk secretion, lipoprotein lipase activity in mammary gland and adipose tissue, and body weight gain in hypophysectomized lactating rats[a].

Treatment	No. of rats	Milk secretion index[b]	Lipoprotein Lipase Activity		Body weight gain during 2nd d
			Mammary gland	Adipose tissue	
			units/g	units/g	g
None	4	0	6 ± 1	13 ± 1	10 ± 3
GH + T + D	7	12 ± 6	15 ± 4	4 ± 1	9 ± 2
D	2	0	27 ± 2	3 ± 1	-5 ± 2
P	4	50 ± 12	50 ± 5	4 ± 2	7 ± 5
P + GH +T	5	75 ± 12	40 ± 12	2 ± 0.5	5 ± 5
P + D	2	75 ± 12	96 ± 22	1 ± 0.4	5 ± 2
P + GH + T + D	10	87 ± 2	70 ± 9	1 ± 0.2	15 ± 2

Rats were hypophysectomized on the 5th–6th d of lactation and given hormone injections, starting 2 h after surgery, every 6 h for 2 d. Tissues were taken for lipoprotein lipase analyses 46 h after hypophysectomy. All rats were given oxytocin 1 U/d. The other hormones and amounts injected were: GH, growth hormone 80 μg/d; T, thyroxine 4 μg/d; D, dexamethasone 4 μg/d; and P, prolactin 2 mg/d. One unit of activity = 1 μmol of glycerol released per h. The values given are means ± SE.

[a]Data for untreated hypophysectomized lactating rats are presented in Fig. 2.

[b]Milk secretion index: percent of pups in each litter that had milk in the stomach at the end of the experiment. [From Zinder et al. (43).]

cretion. Because of the body weight loss during the second 24 hours after surgery, the effect of dexamethsone on LPL activity in adipose tissue could be secondary to a suppressing effect on food intake and body weight gain. Administration of dexamethasone with growth hormone and thyroxine, however, maintained LPL activity in adipose tissue at a low level in animals that gained weight during the second 24 hours, suggesting that dexamethasone may have a direct effect on LPL activity in adipose tissue. Administration of the four hormones together produced the largest increases in LPL activity in mammary gland, milk secretion and body weight gain. Milk secretion occurred only in rats given prolactin, with or without other hormones, and it was always associated with high LPL activity in mammary gland and low activity in adipose tissue (Table II).

Bromocriptine (2-Br-α-ergocryptine), which inhibits release of prolactin from the pituitary gland (45), decreased LPL activity in mammary gland and increased LPL activity in adipose tissue in suckled lactating rats within 2 days (23). Prolactin injections prevented these effects of bromocriptin, demonstrating again the important role of prolactin in the regulation of LPL activity during lactation. Prolactin injections did not block in lactating rats the effect of nonsuckling on LPL activity in either mammary gland or adipose tissue (23). The lack of effect of prolactin in unsuckled lactating rats can be explained by engorgement of mammary gland, with impaired delivery of hormones and nutrients to mammary cells, as observed above in duct-ligated glands (22). Since engorgement would not be expected in adipose tissue, the findings suggest that the suppressing effect of prolactin on LPL activity in adipose tissue may be mediated through, or possible requires, a substance released by functional lactating mammary gland.

Hormonal Control During Late Pregnancy. The above studies demonstrated that prolactin plays a major role in the maintenance of high LPL activity in mammary gland and low activity in adipose tissue during lactation. Furthermore, fluctuations in LPL activities during periods of suckling and nonsuckling can be related to concurrent changes in prolactin concentration in the blood stream (46). Since serum prolactin concentration in pregnant rats increases markedly 2–3 days before parturition (46–48), it seemed possible that changes in LPL activities at that time could be due to prolactin. However, bovine pituitary prolactin injected for 2 days into late pregnant rats, starting on the 18th day of gestation, had no effect on LPL activity in either mammary gland or adipose tissue (49). Since release of prostaglandin F from the uterus to the blood stream in pregnant rats is markedly increased 2–3 days before parturition (50), and lactation occurs when early parturition is induced by prostaglandin $F_{2\alpha}$ in rats (51,52) and humans (53), we studied the effect of this substance on LPL activity during late pregnancy in rats (49).

Prostaglandin $F_{2\alpha}$ injected for 2 days in late pregnant rats, starting on the 18th day of gestation, increased LPL activity in mammary gland, decreased the activity in adipose tissue, and reduced plasma triglyceride concentration to levels characteristic of lactating rats, and induced early lactation (Table III). It also increased the concentration of pituitary prolactin and decreased the concentration of progesterone in serum, suggesting that one or both might be responsible for the changes in mammary gland and adipose tissue. Blocking the rise in serum pituitary prolactin concentration in prostaglandin $F_{2\alpha}$-treated rats with bromocriptine did not alter the effects of prostaglandin $F_{2\alpha}$ on mammary gland, adipose tissue, or serum triglyceride, indicating that the effects of prostaglandin were not mediated through the pituitary gland (Table III). Although these findings might suggest that prolactin was not involved, they do not rule out placental prolactin (chorionic mammotrophin) (55,56). The placenta in pregnant rats secretes large amounts of prolactin during the last half of pregnancy (57), resulting in serum concentrations of placental prolactin 10-40 times that of pituitary prolactin (54,58). Unfortunately, the radioimmunoassay used for measuring rat pituitary prolactin did not measure rat placental prolactin (53,58). Earlier studies showed that mammary gland development was normal in pregnant rats hypophysectomized on or after the 11th day of pregnancy (59). Since bromocriptine did not inhibit prolactin secretion by placental (decidual) tissue *in vitro* (60), it seems likely that placental prolactin may be involved in the action of prostaglandin $F_{2\alpha}$ on LPL activity in pregnant rats.

Administration of progesterone completely blocked the effects of prostaglandin $F_{2\alpha}$ on LPL activity in late pregnant rats (Table III), suggesting that the effects of prostaglandin $F_{2\alpha}$ may be related to its inhibitory action on progesterone secretion (50). Progesterone injected into normal pregnant rats for 3 days, starting on the 20th day of gestation, prolonged pregnancy several days and prevented the expected increases in LPL activity in mammary gland and serum prolactin, but did not prevent the decrease in LPL activity in adipose tissue (61). Since LPL activity in adipose tissue is also affected by factors unrelated to lactation (62), it is difficult to evaluate the findings in adipose tissue of progesterone-treated pregnant rats.

It seems evident that placental prolactin is involved in the development of LPL activity in mammary gland in pregnant rats, but its effect is not manifested until progesterone secretion is reduced several days before parturition (47,48). Endogenous prostaglandin $F_{2\alpha}$ is probably not involved because the rise in prostaglandin F secretion occurs several days after the fall in progesterone production (48). It is possible that reduced progesterone secretion results from decreased secretion of placental (decidual) luteotropin during late pregnancy (48,56,63–65). The role of the anterior pituitary gland in the regulation of LPL begins as soon as the newborns commence to suckle, stimulating secretion of prolactin by the pituitary and preventing engorgement of mammary gland (44,46,66).

Source of Lipoprotein Lipase in Mammary Gland. The half-life of LPL activity in mammary gland of lactating rats was about 3.5 hours after re-

TABLE III Effects of Prostaglandin $F_{2\alpha}$, 2-Br-α-ergocryptine and Progesterone in Near-term Pregnant Rats

Treatment	No. of rats	Lipoprotein lipase activity: Mammary gland	Lipoprotein lipase activity: Adipose tissue	Serum triglyceride concentration	Milk formation index[a]	Serum concentration of: Pituitary prolactin[b]	Serum concentration of: Progesterone
		U/g	U/g	mM		ng/ml	ng/ml
Untreated	5	0.8 ± 0.2	1.6 ± 0.5	2.6 ± 0.4	0	72 ± 16	69 ± 7
$PGF_{2\alpha}$	6	2.0 ± 0.4[c]	0.6 ± 0.08[c]	1.1 ± 0.2[c]	100[c]	248 ± 43[c]	4 ± 1[c]
$PGF_{2\alpha}$ + 2-Br-α-ergocryptine	6	1.4 ± 0.3[c]	0.3 ± 0.03[c]	1.5 ± 0.3[c]	100[c]	39 ± 7[c]	9 ± 2[c]
$PGF_{2\alpha}$ + Progesterone	6	0.6 ± 0.09	1.0 ± 0.2	2.6 ± 0.3	0	59 ± 12	209 ± 24[c]

Treated rats were given i.m. 250 μg of $PGF_{2\alpha}$ tromethamine salt with or without 0.5 mg of 2-Br-α-ergocryptine or 5 mg of progesterone twice daily on the 18th and 19th d of pregnancy, and tissues and blood were taken on the 20th d for analyses. One unit of activity = 1 μmol of fatty acids released per min. [From Spooner et al. (49).]

[a]Milk formation index indicates percent of animals in which mammary gland contained milk at autopsy.

[b]Measured by double-antibody radioimmunoassay with methods and materials provided by the NIAMDD Rat Pituitary Program. This assay does not measure rat placental prolactin (chorionic mammotropin) (58).

[c]Significantly different from value for untreated group by Student's t test for unpaired data ($P < 0.001$).

moval of the anterior pituitary gland (Fig. 2). Prolactin injected subcutaneously, starting 2 hours after hypophysectomy, had a latent period of 10 hours, and then increased LPL activity in mammary gland in the next 36 hours to the same level as that in normal lactating rats (Table I). Prolactin injected into the mammary ducts of pseudopregnant rabbits also increased LPL activity in mammary gland (67). Although a small increase occurred at 24 hours, the major response began after 2 days. The half-life of LPL activity in rabbit mammary gland injected with prolactin was 2.2 hours after injection of actinomycin D and 1.1 hours after injection of cycloheximide (67). These findings indicate that LPL is rapidly inactivated in mammary gland, and that the prolactin-induced increase in lipase activity in the gland requires the continued production of a short-lived messenger-RNA (67).

LPL has been found in the milk of several species (20,21,37,68,69), suggesting that mammary alveolar cells may be the site of synthesis of LPL in mammary gland. Recent studies of synthesis of LPL in incubated mammary tissue from lactating guinea pigs suggest that LPL is secreted into milk as effectively as other milk proteins (70). A lipolytic activity that was partially dependent on serum and partially inhibited by protamine sulfate, presumably LPL activity, has been found on the surfaces of mammary cells and in plasma membrane-enriched and endoplasmic reticulum-enriched fractions isolated from lactating rat mammary gland (71,72), indicating that mammary epithelial cells are probably the source of LPL activity in rat mammary gland. LPL may be transported from mammary cells to the capillary lumen by lateral movement in an interfacial continuum of cell membranes (17).

LPL isolated from milk has a high affinity for heparin (23,69), and heparin infused intravascularly released LPL activity from capillaries of perfused lactating rat mammary gland (74). However, heparin did not release lipolytic activity from either isolated cells or subcellular fractions of lactating rat mammary gland (71,72). This unexpected finding requires verification with immunochemical techniques.

Effect of Prolactin on Lipoprotein Lipase Activity in Pigeon Crop Sac. Prolactin stimulates the production of crop milk in pigeons and doves (75–77). Crop milk, which is used to feed the young, consists of cells containing 10% fat that are sloughed from the epithelium of the crop sac (76,78,79). The responses of crop sac to prolactin, hyperplasia of epithelium lining the lateral lobes and gain in weight (Fig. 4), are widely used for assaying lactogenic hormones (77,78,80). Electron microscopic study of crop sac from pigeons treated with prolactin (1 mg/d) showed small lipid droplets in epithelial cells of the nutritive (stratum spinosus) layer at 12 hours, numerous large droplets in the proliferative (stratum basale) and nutritive layers at 2 days, and large lipid droplets in all layers, including the layer (stratum disjunctum) near the lumen, at 4 days (76).

The fatty acid composition of triglyceride in crop sac of prolactin-treated pigeons is similar to that in adipose tissue (79), suggesting that these tissues

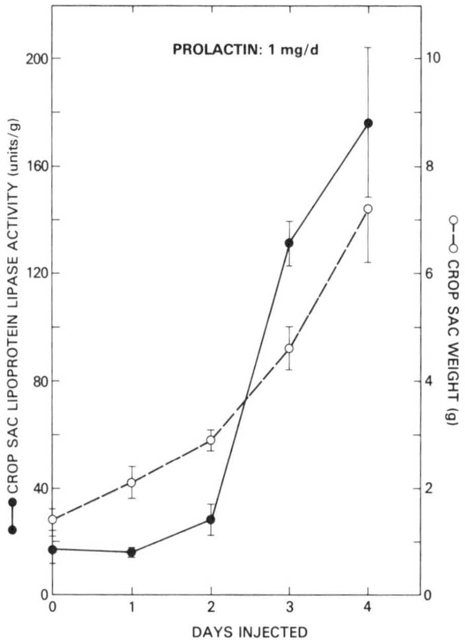

FIGURE 4 Effect of prolactin, 1 mg/d, on lipoprotein lipase activity and weight of crop sac in pigeons. Enzyme activity was measured 20 h after last injection of hormone. One unit of activity = 1 μmol of glycerol released per h. The vertical line through each point represents ± 1 S.E. [From Garrison and Scow (83), with permission].

have a common source of fatty acids. The diet of pigeons is low in fat and high in carbohydrates (81). Fatty acid synthesis in liver is the main source of fatty acids in pigeons (82). Prolactin injected in pigeons increases food intake (77), stimulates fatty acid synthesis in liver (82), increases triglyceride synthesis in crop sac epithelium (76,79), and augments storage of fat in adipose tissue (82). Fatty acids are transported from liver to other tissues as triglyceride in very low density lipoproteins (16). For these reasons, we studied the effect of prolactin on LPL activity in crop sac and adipose tissue in pigeons (83).

Prolactin injections increased LPL activity in crop sac of pigeons 10 fold in 4 days (Fig. 4). The activity increased slowly during the 2nd day, and then increased rapidly during the 3rd and 4th day of injections. Prolactin had no effect on LPL activity in esophagus (83). Prolactin increased the crop sac weight four fold in 4 days (Fig. 4).

Prolactin also increased LPL activity in omental adipose tissue, from 49 to 118 U/g, but not until the 4th day of injections (83). This effect in pigeons is opposite to its inhibitory action in adipose tissue in lactating rats (Table I). Stimulation of LPL activity in avian adipose tissue by prolactin may be an important action in the promotion of pre-migratory fattening in white-crowned sparrows (77,84). Other effects of prolactin in this process would be augmentation of food intake and acceleration of fatty acid synthesis in liver.

The presence of LPL activity in crop milk indicates that the enzyme is present, if not synthesized, in epithelial cells of the crop sac. The site of action of LPL in crop sac is probably at the luminal surface of capillaries near crop epithelium.

Action of Lipoprotein Lipase on Chylomicrons

Action of Lipoprotein Lipase in Capillaries

Perfused mammary tissue of lactating rats was used to study the action of LPL on chylomicrons in capillaries (74,85–88). Rat chylomicrons containing triglyceride labeled in both acyl and glyceryl moieties and [^{32}P]phosphatidylcholine or [^{14}]cholesterol were used in these studies. The chylomicrons were isolated from thoracic duct lymph collected from rats tube-fed corn oil containing appropriate radioactive lipids (89,90). Radioactive phosphatidylcholine was isolated from liver of rats injected 4 hours earlier with disodium hydrogen [^{32}P]phosphate (89). The mammary tissue was perfused *in situ* with a mixture of 1 volume of triply washed bovine red blood cells and 4 volumes of 0.6 mM albumin and 5.5 mM glucose in Tyrode's solution (85).

Uptake of Triglyceride. Perfused mammary gland of suckled lactating rats removed 11–19% of the triglyceride in chylomicrons on a single pass through the tissue (Table IV) (85,91). About 30–40% of the acyl and glyceryl moieties removed were recovered in venous perfusate as fatty acids and glycerol, respectively, and the rest was recovered as acylglycerol in the tissue. Uptake and hydrolysis of chylomicron triglyceride was reduced more than 85% in perfused mammary tissue from lactating rats unsuckled for 18 hours (85) or hypophysectomized for 48 hours (91) (Table IV). Since nonsuckling for 18 hours and hypophysectomy each reduced LPL activity in lactating mammary gland by more than 90% (Fig. 2), these findings demonstrate that uptake of chylomicron triglyceride by mammary gland requires the action of LPL in its capillaries. The presence of LPL in capillaries of lactating rat mammary gland was confirmed by the rapid release of LPL activity to the perfusate when the tissue was perfused with heparin (74).

The ratio of labeled acyl moiety to labeled glyceryl moiety in acylglycerol in mammary gland perfused with chylomicrons was about the same as that in chylomicrons (Table IV). Autoradiographic studies of lactating rat mammary gland perfused with chylomicrons containing acyl-labeled or glyceryl-labeled triglyceride showed that acyl and glyceryl moieties derived from chylomicron triglyceride were both incorporated into milk fat droplets (Fig. 5) (91).

TABLE IV Lipoprotein lipase activity and uptake of triglyceride, phosphatidylcholine and cholesterol from chylomicrons by perfused lactating rat mammary tissue

		Chylomicron						
		Triglyceride				Phosphatidylcholine		Cholesterol
		Oleoyl moiety recovered as		Glyceryl moiety recovered as		Phosphoryl moiety recovered as		
Group[a]	Lipoprotein lipase activity	Fatty acid in venous perfusate	Acylglycerol in tissue	Glycerol in venous perfusate	Acylglycerol in tissue	Lysophosphatidylcholine in venous perfusate	Phospholipid in tissue	Cholesteryl moiety recovered as lipid in tissue
	U/g	% of lipid infused						
Experiment A								
Suckled (2)	n.d.	8.0 ± 2.0	11.2 ± 3.0	6.3 ± 1.3	11.7 ± 3.0	5.4 ± 1.2	4.7 ± 0.7	n.d.
Unsuckled (3)	n.d.	0.8 ± 0.8	1.8 ± 0.2	1.4 ± 0.3	1.4 ± 0.3	1.6 (1)	2.4 ± 0.7	n.d.
Experiment B								
Suckled (4)	0.5	4.1 ± 0.7	8.8 ± 1.8	4.5 ± 1.1	6.6 ± 1.1	n.d.	n.d.	15.1 ± 3.9
Hypophysectomized (4)	0.1	0.1 ± 0.1	0.5 ± 0.2	0.3 ± 0.1	0.4 ± 0.2	n.d.	n.d.	0.8 ± 0.1

Experiment A: Left inguinal-abdominal mammary glands of rats lactating 10 d were perfused 15 min. with perfusing fluid, 30 min with perfusing fluid containing chylomicrons at a triglyceride concentration of 0.5 mM for tissues of suckled rats and 0.4 mM for tissues of unsuckled rats, and then 15 min with perfusing fluid alone. The chylomicrons contained double labeled triglycerides ([^{14}C]oleic acid and [^{3}H]glycerol) and [^{32}P]phosphatidylcholine. Unsuckled rats were separated from their litters for 18 h prior to experiment. (From R. O. Scow and T. R. Fleck, unpublished data.)

Experiment B: Left inguinal-abdominal mammary glands of rats lactating 10–15 d were perfused 15 min with perfusing fluid, 15 min with perfusing fluid containing chylomicrons at a triglyceride concentration of 0.7 mM for tissues of suckled rats and 0.5 mM for tissues of hypophysectomized rats, and then perfused with perfusing fluid alone for 15 min. The chylomicrons contained double labeled triglyceride ([^{3}H]oleic acid and [^{3}H]glycerol) and [^{14}C]cholesteryl moiety. Two-thirds of the [^{14}C]cholesteryl moiety in the chylomicrons was cholesterol and the other third was cholesteryl ester. Hypophysectomized lactating rats were operated on 2 d before experiment, given injections of oxytocin every 6 h, and allowed to suckle. One unit of activity = 1 μmol of glycerol released per h. [From Zinder et al. (91).]

[a]Figure in parenthese indicates number of animals per group.

[b]Lipoprotein lipase activity was measured in contralateral tissue at start of perfusion.

n.d. = not done.

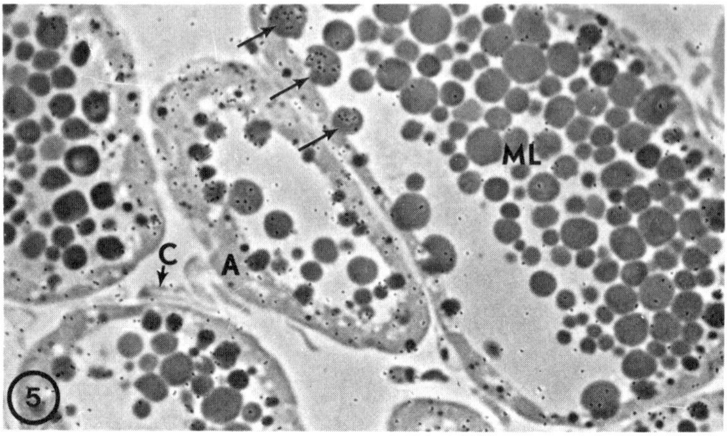

FIGURE 5 Light microscope autoradiograph demonstrating ^{3}H-glyceryl-labeled lipid in alveolar cells (A) and in milk lipid droplets (ML) in the lumen of alveoli of perfused lactating rat mammary gland. Note the high concentration of silver grains overlying lipid droplets adjacent to alveolar cells (arrows). The tissue was perfused 20 min with perfusing fluid and chylomicrons containing triacyl[2-^{3}H]glycerol and then 15 min with perfusing fluid only. 92% of the [^{3}H]glyceryl moiety retained by the tissue was found in triglyceride, 3% in diglyceride, 0.5% in monoglyceride and 2.6% in phospholipid. C, capillary. X 800. [From Zinder et al. (91), with permission.]

The appearance of labeled glycerol in venous perfusate (Table IV) indicates that some of the triglyceride was hydrolyzed completely to fatty acids and glycerol. Fatty acids, however, were released to the perfusate much earlier than glycerol, and the molar ratio of fatty acid to glycerol in the perfusate was several times larger than 3 during the first 4 minutes of infusion of chylomicrons (Fig. 6), indicating that fatty acid and di- or monoglyceride were formed in capillaries from chylomicrons, and fatty acid was released to the perfusing fluid. The continued release of glycerol to the venous perfusate and the decrease in molar ratio of fatty acid to glycerol in venous perfusate to less than 3 after infusion of chylomicrons was stopped (Fig. 6), indicate that glycerol was formed from acylglycerol outside of the capillary lumen. Thus, acylglycerol produced by action of LPL in capillaries was transferred into the tissue.

Purified bovine milk LPL readily hydrolyzes triglyceride of rat chylomicrons to fatty acids and glycerol *in vitro* if the medium contains enough albumin to bind all of the fatty acids produced (90). However, there is transient accumulation of monoglyceride in the chylomicrons, as much as 30 mol% of initial acylglycerol content, when the rate of hydrolysis is fast. In contrast, when chylomicrons are incubated with LPL in the presence of 9–20 fold excess albumin, albumin removes up to 65% of the monoglyceride produced, and thereby prevents monoglyceride from being hydrolyzed by LPL (90). These findings can be explained by positional specificity of LPL

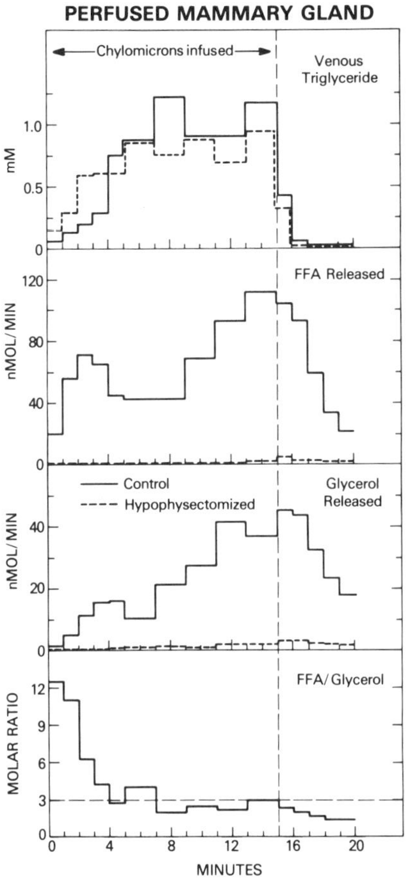

FIGURE 6 Release of fatty acids and glycerol from infused chylomicrons into the venous perfusate by perfused mammary gland of normal and hypophysectomized lactating rats. Operated rats were hypophysectomized 2 d before experiment, given oxytocin every 6 h and allowed to suckle their young. Chylomicrons used in these experiments contained doubly labeled ([^{14}C]oleoyl and [^{3}H]glyceryl moieties) triglyceride. See Table IV for other details of the perfusion technique. [From Scow (87), with permission.]

for the primary ester bonds of triglyceride. The enzyme hydrolyzes triglyceride directly to fatty acids and 2-monoacylglycerol, and hydrolyzes the monoglyceride only after it is isomerized to the 1(3) isomer (92,93). The transient accumulation of monoglyceride in chylomicrons undergoing lipolysis *in vitro* reflects the slowness of isomerization compared to hydrolysis. In view of the rapid hydrolysis of chylomicron triglyceride to 2-monoacylglycerol and fatty acids by LPL *in vitro* (90), 2-monoacylglycerol is probably the chemical form in which acylglycerol is transported from chylomicrons to mammary cells.

Uptake of Phospholipid. Phosphatidylcholine accounts for more than 60% of the lipid in the monolayer surface film surrounding the triglyceride core of chylomicrons (17). Perfused mammary gland of suckled lactating rats removed 10% of the phosphatidylcholine in chylomicrons in a single pass through the tissue (Table IV). About 55% of the phosphatidylcholine removed was recovered in venous perfusate as lysophosphatidylcholine and the rest was recovered as phospholipid in the tissue. Uptake and hydrolysis of chylomicron phosphatidylcholine was reduced at least 50% in perfused mammary gland from lactating rats unsuckled for 18 hours (Table IV). These findings suggest that chylomicron phosphatidylcholine was hydrolyzed to lysophosphatidylcholine by LPL in the capillaries.

Purified bovine LPL hydrolyzes phosphatidylcholine of chylomicrons *in vitro* to lysophosphatidylcholine and fatty acid at the same time it hydrolyzes triglyceride to monoglyceride and fatty acids (89). Although the amount of phosphatidylcholine hydrolyzed per unit time was about 4% of that of triglyceride, the rates were similarly affected when hydrolysis was reduced by limiting either the amount of enzyme present or the number of fatty acid binding sites available on albumin in the medium (89). Analyses of hydrolytic products showed that LPL cleaves the l-acyl ester bond of phosphatidylcholine (89). These findings support our conclusion that LPL in capillaries of mammary gland hydrolyzes chylomicron phosphatidylcholine, and that some of the lysophosphatidylcholine formed is released to the venous perfusate. The chemical form in which phospholipid is transferred from chylomicrons to mammary cells is not known.

Uptake of Cholesterol. Perfused mammary gland of suckled lactating rats removed 15% of the cholesteryl moiety in chylomicrons on a single pass through the tissue (Table IV). The perfused tissue removed at the same time 12% of the triglyceride in the chylomicrons. Uptake of both the cholesteryl moiety and triglyceride from chylomicrons was reduced 95% in perfused mammary tissue from lactating rats hypophysectomized for 48 hours (Table IV). LPL activity in mammary gland of these animals was also reduced by hypophysectomy (Table IV). These findings demonstrate that uptake of the cholesteryl moiety from chylomicrons by mammary gland requires LPL, and is associated with hydrolysis of chylomicron triglyceride and uptake of hydrolytic products by the tissue. The chemical form in which the cholesteryl moiety was transferred to mammary gland was not determined.

Cholesterol accounts for at least 85% of the cholesteryl moiety in milk (9). Studies in several species have shown that 50–85% of the cholesterol in milk is derived from diet (94–96), and cholesterol in chylomicrons is readily taken up by lactating mammary gland *in vivo* (94,97). Perfused mammary gland of suckled lactating rats, described above, removed 15% of the cholesteryl moiety of chylomicrons on a single pass through the tissue (Table IV), and this process was associated with hydrolysis of chylomicron triglyceride by LPL and transfer of hydrolytic products into the tissue (Fig. 5). We also found that mammary glands of suckled lactating rats *in vivo* removed within 11 minutes 12.6% of the cholesteryl moiety of chylomicrons injected intravenously, whereas mammary glands of lactating rats unsuckled for 44 hours removed only 3.8% (Table V). The reduction in LPL activity in mammary gland caused by nonsuckling for 44 hours and the resultant decrease in uptake of chylomicron triglyceride by mammary gland are shown in Fig. 7. Two-thirds of the cholesteryl moiety in the chylomicrons used in our studies was cholesterol and the rest was cholesteryl esters (91). It should be noted that cholesterol is located primarily in the surface film, whereas cholesteryl esters are located in the triglyceride core of chylomicrons (98). Studies in several species have shown that triglyceride in chylomicrons is removed primarily by extrahepatic tissues, whereas the cholesteryl esters are taken up mostly by liver, but only after lipolytic conversion of chylomicrons to remnants (99–104).

Cholesteryl linoleoyl ether, a nondegradable analogue of cholesteryl esters, has been used to study the mechanism of uptake of cholesteryl esters from chylomicrons by extrahepatic tissues and cultured cells (105–109). Uptake by lactating rat mammary gland of [^{3}H]cholesteryl linoleoyl ether in chylomicrons injected *in vivo* was found to be related to LPL activity in the tissue (106). Since uptake of cholesteryl linoleoyl ether by mammary gland was measured 3 hours after injection of chylomicrons, it is not known whether the tracer was taken up from chylomicrons or chylomicron remnants. Subsequent studies showed that various types of cells in culture can take up cholesteryl linoleoyl ether from chylomicron remnants and liposomes, as well as from chylomicrons (105,107–109). Although LPL attached to cell surfaces was required for uptake of cholesteryl linoleoyl ether, uptake of the ether was not dependent on concurrent hydrolysis of triglyceride (105,107–109). The role of LPL in transfer of cholesteryl linoleoyl ether into cells is discussed in Chapter 2. The above findings suggest that cholesteryl linoleoyl ether was taken up by mammary gland *in vivo* after the chylomicrons were converted to remnants.

On the basis of the high requirement for blood-borne cholesterol by lactating mammary gland (94–96), rapid uptake of cholesteryl moiety from chylomicrons by perfused lactating mammary gland (91), dependence of uptake of cholesteryl moiety from chylomicrons on LPL activity in the tissue (91), and negligible uptake by extrahepatic tissues of cholesteryl esters from chylomicrons (99–104), we conclude that cholesterol is the principal chemical form in which cholesteryl moiety is transferred from chylomicrons to lactating mammary gland. In addition, its transfer requires concurrent hydrolysis of chylomicron triglyceride and uptake of hydrolytic products by the tissue.

Effect of Lactation on Distribution of Chylomicron Lipids

Hormonal changes during late pregnancy and lactation cause a marked decrease in LPL activity in adipose tissue and an increase in LPL activity

TABLE V Effect of nonsuckling in lactating rats on amount of [^{3}H]cholesteryl moiety and [^{32}P]phospholipid recovered in their tissues and blood at 11 min after intravenous injection of chylomicrons

Group	Mammary gland		Adipose tissue		Blood		Liver	
	[^{32}P]phospholipid	[^{3}H]cholesteryl moiety	[^{32}P]phospholipid	[^{3}H]cholesteryl moiety	[^{32}P]phospholipid	[^{3}H]cholesteryl moiety	[^{32}P]phospholipid	[^{3}H]cholesteryl moiety
	% of lipid injected							
Suckled	8.2 (5)	12.6 (5)	5.2	2.8	55.8	26.7	16.3	53.8
Unsuckled	3.0 (6)	3.8 (5)	9.0	6.5	72.4	38.8	13.4	50.5

Lactating rats were injected intravenously with rat chylomicrons containing triglyceride labeled with [^{14}C]oleic acid and either [^{32}P]phosphatidylcholine or [^{3}H]cholesteryl moiety. Blood and tissues were taken for analyses 11 min later. The values for recovery of [^{14}C]oleoyl moiety in tissues and blood were similar to those presented in Fig. 7. Unsuckled rats were separated from their litters for 44 h prior to experiment. The figure in parentheses indicates number of animals per group. [From Scow et al. (24).]

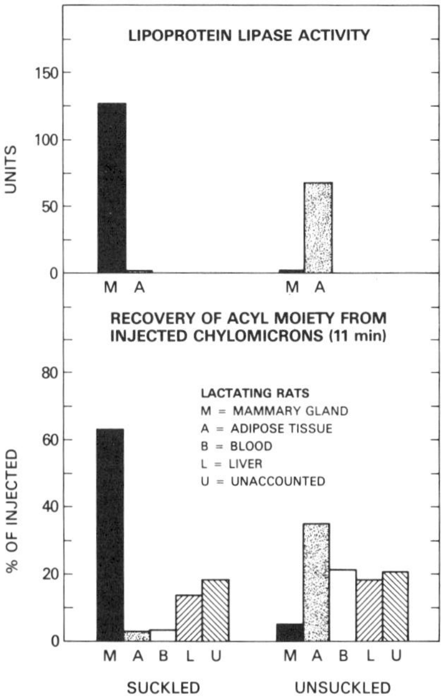

FIGURE 7 Effect of nonsuckling for 44 h on total lipoprotein lipase activity in mammary and adipose tissues, and recovery of acyl moiety of injected chylomicrons in tissues and blood of lactating rats. Chylomicrons containing [^{3}H]oleoyl-labeled triglyceride were injected intravenously, and tissues and blood were taken 11 min later for anlayses. One unit of activity = 1 μmol of fatty acids released per min. [Adapted from Scow et al. (24).]

in mammary gland (Fig. 1). This results in redistribution of chylomicron triglyceride from storage in adipose tissue to milk production in mammary gland (Fig. 7). Nonsuckling in lactating rats for 44 hours caused the disappearance of LPL activity from mammary gland and return of LPL activity to adipose tissue (Fig. 2), resulting in decreased delivery of chylomicron triglyceride to mammary gland and increased delivery of chylomicron triglyceride to adipose tissue (Fig. 7). It is notable that the ratio of amount of chylomicron acyl moiety taken up *in vivo* to LPL activity measured *in vitro* was the same in mammary gland of suckled rats and adipose tissue of unsuckled rats (Fig. 7). The fall in LPL activity in mammary gland retarded clearance of injected chylomicron triglyceride from blood (24) and increased slightly uptake of acyl moiety by liver (Fig. 7).

Nonsuckling also diverted phospholipid and cholesteryl moiety of injected chylomicrons in lactating rats from mammary gland to adipose tissue, and retarded clearance of these substances from blood (Table V). It did not affect the amounts of phospholipid and cholesteryl moiety taken up by liver. Distribution of phospholipid and cholesteryl moiety of chylomicrons during lactation is also regulated by LPL activity. Thus, delivery of dietary lipids to mammary gland for synthesis and secretion of fat globules in milk is effected by reciprocal changes in LPL activity in mammary gland and adipose tissue.

Transport of Lipids and Other Substances from Chylomicrons to Milk

Fatty Acids and Monoglycerides

We have developed a model for transport of fatty acids and monoglycerides from the capillary lumen to endoplasmic reticulum of parenchymal cells by lateral movement in an interfacial continuum of cell membranes (17,110–112) (Fig. 8). The continuum consists of the external (luminal) leaflets of the plasma membrane and membranes lining transcellular channels of endothelial cells and the corresponding leaflets of plasma membrane and membranes of endoplasmic reticulum of parenchymal cells (112). During uptake of lipolytic products from chylomicrons, the continuum would include the surface film of individual chylomicrons (111). We propose that some of the fatty acids formed by action of LPL on chylomicron triglyceride in capillaries of mammary gland are released to albumin in the blood stream (Table IV), whereas the rest of the fatty acids and the monoglyceride produced enter the continuum at sites of lipolysis and move in the continuum to the endoplasmic reticulum of mammary cells where they are reesterified to triglyceride (113) and accumulate as fat droplets between leaflets of the reticulum. Whether the droplets protrude into the lumen of the endoplasmic reticulum or the surrounding cytoplasm as they enlarge is not known. Also, the mechanism of transport of fat droplets from endoplasmic reticulum to the alveolar lumen of mammary gland is not known (9).

Phospholipid and Cholesterol

Uptake of phosphatidylcholine and cholesterol from chylomicrons by mammary gland was always associated with hydrolysis of triglyceride and uptake of lipolytic products by the tissue (Tables IV and V, Fig. 7). About 50% of phosphatidylcholine taken up was recovered in the venous perfusate as lysophosphatidylcholine and the other half was recovered as unidentified phospholipid in the tissue, whereas all of the cholesteryl moiety taken up was recovered in the tissue (Table V). Electron microscopic studies of lipid particles in venous perfusate from lactating mammary glad showed markedly depleted chylomicron remnants in the venous perfusate 2–3 minutes after starting the infusion of chylomicrons (74), indicating very rapid removal of triglyceride from chylomicrons by mammary gland. Since the surface film of chylomicrons becomes redundant as the triglyceride core is reduced by hydrolysis and transfer of lipolytic products to tissue and circulating albumin (74), excess phospholipid and cholesterol in the surface film could be expected to be transported with fatty acids and monoglycerides

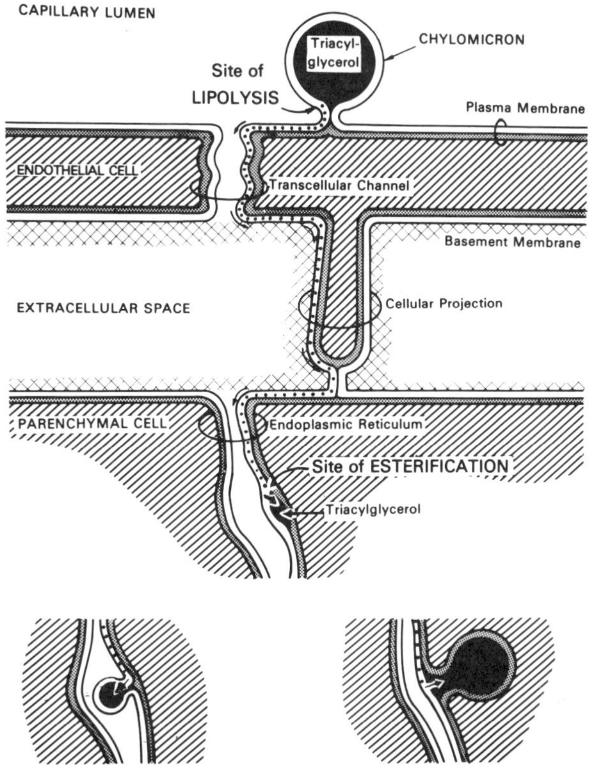

FIGURE 8 Route proposed for transport of fatty acids and monoglycerides from a chylomicron in the capillary lumen to an alveolar cell in mammary gland by lateral movement in an interfacial continuum of cell membranes. The interfacial continuum, represented by the broad white line, is composed of the external (luminal) leaflets of plasma and intracellular membranes of the endothelial cell, the corresponding leaflets of plasma membrane and endoplasmic reticulum of the alveolar (parenchymal) cell, and the surface film of the chylomicron. Lipolytic products formed by action of lipoprotein lipase on triglyceride in the chylomicron enter the continuum in the capillary lumen, and move (shown by black dots) in the continuum to endoplasmic reticulum where they are reesterified to triglyceride and accumulate as a lipid droplet between leaflets of the reticulum. It is not known whether the enlarging droplet protrudes into the lumen of endoplasmic reticulum or surrounding cytoplasm. [From Scow et al. (111).]

into the tissue by lateral movement in an interfacial continuum of cell membranes (17,112).

Fat-soluble Vitamins

The fat-soluble vitamins are usually present in milk (Table VI). The concentrations of vitamins A and E (2,114,115), 0.7–2.5 μM and 2.5–15 μM respectively, are much higher than those of vitamins D (2,115,116) and K

(117), 0.4–0.9 nM and 4–16 nM respectively. The amounts of vitamins A and E in milk are usually sufficient for the needs of the suckling (115), while the amount of vitamin D in milk is often inadequate (116,118–120). Little is know about vitamin K in milk (2,121).

Although fat-soluble vitamins are transported from the small intestines in chylomicrons (Table VI), vitamin E, because of its strongly amphipathic properties (122,123), is probably the only one transported in the chylomicron surface film. The concentration of vitamin E in milk is readily altered by changes in dietary intake of the vitamin (2,121,124,125), whereas the concentrations of vitamins A, D and K change very little and slowly with diet (116,119–121,124,126). LPL activity is involved, directly or indirectly, in the delivery of fat-soluble vitamins to mammary gland and milk.

Vitamin A. Dietary β-carotene and retinol, and retinol produced by hydrolysis of dietary retinyl esters, are taken up by intestinal cells, and most, if not all, of the β-carotene taken up is converted to retinol (126,127). Retinol is then esterified and incorporated, with cholesteryl esters, into the triglyceride core of chylomicrons (Table VI). After chylomicrons are depleted of triglyceride by LPL activity in extrahepatic tissues, retinyl esters in the remnants are taken up by liver, hydrolyzed, and either esterified for storage, or released to the circulation as retinol bound to retinol-binding protein (127). Studies in lactating monkeys (128) showed that retinol taken up from plasma retinol-binding protein accounts for 90% of vitamin A in milk. Since retinol is strongly amphipathic (129), it too could be transported from capillaries into mammary cells by lateral movement in an interfacial continuum of cell membranes (112). Vitamin A is present in milk primarily as retinyl esters (126).

β-Carotene colors the milk and adipose tissue of certain species, such as bovine and human (121,126). Since β-carotene is a hydrocarbon with 40 carbon atoms, it would be transported in the triglyceride core of chylomicrons from the small intestines, and probably delivered directly to mammary gland (121) (Table VI) and adipose tissue, during uptake of lipolytic products, by the mechanism proposed below for lipophilic xenobiotic compounds (112,130).

Vitamin D. Vitamin D_3 (cholecalciferol) absorbed from the intestines is transported in the blood stream in chylomicrons, probably in the core, and taken up primarily by liver (131). Since chylomicrons are not metabolized directly by liver (99), uptake of vitamin D_3 by liver probably occurs after conversion of chylomicrons to remnants. Vitamin D_3 is converted in liver to 25-OH-vitamin D_3 and immediately transported by the vitamin D transport protein in blood to the kidney where it undergoes further modification (131). Very small amounts of 25-OH-vitamin D have been found in human milk (116), suggesting that 25-OH-vitamin D_3 may be the chemical form in which vitamin D_3 is transported to mammary gland. However, 25-OH-vitamin D_3 accounted for only 8%, while vitamin D_3 accounted for

TABLE VI Probable mechanisms for transport in blood of fat-soluble vitamins from small intestines to mammary gland

Principal chemical form in diet	Transport from small intestines			Transport to mammary gland		Principal chemical form in milk
	Form	Carrier	Conversion in liver	Form	Carrier	
VITAMIN A						
β-Carotene	Retinyl esters	Chylomicron core	Retinyl esters $\rightarrow$ retinol	Retinol	Retinol-binding protein	Retinyl esters
Retinol	β-Carotene	Chylomicron core	—	β-Carotene	Chylomicron core	β-Carotene
Retinyl esters						
VITAMIN D						
Vitamin D_3	D_3	Chylomicron core	—	D_3	Chylomicron core	D_3
VITAMIN K						
Vitamin K	K	Chylomicron core	—	K	Chylomicron core	K
VITAMIN E						
α-Tocopherol	α-Tocopherol	Chylomicron surface film	—	α-Tocopherol	Chylomicron surface film	α-Tocopherol

90%, of the radioactivity in rat mammary gland derived from administered radiolabeled vitamin D_3 (132). This finding suggests that vitamin D_3 is the chemical form taken up from blood by mammary gland. Accordingly, vitamin D_3 derived from the diet would be delivered directly to mammary gland by chylomicrons (Table VI), and the uptake process would be similar to that described above for β-carotene. The low concentration of vitamin D_3 in milk (116,118–120) implies that this delivery process is not efficient.

Vitamin K. Since vitamin K is weakly amphipathic (122,133), it is transported from the intestines in the core of chylomicrons (117,134,135) and delivered mostly to liver (136), its primary site of action, after conversion of chylomicrons to remnants. Vitamin K is probably delivered to mammary gland by chylomicrons (Table VI), and the uptake process would be similar to that proposed for vitamin D_3 and β-carotene.

Vitamin E. Vitamin E (α-tocopherol) is readily transferred from maternal dietary sources into milk (114,125). It is transported from the small intestines in chylomicrons (134,137,138), and taken up from blood by heart, muscle, adipose tissue and liver, as well as lactating mammary gland (138–140) (Table VI). All of these tissues except liver have LPL activity and take up triglyceride from chylomicrons. Most of the α-tocopherol in chylomicrons, however, is taken up by liver (138), with cholesterol and cholesteryl esters (Table V), after conversion of chylomicrons to remnants. Recent studies with cultured human fibroblasts showed that transfer of α-tocopherol from chylomicrons into cells *in vitro* required active LPL on the surface of the cells (141). Transfer of tocopherol occurred only during hydrolysis of chylomicron triglyceride and uptake of fatty acids by the cells. α-Tocopherol is strongly amphipathic (123,129), and thus would be located mostly in the surface film with phospholipids and cholesterol (17,98). We propose that α-tocopherol is transported from chylomicrons into mammary gland, with fatty acids, monoglyceride, phospholipids and cholesterol, by lateral movement in an interfacial continuum of cell membranes (Fig. 8). A similar process is probably involved in uptake of α-tocopherol and lipolytic products from chylomicrons by cultured cells (141,142).

Summary. The mechanisms proposed above for transport in blood of fat-soluble vitamins from small intestines to mammary gland are summarized in Table VI. Vitamin A is the only fat-soluble vitamin that is not delivered directly to mammary gland by chylomicrons. Nonetheless, LPL is involved, converting chylomicrons to remnants and thereby facilitating uptake of retinyl esters by liver and subsequent binding of the hydrolytic product, retinol, to retinol-binding protein for transport to mammary gland. β-Carotene, vitamin D_3 and vitamin K, which are transported in the chylomicron core with cholesteryl esters, are taken up poorly by mammary gland, perhaps during transfer to mammary gland of fatty acids and monoglyceride produced by the action of LPL on chylomicrons. Vitamin E is carried in the chylomicron surface film, and consequently could be swept, with cholesterol and phospholipids, by the flow of lipolytic products in the surface film and membrane continuum into mammary cells.

Other Fat-soluble Substances (Hormones and Xenobiotics)

When lactating rats were fed fat stained with sudan III or IV, chylomicrons, body fat and milk of these animals were stained pink within several hours, and if they were allowed to suckle their young, chylomicrons and body fat in the young were also stained pink within a few hours (143). In view of the marked solubility of these dyes in fat and hydrocarbons, it is likely that these dyes were transferred from the intestinal lumen of the mother to adipose tissue of the suckling animals within a continuous hydrocarbon domain (112,144). The dye, soluble in triglyceride, was transported in chylomicrons in the maternal blood stream, in milk fat droplets between the mother and suckling, and in chylomicrons in the blood stream of the young. Transfer of fatty acids and monoglycerides from dietary fat into intestinal cells and from chylomicrons in capillaries into mammary cells or adipocytes requires lipolysis outside the cells and lateral movement of lipolytic products in an interfacial continuum composed of the monolayer surrounding the triglyceride droplet (in intestinal or capillary lumen) and the external leaflets of plasma and intracellular membranes (112,145) (Fig. 8). It is likely that the dye molecules were transported into cells via the hydrocarbon domain of lipid molecules in the continuum. The dye molecules could locate among the hydrocarbon tails of fatty acids and monoglycerides flowing in the continuum, and thereby be swept into the cells (112). Other fat-soluble substances, such as vitamins, drugs, and xenobiotics (e.g., DDT), could also be transported into cells by the same mechanism (112,130,144). This process, however, could deliver these substances only to cells of tissues that have LPL activity and utilize chylomicron triglyceride (heart, red skeletal muscle, adipose tissue, lung, and lactating mammary gland), or cells of liver that metabolize chylomicron remnants, or intestinal cells during absorpotion of dietary fat.

Since the interfacial continuum involved in fatty acid-monoglyceride transport is connected with the luminal leaflet of the nuclear envelope of parenchymal and endothelial cells (19,146), this mechanism could also transport other amphipathic substances, such as steroid and thyroid hormones and carcinogens, from blood to nuclei of cells in these tissues.

Combined Lipase Deficiency (*cld/cld*) in Mice

A Lethal Recessive Mutation (cld)

Extreme hyperchylomicronemia, with plasma concentrations of triglyceride as high as 20,000 mg/dl and cholesterol as high as 480 mg/dl, develops and results in death within 3 days in suckling newborn mice that are homozygous for the recessive mutation called combined lipase deficiency (*cld*)

(25). The mutation, at the T/t complex of mouse chromosome 17, causes taillessness and a deficiency of both LPL and hepatic lipase activities (25). During the first 12 hours of life, *cld/cld* mice appear normal, except for taillessness, and keep their stomachs filled with milk. Later, they become less active and pale, due to hyperlipemia, and several hours before death they become cyanotic and cold (147).

Morphological Studies

Capillaries in tissues of suckled *cld/cld* mice were packed with numerous abnormally shaped chylomicrons (Fig. 9), and the subendothelial spaces in heart, lung and liver and the lumen of lung alveoli contained extravasated chylomicrons (147). In contrast, capillaries in tissues of suckled unaffected mice contained very few chylomicrons (Fig. 10), and the subendothelial spaces and lung alveoli were free of chylomicrons. Myocytes of diaphragm muscle (Fig. 9) and heart in suckled *cld/cld* mice did not contain lipid droplets, and adipocytes of brown adipose tissue contained a few small droplets, which were probably acquired *in utero* (147). Lipid-containing-Type II alveolar cells in lung were not prominent in *cld/cld* mice. The

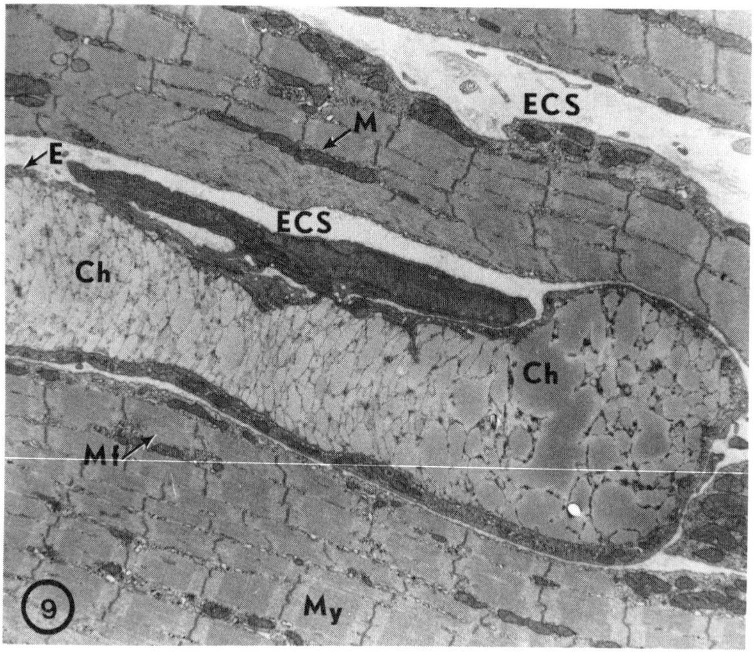

FIGURE 9 A section of diaphragm muscle from an 18-hour-old suckled *cld/cld* mouse, showing a portion of a capillary and three myocytes. Note that the capillary lumen is packed with chylomicrons (Ch), while the myocytes (My) contain no lipid droplets. E, endothelial cell; ECS, extracellular space; M, mitochondria, Mf, myofibril. X 6,000. [From Blanchette-Mackie et al. (147), with permission.]

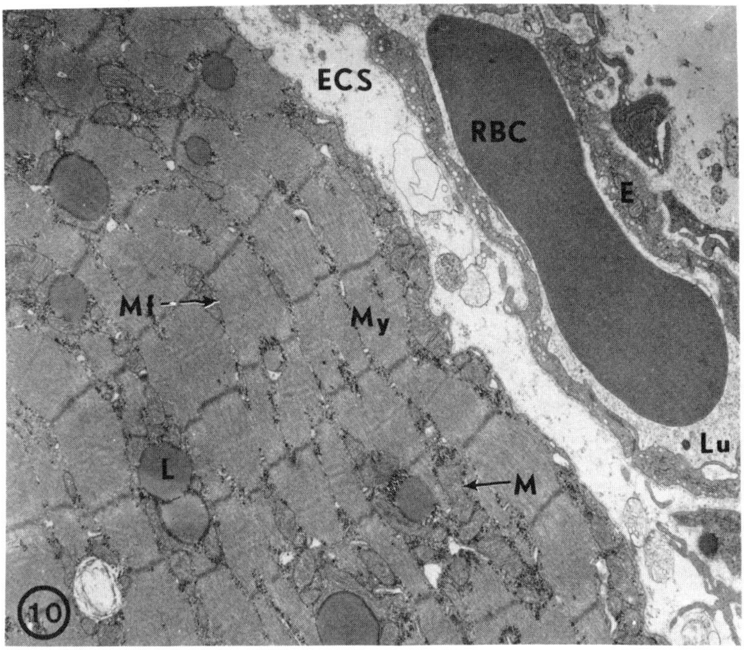

FIGURE 10 A section of diaphragm muscle from an 18-hour-old suckled unaffected mouse, showing a portion of a capillary and a myocyte. Note the large lipid droplets (L) in the myocyte (My) and the absence of chylomicrons in the capillary lumen (Lu). E, endothelial cell; ECS, extracellular space; M, mitochondria; Mf, myofibrils; RBC, red blood cell. X 7,000. [From Blanchette-Mackie et al. (147), with permission.]

opposite was seen in suckled unaffected mice (Fig. 10), in which the parenchymal cells in these tissues contained numerous large lipid droplets (147). The large amount of chylomicrons in capillaries and the virtual absence of lipid droplets in tissues of *cld/cld* mice reflect vividly the deficiency of LPL activity in these animals.

Hepatocytes in suckled unaffected mice contained large lipoprotein particles (d = 400 A) in endoplasmic reticulum and Golgi, large lipid droplets, and very few lysosomes (147). Hepatocytes of suckled *cld/cld* mice, however, contained much smaller lipoprotein particles (d = 100 A), numerous large lysosomes filled with lipoprotein particles, lipid spheres and lamellar structures, and no lipid droplets. The extent to which uptake of chylomicron remnants, or intracellular degradation of nascent lipoproteins, could contribute to lysosomal proliferation in liver of *cld/cld* mice is not known (147).

Inactive Lipoprotein Lipase

LPL activity in diaphragm muscle, heart, brown adipose tissue and lung of *cld/cld* mice was less than 5% of that in tissues of unaffected mice (Table VII) (26). LPL activity in liver of *cld/cld* mice, however, was only 60% less

TABLE VII Effect of combined lipase deficiency (*cld/cld*) on lipoprotein, hepatic, lingual and pancreatic lipase activities in tissues of newborn mice

Group	Lipoprotein lipase activity in: Diaphragm muscle	Heart	Brown adipose tissue	Lung	Liver	Hepatic lipase activity in liver	Lingual lipase activity in tongue	Pancreatic lipase activity in pancreas
			mU/g			mU/g	mU/tongue	U/g
cld/cld	15 ± 18	7 ± 4	19 ± 2	2 ± 1	75 ± 3	5 ± 2	29 ± 5	238 ± 33
Unaffected	313 ± 41	333 ± 75	582 ± 136	73 ± 13	187 ± 5	228 ± 5	62 ± 9	265 ± 40

Mice used in these studies were 3–24 h old. Data on lipoprotein lipase activity in diaphragm muscle, heart, brown adipose tissue and lung, with 3–5 assays per group, are from Olivecrona et al. (26). Data on lipoprotein lipase and hepatic lipase activities in liver, with 5 assays per group, are from Olivecrona et al. (26). Data on lingual and hepatic lipase activities, with 10–12 assays per group, are unpublished observations of R. O. Scow and S. S. Chernick. Lingual lipase activity was measured in homogenates of tongue at pH 5.4 by the procedure of Field and Scow (150). Pancreatic lipase activity was measured in homogenates of pancreas at pH 8.1 by the same procedure (150). One unit of activity = 1 μmol of fatty acids released per min. Values given are means ± S. E.

than that in liver of unaffected mice (26). This suggests that regulation of LPL activity in liver of neonatal rodents (27,61) is different from that in other tissues (27). Heparin injected intraperitoneally increased plasma LPL activity in *cld/cld* mice, but the increment was less than 10% of that in unaffected mice (27).

There was 2–6 times more LPL protein (determined by radioimmunoassay) in diaphragm muscle, heart, and brown adipose tissue of *cld/cld* mice than in corresponding tissues of unaffected mice (Fig. 11) (26). Diaphragm muscle, heart, brown adipose tissue, and liver of 1-day-old *cld/cld* and unaffected mice incorporated *in vivo* [^{35}S]methionine into a protein that could be immunoprecipitated by anti-LPL serum (26). The proportion of radioactivity in LPL to that in total protein was 0.02% in tissues of *cld/cld* mice and 0.01% in tissues of unaffected mice. The immunoprecipitated protein in all tissues of both groups of animals had the same M_r as bovine LPL when determined by sodium dodecyl sulfate-polyacrylamide gel electrophoresis (26), indicating that LPL in tissues of *cld/cld* mice is not grossly

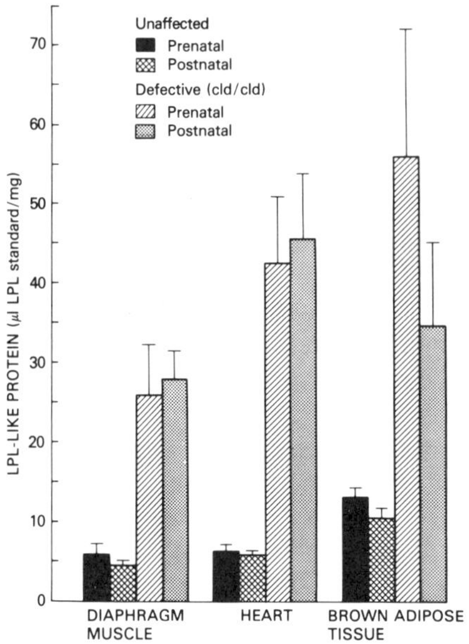

FIGURE 11 Amounts of lipoprotein lipase protein, determined by radioimmunoassay, in tissues of *cld/cld* and unaffected mice. The mice in the prenatal group were either delivered by Caesarian section on the expected day of birth or naturally born less than 2 h before experiment; none were allowed suckle. The postnatal mice were 18–36 h old and allowed to suckle. Tissues of postnatal mice were analyzed separately, while tissues from two or three prenatal mice were pooled for each assay. The vertical bars represent the means of 4–6 assays and the vertical lines represent 1 S. E. [From Olivecrona et al. (26), with permission.]

abnormal. The findings demonstrate that the tissues in *cld/cld* mice synthesize and retain an inactive form of LPL.

Other mutations in the T/t complex of chromosome 17, such T^{12}, affect glycosylation of cell surface glycoproteins (148). Since LPL is a glycoprotein, it is possible that defective glycosylation could result in synthesis of a form of LPL lacking the proper compliment of carbohydrates required for full activity and transport of the enzyme in tissues (26).

Lack of Hepatic Lipase Activity

Hepatic lipase activity in liver of *cld/cld* mice was less than 2% of that in liver of unaffected mice (Table VII). The plasma of unaffected mice contained a high level of hepatic lipase activity, 244 mU/ml, but practically no LPL activity (27). Heparin injected intraperitoneally increased plasma LPL activity to 152 mU/ml, but had no effect on plasma hepatic lipase activity in unaffected mice. Heparin had no significant effect on plasma hepatic lipase activity in defective mice. These findings establish that hepatic lipase activity is markedly reduced in liver and plasma of combined lipase deficient (*cld/cld*) mice (25,27). Lysosomal proliferation in liver of *cld/cld* mice (147) could result from the severe deficiency of hepatic lipase activity in these animals.

Decreased Lingual Lipase Activity

Chylomicrons appear in intestinal lymph of *cld/cld* mice soon after they begin to suckle, and the plasma concentration of triglyceride increases continuously during the first 12–16 hours of life (25), suggesting that intestinal absorption of fat is not impaired in these animals. Since lingual lipase in rat (149) and pancreatic lipase in certain species (porcine, human) (145) are glycoproteins, we measured the activity of these enzymes in *cld/cld* mice to determine if these enzymes were affected. Lingual lipase activity was 50% less in tongue of *cld/cld* mice than that in tongue of unaffected mice (Table VII), whereas pancreatic lipase activity in pancreas was unaffected. Possibly murine pancreatic lipase, like bovine and ovine pancreatic lipases (145), is not a glycoprotein. The effect of combined lipase deficiency on lingual lipase requires further study.

Summary

LPL is essential for the delivery of dietary lipids and fat-soluble vitamins to mammary gland for milk production. LPL activity increases in mammary gland during late pregnancy and continues at a high level throughout lactation. Although LPL activity in mammary gland is dependent on several hormones, it is regulated primarily by prolactin, secreted by placenta during late pregnancy and by anterior pituitary gland during lactation. Suckling stimulates secretion of prolactin by the pituitary, as well as prevents engorgement of mammary gland. LPL activity in adipose tissue is markedly suppressed, during late pregnancy and lactation, by prolactin in conjunction with an unknown substance, possibly produced by lactating mammary gland. These reciprocal changes in LPL activity, in adipose tissue and mammary gland, divert plasma triglyceride from storage in body fat to milk production in mammary gland.

Transport of fatty acids and monoglycerides from chylomicrons to milk involves lateral movement of these amphipathic substances in an interfacial continuum of cell membranes, extending from the surface of chylomicrons to sites of triglyceride synthesis in mammary cells. Phospholipids, cholesterol, and lipophilic vitamins and xenobiotics are probably transported from chylomicrons to milk by the same mechanism.

An inactive but normal-sized LPL is synthesized and retained in tissues of mice homozygous for the mutation called combined lipase deficiency (*cld*). *cld/cld* mice develop extreme hyperchylomicronemia and die within 3 days if allowed to suckle. This mutation, which also causes deficiency of hepatic lipse and lingual lipase activities, is located in the T/t complex of mouse chromosome 17, suggesting it could act by impairing glycosylation of specific enzymes.

References

1. Breckenridge, W. C. and A. Kuksis. 1967. *J. Lipid Res.* 8:473–478.
2. Jenness, R. 1974. *In:* Lactation. B. L. Larson and V. R. Smith, editors. Academic Press, New York. Vol. III, 3–107.
3. Jensen, R. G., R. M. Clark and A. M. Ferris. 1980. *Lipids* 15:345–355.
4. Patton, S. and F. M. Fowkes. 1967. *J. Theor. Biol.* 15:274–281.
5. Huang, T. C. and A. Kuksis. 1967. *Lipids* 2:453–460.
6. Garton, G. A. 1963. *J. Lipid Res.* 4:237–254.
7. Insull, W., Jr., J. Hirsch, T. James and E. H. Ahrens, Jr. 1959. *J. Clin. Invest.* 38:443–450.
8. Beare, J. L., E. R. W. Gregory, D. M. Smith and J. A. Campbell. 1961. *Canad. J. Biochem. Physiol.* 39:195–201.
9. Patton, S. and T. W. Keenan. 1975. *Prog. Chem. Fats and other Lipids* 14:167–277.
10. Jensen, R. G., M. M. Hagerty and K. E. McMahon. 1978. *Am. J. Clin. Nutr.* 31:990–1016.
11. Patton, S. and T. W. Keenan. 1975. *Biochim. Biophys. Acta* 410:273–309.
12. Annison, E. F., J. L. Linzell, S. Fazakerley and B. W. Nichols. 1967. *Biochem. J.* 102:637–647.
13. Bishop, C., T. Davies, R. F. Glascock and V. A. Welch. 1969. *Biochem. J.* 113:629–633.
14. West, C. E., R. Bickerstaffe, E. F. Annison and J. L. Linzell. 1972. *Biochem. J.* 126:477–490.
15. Carey, E. M. and R. Dils. 1972. *Biochem. J.* 126:1005–1007.
16. Robinson, D. S. 1970. *In:* Comprehensive Biochemistry. M. Florkin and E. H. Stotz, editors. Academic Press, New York. Vol. 18, 51–116.
17. Scow, R. O., E. J. Blanchette-Mackie and L. C. Smith. 1976. *Circ. Res.* 39:149–162.
18. Scow, R. O., M. Hamosh, E. J. Blanchette-Mackie and A. J. Evans. 1972. *Lipids* 7:497–505.
19. Wetzel, M. G. and R. O. Scow. 1984. *Am. J. Physiol.* 246:C467–C485.
20. McBride, O. W. and E. D. Korn. 1963. *J. Lipid Res.* 4:17–20.
21. Robinson, D. S. 1963. *J. Lipid Res.* 4:21–23.

22. Hamosh, M., T. R. Clary, S. S. Chernick and R. O. Scow. 1970. *Biochim. Biophys. Acta* 210:473–482.
23. Flint, D. J., R. A. Clegg and R. G. Vernon. 1981. *Molec. Cell. Endocrinology* 22:265–275.
24. Scow, R. O., S. S. Chernick and T. R. Fleck. 1977. *Biochim. Biophys. Acta* 487:297–306.
25. Paterniti, J. R., Jr., W. V. Brown, H. N. Ginsberg and K. Artzt. 1983. *Science* 221:167–169.
26. Olivecrona, T., S. S. Chernick, G. Bengtsson-Olivecrona, J. R. Paterniti, Jr., W. V. Brown and R. O. Scow. 1985. *J. Biol. Chem.* 260:2552–2557.
27. Olivecrona, T., G. Bengtsson-Olivecrona, S. S. Chernick and R. O. Scow. 1986. *Biochim. Biophys. Acta* 876:243–248.
28. Boyd, E. M. 1935. *Am. J. Obst. Gynec.* 29:797–805.
29. Brown, W. D. 1952. *Quart. J. Expt. Physiol.* 37:119–129.
30. Scow, R. O., S. S. Chernick and B. -B. Smith. 1958. *Proc. Soc. Exp. Biol. Med.* 98:833–835.
31. Scow, R. O., S. S. Chernick and M. S. Brinley. 1964. *Am. J. Physiol.* 206:796–804.
32. Otway, S. and D. S. Robinson. 1968. *Biochem. J.* 37:119–129.
33. Chernick, S. S. and M. Novak. 1970. *Diabetes* 19:563–570.
34. Barry, J. M., W. Bartley, J. L. Linzell and D. S. Robinson. 1963. *Biochem. J.* 89:6–11.
35. Askew, E. W., R. S. Emery and J. W. Thomas. 1970. *J. Dairy Sci.* 53:1415–1423.
36. Shirley, J. E., R. S. Emery, E. M. Convey and W. D. Oxender. 1973. *J. Dairy Sci.* 56:569–574.
37. Hernell, O. and T. Olivecrona. 1974. *J. Lipid Res.* 15:367–374.
38. Chillard, Y., D. Sauvant, J. Hervieu, M. Dorleans and P. Morandfehr. 1977. *Ann. Biol. Animal Bioch. Biophys.* 17:1021–1033.
39. Jones, E. H. 1968. *Biochim. Biophys. Acta* 177:158–160.
40. McLean, P. 1964. *Biochem. J.* 90:271–278.
41. Lyons, W. R., C. H. Li and R. E. Johnson. 1958. *Recent Prog. Hormone Res.* 14:219–248.
42. Cowie, A. T. 1969. *In:* Lactogenesis: The Initiation of Milk Secretion at Parturition. M. Reynolds and S. J. Folley, editors. University of Pennsylvania Press, Philadelphia. 157–169.
43. Zinder, O., M. Hamosh, T. R. C. Fleck and R. O. Scow. 1974. *Am. J. Physiol.* 226:744–748.
44. Cross, B. A. 1961. *In:* Milk: The Mammary Gland and its Secretion. S. K. Kon and A. T. Cowie, editors. Academic Press, New York. Vol. I, 229–277.
45. Parkes, D. 1977. *Adv. Drug Res.* 12:248–344.
46. Amenomori, Y., C. L. Chen and J. Meites. 1970. *Endocrinology* 86:506–510.
47. Morishige, W. K., G. J. Pepe and I. Rothchild. 1973. *Endocrinology* 92:1527–1531.
48. Labhsetwar, A. P. and D. J. Watson. 1974. *Biol. Reprod.* 10:103–110.
49. Spooner, P. M., M. M. Garrison and R. O. Scow. 1977. *J. Clin. Invest.* 60:702–708.
50. Labhsetwar, A. P. 1974. *Federation* Proc. 33:61–77.
51. Deis, R. P. 1971. *Nature* 229:568.
52. Vermouth, N. J. and R. P. Deis. 1972. *Nature* 238:248–250.
53. Smith, I. D., R. P. Shearon and A. R. Korda. 1972. *Nature* 240:411–412.
54. Daughaday, W. H., B. Trivedi and M. Kapadia. 1979. *Endocrinology* 105:210–214.
55. Ray, E. W., S. C. Averill, W. R. Lyons and R. E. Johnson. 1955. *Endocrinology* 56:359–373.
56. Kelly, P. A., R. P. C. Shiu, M. C. Robertson and H. G. Friesen. *Endocrinology* 96:1187–1195.
57. Riddick, D. H. 1985. *In:* Prolactin: Basic and Clinical Correlates. R. M. McLeod, M. O. Thorner and U. Scapagnini, editors. Liviana Press, Padova. 464–473.
58. Shiu, R. P. C., P. A. Kelly and H. G. Friesen. 1973. *Science* 180:968–971.
59. Anderson, R. R. 1976. *Proc. Soc. Exptl. Biol. Med.* 148:283–287.
60. Golander, A., J. Barrett, T. Hurley, S. Barry and S. Handwerger. 1979. *J. Clin. Endocrinol. Metab.* 49:787–789.

61. Ramirez, I., M. Llobera and E. Herrera. 1983. *Metabolism* 32:333–341.
62. Robinson, D. S., S. M. Parkins, B. K. Speake and J. A. Little. 1983. *In:* The Adipocyte and Obesity: Cellular and Molecular Mechanisms. A. Angel, C. H. Hollenberg and D. A. K. Roncari, editors. Raven Press, New York. 127–136.
63. Linkie, D. M. and G. D. Niswender. 1973. *Biol. Reprod.* 8:48–57.
64. Glaser, L. A., I. Khan, G. J. Pepe, P. A. Kelly and G. Gibori. 1985. *In:* Prolactin. Basic and Clinical Correlates. R. M. McLeod, M. O. Thorner and U. Scapagnini, editors. Liviana Press, Padova. 495–499.
65. Jayatilak, P. G., L. A. Glaser, R. Basuray, P. A. Kelly and G. Gibori. 1985. *In:* Prolactin: Basic and Clinical Correlates. R. M. Mcleod, M. O. Thorner and U. Scapagnini, editors. Liviana Press, Padova. 475–480.
66. Terkel, J., C. A. Blake and C. W. Sawyer. 1972. *Endocrinology* 91:49–53.
67. Falconer, I. R. and T. J. Fiddler. 1970. *Biochim. Biophys. Acta* 218:508–514.
68. Hamosh, M. and R. O. Scow. 1971. *Biochim. Biophys. Acta* 231:283–289.
69. Egelrud, T. and T. Olivecrona. 1972. *J. Biol. Chem.* 247:6212–6217.
70. Semb, H. and T. Olivecrona. 1986. *Biochim. Biophys. Acta* In press.
71. Clegg, R. A. 1981. *Biochim. Biophys. Acta* 663:598–612.
72. Clegg, R. A. 1981. *Biochim. Biophys. Acta* 664:397–408.
73. Olivecrona, T., T. Egelrud, P. -H. Iverius and U. Lindahl. 1971. *Biochem. Biophys. Res. Commun.* 43:524–529.
74. Scow, R. O., C. R. Mendelson, O. Zinder, M. Hamosh and E. J. Blanchette-Mackie. 1973. *In:* Dietary lipids and Postnatal Development. C. Galli, G. Jacini and A. Pecile, editors. Raven Press, New York. 91–114.
75. Riddle, O., R. W. Bates, and S. W. Dykshorn. 1933. *Am. J. Physiol.* 105:191–216.
76. Dumont, J. N. 1965. *Z. Zellforsch.* 68:755–782.
77. Ensor, D. M. 1978. Comparative Endocrinology of Prolactin. Chapman and Hall, London. 112–115; 120–125.
78. Lyons, W. R. and J. S. Dixon. 1966. *In:* The Pituitary Gland. G. W. Harris and B. T. Donavan, editors. University of California Press, Berkeley. Vol. 1, 527–581.
79. Chadwick, A. and B. J. Jordan. 1971. *Endocrin. J.* 49:51–58.
80. Bates, R. W., M. M. Garrison and J. Cornfield. 1963. *Endocrinology* 73:217–223.
81. Whitney, L. F. Keeping Your Pigeons Flying. Erickson, New York. 68–85.
82. Goodridge, A. G. and E. G. Ball. 1967. *Biochemistry* 6:2335–2343.
83. Garrison, M. M. and R. O. Scow. 1975. *Am. J. Physiol.* 228:1542–1544.
84. Meier, A. H. and D. S. Farner. 1964. *Gen. Comp. Endocrin.* 4:584–594.
85. Mendelson, C. R. and R. O. Scow. 1972. *Am. J. Physiol.* 223:1418–1423.
86. Scow, R. O., E. J. Blanchette-Mackie, C. R. Mendelson, M. Hamosh and O. Zinder. 1975. *Mod. Probl. Paediat.* 15:31–45.
87. Scow, R. O. 1977. *Federation Proc.* 26:182–185.
88. Mendelson, C. R., O. Zinder, E. J. Blanchette-Mackie, S. S. Chernick and R. O. Scow. 1977. *J. Dairy Sci.* 60:666–676.
89. Scow, R. O. and T. Egelrud. 1976. *Biochim. Biophys. Acta* 431:538–549.
90. Scow, R. O. and T. Olivecrona. 1977. *Biochim. Biophys. Acta* 487:472–486.
91. Zinder, O., C. R. Mendelson, E. J. Blanchette-Mackie and R. O. Scow. 1976. *Biochim. Biophys. Acta* 431:526–537.
92. Nilsson-Ehle, P., T. Egelrud, P. Belfrage, T. Olivecrona and B. Borgstrom. 1973. *J. Biol. Chem.* 248:6734–6737.
93. Morley, N., A. Kuksis, D. Buchnea and J. J. Myher. 1975. *J. Biol. Chem.* 250:3413–3418.
94. Clarenburg, R. and I. L. Chaikoff. 1966. *J. Lipid Res.* 7:27–37.
95. Conner, W. E. and D. S. Lin. 1967. *Am. J. Physiol.* 213:1353–1358.
96. Patton, S. 1973. *J. Am. Oil Chemists Soc.* 50:178–185.
97. McBride, O. W. and E. D. Korn. 1964. *J. Lipid Res.* 5:459–467.
98. Zilversmit, D. B. 1969. *In:* Structural and Functional Aspects of Lipoproteins in Living Systems. E. Tria and A. N. Scanu, editors. Academic Press, New York. 209–229.

99. Goodman, D. S. 1962. *J. Clin. Invest.* 41:1886–1896.
100. Quarfordt, S. H. and D. S. Goodman. 1967. *J. Lipid Res.* 8:264–273.
101. Redgrave, T. G. 1970. *J. Clin. Invest.* 49:465–471.
102. Bergman, E. M., R. J. Havel, B. M. Wolfe and T. Bohmer. 1971. *J. Clin. Invest.* 50:1831–1839.
103. Redgrave, T. G. 1973. *Biochem. J.* 136:109–113.
104. Mjos, O. D., O. Faergman, R. L. Hamilton and R. J. Havel. 1975. *J. Clin. Invest.* 56:603–615.
105. Chajek-Shaul, T., G. Friedman, G. Halperin, O. Stein and Y. Stein. 1981. *Biochim. Biophys. Acta* 666:147–155.
106. Chajek-Shaul, T., G. Friedman, G. Halperin, O. Stein and Y. Stein. 1981. *Biochim. Biophys. Acta* 666:216–222.
107. Friedman, G., T. Chajek-Shaul, O. Stein, T. Olivecrona and Y. Stein. 1981. *Biochim. Biophys. Acta* 666:156–164.
108. Chajek-Shaul, T., G. Friedman, O. Stein, T. Olivecrona and Y. Stein. 1982. *Biochim. Biophys. Acta* 712:200–210.
109. Stein, O., G. Friedman, T. Chajek-Shaul, G. Halperin, T. Olivecrona and Y. Stein. 1983. *Biochim. Biophys. Acta* 750:306–316.
110. Smith, L. C. and R. O. Scow. 1979. *Prog. Biochem. Pharmacol.* 15:109–138.
111. Scow, R. O., E. J. Blanchette-Mackie and L. C. Smith. 1980. *Federation Proc.* 39:2610–2617.
112. Scow, R. O. and E. J. Blanchette-Mackie. 1985. *Prog. Lipid Res.* 24:197–241.
113. Stein, O. and Y. Stein. *J. Cell Biol.* 34:251–263.
114. Wright, S. W., L. J. Filer, Jr. and K. E. Mason. 1951. *Pediatrics* 7:386–393.
115. Macy, I. G. and H. J. Kelly. 1961. *In:* Milk: The Mammary Gland and Its Secretion. S. K. Kon and A. T. Cowie, editors. Academic Press, New York. Vol. II, 265–304.
116. Greer, F. R., M. Ho, D. Dodson and R. C. Tsang. 1981. *J. Pediatr.* 99:233–235.
117. Shearer, M. J., V. Allan, Y. Haron and P. Barkhan. 1980. *In:* Vitamin K Metabolism and Vitamin K-Dependent Poteins. J. W. Suttie, editor. University Park Press, Baltimore. 317–327.
118. Drumond, J. C., C. H. Gray and N. E. G. Richardson. 1939. *Brit. Med. J.* 2:757–760.
119. Hyten, F. E. and A. M. Thomson. 1961. *In:* Milk: The Mammary Gland and Its Secretion. S. K. Kon and A. T. Cowie, editors. Academic Press, New York. Vol. II, 3–46.
120. Finberg, L. 1981. *J. Pediatr.* 99:228–229.
121. Ling, E. R., S. K. Kon and J. W. G. Porter. 1961. *In:* Milk: The Mammary Gland and Its Secretion. S. K. Kon and A. T. Cowie, editors. Academic Press, New York. Vol. II, 195–263.
122. Weitzel, G., A. -M. Fretzdorff and S. Heller. 1956. *Hoppe Seyler's Z. Physiol. Chem.* 303:14–26.
123. Maggio, B., A. T. Diplock and J. A. Lucy. 1977. *Biochem. J.* 161:111–121.
124. Reid, J. T. 1961. *In:* Milk: The Mammary Gland and Its Secretion. S. K. Kon and A. T. Cowie, editors. Academic Press, New York. Vol. II, 47–87.
125. Martin, M. M. and L. S. Hurley. 1977. *Am. J. Clin. Nutr.* 30:1629–1637.
126. Wallingford, J. C. and B. A. Underwood. 1986. *In:* Vitamin A Deficiency and Its Control. J. C. Bauernfeind, editor. Academic Press, New York. 101–151.
127. Goodman, D. S. and W. S. Blaner. 1984. *In:* The Retinoids. M. B. Sporn, A. B. Roberts and D. S. Goodman, editors. Academic Press, Orlando. Vol. 2, 1–39.
128. Vahlquist, A. and S. Nilsson. 1979. *J. Nutr.* 109:1456–1463.
129. Weitzel, G., A. -M. Fretzdorff and S. Heller. 1952. *Hoppe Seyler's Z. Physiol. Chem.* 290:32–47.
130. Patton, J. S. 1986. *In:* Human Lactation: Maternal-environmental Effects. M. Hamosh and A. S. Goldman, editors. Plenum Press, New York. 469–491.
131. De Luca, H. F. 1979. Vitamin D Metabolism and Function. Springer-Verlag, Berlin. 11–23.

132. Weisman, Y., R. Sapir, A. Harrell and S. Edelstin. 1976. *Biochim. Biophys. Acta* 428:388–395.
133. Gaines, G. L., Jr., A. G. Tweet and W. D. Bellamy. 1965. *J. Chem. Phys.* 42:2193–2199.
134. McCormick, E. C., D. G. Cornwell and J. B. Brown. 1960. *J. Lipid Res.* 1:221–228.
135. Blomstrand, R. and L. Forsgren. 1968. *Internat. Z. Vit. Forschung.* 38:45–64.
136. Wiss, O. and Gloor, H. 1966. *Vitamins and Hormones* 24:575–586.
137. Bjornson, L. K., H. J. Kayden, E. Miller and A. N. Moshell. 1976. *J. Lipid Res.* 17:343–352.
138. Peake, I. R., H. G. Windmueller and J. G. Bieri. 1972. *Biochim. Biophys. Acta* 260:679–688.
139. Kayden, H. J. 1983. *In:* Biology of Vitamin E. R. Porter and J. Wheelan, editors. Ciba Foundation Symposium 101. Pitman, London. 70:70–85.
140. Kayden, H. J., L. J. Hatam and M. G. Traber. 1983. *J. Lipid Res.* 24:652–656.
141. Traber, M. G., T. Olivecrona and H. J. Kayden. 1985. *J. Clin. Invest.* 75:1729–1734.
142. Blanchette-Mackie, E. J., T. Briggs, S. S. Chernick and R. O. Scow. 1986. *Cell Tissue Res.* 244:95–105.
143. Gage, S. H. and P. A. Fish. 1924. *Am. J. Anat.* 34:1–85.
144. Patton, J. S. 1981. *In:* Physiology of the Gastrointestinal Tract. L. R. Johnson, editor. Raven Press, New York. 1123–1146.
145. Verger, R. 1984. *In:* Lipases. B. Borgstrom and H. L. Brockman, editors. Elsevier, Amsterdam. 84–150.
146. Blanchette-Mackie, E. J., and R. O. Scow. 1981. *J. Ultrastruct. Res.* 77:295–318.
147. Blanchette-Mackie, E. J., M. G. Wetzel, S. S. Chernick, J. R. Paterniti, Jr., W. V. Brown and R. O. Scow. 1986. *Lab. Invest.* 55:347–362.
148. Cheng, C. C. and D. Bennett. 1980. *Cell* 19:537–543.
149. Docherty, A. J. P., M. W. Bodner, S. Angal, R. Verger, C. Riviere, P. A. Lowe, A. Lyons, S. S. Entage and T. J. R. Harris. 1985. *Nucleic Acid Res.* 13:1891–1903.
150. Field, R. B. and R. O. Scow. 1983. *J. Biol. Chem.* 258:14563–14569.

Chapter 7

ROLE OF LIPOPROTEIN LIPASE IN METABOLIC ADAPTATION TO EXERCISE AND TRAINING

Esko A. Nikkilä

Any form of physical activity will cause a change in the body energy balance compared to a resting state. Additional fuel is needed not only for the contracting muscles, but also for the increased work demand of circulation and respiration. Both skeletal and respiratory muscles and the heart must be supplied by oxidative substrates in amounts which, during exercise, exceed several times the needs at rest. The two immediately available sources of energy are glucose and fatty acids. The proportion of utilization of these substrates depends on many factors like work intensity and duration, feeding status, previous diet, physical fitness, training, body composition, environmental conditions, sex, and hormonal balance. The effect of each of these factors, alone or in combination, on the metabolic adaptation to exercise has been subject to a large number of studies in both experimental animals and man. The exercise-induced changes in the flux rates of various substrates through intravascular or extracellular space are relatively well characterized. However, the mechanisms of body adaptation to exercise and training at the cellular level are far from resolved as regards both substrate production and utilization. This is particularly true in man even though analytical microtechniques have been recently developed for a reliable study of small tissue samples obtained by needle biopsies.

Fatty Acids as Energy Substrates During Exercise

A major part of the energy requirement of exercise is covered by the oxidation of fatty acids. Their proportion from the total fuel consumption is dependent on duration and intensity of the work and on training. The fatty acids utilized by the muscles can be derived from three different triglyceride depots, *viz.* adipose tissue, working muscle itself, or plasma chylomicrons and very low-density lipoproteins (VLDL). Before entering the oxidative pathway, the fatty acids must be released from the triglycerides and, therefore, lipolysis is an obligatory first step of all fatty acid utilization. In adipose tissue, the triglycerides are hydrolyzed by an enzyme called hormone-sensitive lipase. The liberated fatty acids are released into the plasma where they circulate as "free" or non-esterified fatty acids (FFA, NEFA) bound to albumin. Lipolysis of circulating chylomicron and VLDL triglycerides, on the other hand, is performed by lipoprotein lipase (LPL) located at the luminal surface of capillary endothelial cells. The fatty acids liberated in this latter reaction are probably transferred directly to the cells by lateral movement in the cell membranes (1) without being circulated through the plasma FFA pool. In contrast to these two lipases, the enzymes responsible for the lipolysis of intramuscular triglycerides are less well characterized. In addition to the endothelial LPL, both cardiac and skeletal muscle contain acid (lysosomal) and neutral lipases of which the latter may be the intramuscular precursor of LPL (2–7). It is not known, however, which of these lipases releases the fatty acids from intramuscular triglycerides for direct oxidation in myocytes (7).

At the very beginning of exercise, the working skeletal muscles utilize preferentially their own glycogen stores. Due to the increased blood flow to exercising muscle, the muscular uptake of plasma FFA is increased even though the fractional FFA uptake is even less than at rest (8,9). Plasma FFA levels will first decrease, but upon continuation of the exercise, an increased release of catecholamines activates the hormone-sensitive lipase of adipose tissue and the accelerated lipolysis results in an increased flux and concentration of plasma FFA levels. Depending on the duration and intensity of the exercise, the muscles and heart derive up to 80% of their energy requirement from fatty acids. Of these, only one-third to one-half is taken directly from plasma FFA (and ultimately from adipose tissue) (10–12) while the rest is contributed by the intramuscular triglycerides. It is possible that the muscle already begins to utilize its own triglycerides at the very beginning of exercise (along with glycogen), the loss being more or less replaced by the influx from plasma FFA. In fact, it has been suggested that at rest, a major part of the FFA taken up by the muscle is first esterified and incorporated into some of the intramuscular triglyceride pools before entering the mitochondrial oxidation (13,14). At greater work loads or during prolonged exercise, the plasma FFA is turned over at a high rate and the muscles get progressively more of their energy directly from plasma FFA (10,12). In exhaustive work, the amount of muscle triglycerides decreases (12–17), indicating a net utilization of the muscles' own triglycerides. This decrease may ultimately be the factor which puts a limit on continued exercise and thus determines the total work performance (12).

Role of Plasma Triglycerides as a Source of Fatty Acids During Exercise

Plasma triglycerides represent a potential source of fatty acid substrate for moderate exercise. Their circulating mass is much greater than that of FFA and although they have a much slower fractional turnover rate than the FFA, the plasma triglyceride fatty acid flux is still substantial. This is particularly the case for chylomicrons which have a half-life of only 5 to 15 minutes. Moreover, both myocardium and skeletal muscles possess a high activity of LPL for utilization of lipoprotein triglycerides. In spite of these facts, it seems that at least VLDL triglycerides do not form any significant source of fatty acid for working muscles. The concentration of plasma triglycerides will not decrease during exercise even when it is exhausting and lasts for several hours like a marathon run (18–22). A significant fall of plasma triglyceride levels is observed only after the exercise has continued for 7 to 9 hours (23–25). Kinetic studies have uniformly shown that in spite of the increased blood flow, the rate of removal of endogenous plasma triglycerides is not increased during exercise (11,24). In an exercising human leg, the contribution of plasma triglycerides to total oxidized fatty acids has been estimated to be less than 10% (9).

Chylomicron triglycerides may be utilized more readily than VLDL by the exercising muscles. Exercise during the postprandial period diminishes the height of alimentary lipemia in man (26). Consistent with this, the removal of intravenously injected labeled chylomicrons is accelerated during exercise in rats (27,28), and induced muscular contractions in rat hindlimb preparation increase the uptake of chylomicron fatty acids by all skeletal muscle fiber types (29). On the other hand, exercise has not been found to increase the disappearance rate of intravenously injected Intralipid in man (30). This observation does not exclude the possibility, however, that the site of the principal removal of Intralipid during exercise is shifted from adipose tissue to the working skeletal muscles and heart. Indeed, such a change has been documented in rats (27,28). However, direct evidence for a significant role of chylomicron fat in the energy metabolism of exercising muscles is still lacking.

After the end of acute exercise, the plasma triglyceride levels start to decrease, reaching a nadir about 24 hours later (next morning). This change is accounted for by a fall of VLDL concentration (21) and it is observed not only after a strenuous prolonged exercise (20,21,25,31), but also following a one- or two-hour work at a well submaximal load level (22,32). This decrease may be a consequence of reduced hepatic FFA uptake (27,33) and the concomitant fall of VLDL synthesis during the exercise. However, there is also evidence of an accelerated removal of exogenous fat (Intralipid) from plasma during the post-exercise period in man (21). Thus, plasma triglycerides could contribute to the restoration of fat stores both in muscles and in adipose tissue after exercise rather than acting as a direct source of fuel during exercise.

Lipoprotein Lipase in Muscles

LPL is the key enzyme in the uptake of plasma triglycerides by various tissues. It represents an obligatory step in the utilization of all dietary fats. A great part of the body LPL activity is present in heart and skeletal muscles. The quantities of exogenous fat taken up by these tissues are quite substantial (34,35) and may correspond up to 50% of the energy requirement, e.g. in the human heart at rest (35). The uptake of chylomicron fatty acids by various muscles is closely related to their LPL activity (36,37), and removal of the endothelial lipoprotein lipase by heparin perfusion is followed by an abrupt fall in chylomicron uptake (38,39).

The LPL of heart and skeletal muscles resides in two separate pools. Capillary endothelial cells contain the enzyme which is responsible for the hydrolysis of plasma chylomicron and VLDL triglycerides. This enzyme is released by heparin and appears in heparin perfusate or postheparin plasma. The other pool is located in muscle cells and may represent the precursor of the endothelial enzyme. The muscle nonendothelial LPL has a low affinity for chylomicrons (40) and it has been suggested that this enzyme species has a physiological function in the hydrolysis of the intramuscular triglyceride stores (41). The endothelial and intramuscular forms of LPL in heart share many properties including common antigenic sites (42,43). The activities of both enzymes may be incresed by catecholamines (4,43,44) and by glucagon (45). The results of LPL assays from tissues may vary depending on whether the measurement is made from whole tissue homogenates or from heparin eluates. The former method includes both enzyme species present in muscle, whereas the latter measures mainly the endothelial LPL activity.

Response of Lipoprotein Lipase to Acute Exercise

Acute exercise modulates the LPL activity of muscles and adipose tissue in a manner which serves as a meaningful redistribution of circulating triglycerides. This was first demonstrated in a 1963 experiment where fed rats were forced to run on a treadmill for one hour and tissues were anlyzed for heparin-releasable LPL activity immediately after the exercise (46). The activity was increased in heart but reduced in adipose tissue, while no significant change was observed in skeletal muscle. The findings were confirmed in a later study (47) where a relationship was demonstrated between the increases of LPL activity and norepinephrine content of the heart muscle during exercise. The enzyme response was not dependent on catecholamines, however, since depletion of the myocardial catecholamine stores by reserpine treatment did not prevent the rise of LPL during exercise (47). A more prolonged or exhaustive muscular work will also increase the skeletal muscle LPL activity of experimental animals (48–50). In dogs, this response is observed in the fasting state, but it is completely abolished after a meal (50). The exercise-induced increase in the activity of the heparin-releasable muscle LPL of dogs is directly correlated to the duration of exercise and to the intensity of the work load (51). A dose-response relationship has been also observed in heart LPL of rats after swimming (41). Interestingly, the LPL activity remains high for as long as 24 to 48 hours after a single exercise bout in both heart (41,52) and skeletal muscle (41).

Fractionation of the muscle LPL into endothelial (heparin-releasable) and intramuscular (heparin-nonreleasable) enzyme types has increased our understanding of the mechanism of the lipase response to exercise. Oscai et al. (41) found that in rats studied 24 hours after a two-hour swimming, both the endothelial and intramuscular lipase activities of heart were increased. In another study, both fractions of myocardial LPL were already shown to be elevated at the end of exhaustive exercise in rats (53). Budohoski (51) followed the lipase responses in the working femoral muscle of dogs by sequential biopsies taken during a three-hour exercise period and found a reciprocal change of the two LPL species within two hours. The endothelial enzyme activity increased, whereas there was a remarkable decline in the intramuscular lipase activity. On continuation of exercise, the activity of the intramuscular enzyme returned to the pre-exercise level (51). A close inverse correlation was found to be present between the two lipase activities during the first two hours of exercise. In a non-exercising muscle of the same animals, the LPL activity decreased slightly (51). All these results suggest that exercise first stimulates the translocation of the intramuscular enzyme into endothelium and later induces synthesis of new enzyme molecules in myocytes. It is of interest that in perfused rat heart, catecholamines and glucagon cause exactly similar reciprocal changes as exercise in the activity of the two forms of LPL (43,44).

In the adipose tissue of experimental animals, exercise stimulates both basal and epinephrine-induced lipolysis in vitro (48,52,54). In contrast, the adipose tissue LPL activity is reduced (46,47,52,54). This is consistent with the enhanced lipolysis of the tissue's own triglycerides and may be accounted for by an increased intracellular concentration of free fatty acids in adipocyte (55,56). The suppression of LPL activity lasts for at least 24 hours after the exercise (52).

In *human subjects,* the response of muscle LPL to acute exercise is similar to that of animals, but adipose tissue seems to behave differently. A significant twofold average increase in the heparin-releasable LPL activity of skeletal muscle was observed when trained men run 20 km in fasting state (19). In contrast, no change of this activity could be found when an approximately similar exercise was performed in a postprandial state (57). Thus, as with the experience on dogs (50), meal intake also prevents the exercise-induced rise of muscle LPL in man. On the other hand, a prolonged and exhaustive exercise presented by an 85 km 8-hour ski race was followed by three-fold average increase in the muscle heparin-releasable LPL activity in spite of a repeated intake of food during the exercise (17). The magnitude of the lipase response was inversely correlated to fitness level (VO_2 max), being as much as 6-fold in the least fit men (17). The increase of LPL activity also showed an inverse relationship to the amount of visible fat in muscle fibers (17). The relative increase of muscle LPL during exercise is positively correlated with the relative decrease of plasma insulin/glucagon ratio (19).

In the adipose tissue of man, unlike the response in animals, exercise results in an increase of the heparin-released LPL activity (19,57). However, this change is quantitatively much less remarkable than that occurring in working muscle. The rise in the endothelial portion of tissue LPL activity upon strenuous exercise is also reflected in values measured from postheparin plasma (31). These still remain elevated 18 hours after cessation of the work (31).

The mechanism by which muscular work leads to the increase in LPL activity of heart and skeletal muscle and to the changes of the activity in adipose tissue is not clear. Since both glucagon and catecholamines are known to increase during exercise and, also, to stimulate the muscle LPL activity, they could afford one possible explanation. The increase in insulin sensitivity which regularly accompanies acute exercise does not account for the increment in muscle LPL because this enzyme does not seem to be insulin-dependent. On the other hand, the adipose tissue LPL is insulin-dependent and, therefore, its up-regulation by exercise in human subjects could be explained by the increase in insulin sensitivity and in glucose transport during acute exercise.

Physiological Function of Lipoprotein Lipase in Exercise

As stated above, it is generally agreed that working skeletal muscle and heart derive their fatty acids from circulating FFA and from intramuscular triglyceride stores. The role of VLDL triglyceride fatty acids as a fuel for exercising muscle is minimal, but chylomicron fatty acids may be utilized to some extent during the postprandial period. Thus, the exercise-induced rise of the functional LPL activity of skeletal muscle and heart does not seem to serve the increased energy requirements during exercise. It is, therefore, likely that a high activity of LPL is needed for the postexercise refilling of the triglyceride depots in muscle and fat cells. The rapid restoration of intramuscular triglyceride stores may be particularly important for the recovery of muscle after strenuous exercise. This adaptation enables the muscle to start a new working period more quickly and to continue it for a longer time. The abolishment of the LPL response to acute exercise by the intake of carbohydrates is appropriate because in this situation, the muscle can increase its glycogen stores and become less dependent on fatty acids.

Effects of Training on Fat Metabolism

Regularly repeated exercise induces metabolic adaptations which increase the maximal working capacity and enable the individual to maintain a submaximal level of exercise for longer periods of time than before training. In exercising skeletal muscle cells, the essential consequences of training are the increase of the mitochondrial content and of respiratory capacity (58). The trained muscles have a markedly enhanced potential to utilize fatty acids during exercise and consequently to spare glycogen and produce less lactate. Training also increases the synthesis of triglycerides in the muscles (59,60), but reports on the triglyceride content of trained *vs.* untrained muscle are controversial (61,62).

Training decreases the amount of adipose tissue and the size of fat cells (59,63). Both basal and hormone-stimulated lipolysis are increased (63–65) in the adipose tissue of exercise trained *vs.* sedentary rats. Thus, endurance training may enhance the mobilization of FFA from adipose tissue both at rest and during exercise. Simultaneously, the triglyceride synthesis is also increased (59,60).

Serum lipid and lipoprotein concentrations are also influenced by training. Well-trained subjects have lower mean levels of serum triglycerides and very low density lipoproteins, and higher concentrations of HDL (for review of this topic see references 66 and 67). The decrease of triglycerides may be mainly due to an accelerated clearance from the plasma, but training also decreases the secretion of new VLDL into plasma (68,69).

Effect of Training on Lipoprotein Lipase Activity Levels

The studies on the effect of exercise training on tissue LPL activities of experimental animals have given somewhat inconsistent results. Borenstzajn et al. (70) measured the lipoprotein lipase from tissue homogenates of trained rats and found a significant increase of the activity in all fiber types of skeletal muscle, but no change in the lipase activity of myocardium. In contrast, several other investigators were unable to find any difference between the muscle, heart or adipose tissue LPL activities of trained and sedentary rats (48,71–73). Oscai et al. (41,43) found a significant increase of the activity of the intracellular portion of muscle LPL but no change in the endothelial enzyme activity during strenuous training of rats. Walberg et al. (74) on the other hand, could demonstrate a rise in muscle, heart and adipose tissue heparin-releasable (endothelial) LPL activity during swim training of obese Zucker rats. The reasons for these relatively large discrepancies are not readily apparent.

Human studies have consistently shown that endurance training is associated with striking increases of the endothelial LPL activity both in skeletal muscle and adipose tissue (75). Moreover, these changes appear to provide an obvious explanation for the low VLDL and elevated HDL levels of physically active people (75). In a cross-sectional study of competitive runners, we showed that endurance trained male and female subjects had significantly higher heparin-releasable LPL activity in skeletal muscle than matched sedentary controls (75). Male runners showed an increased LPL activity also in adipose tissue. A similar trend was also present in female runners, but the difference from controls was not significant. Estimated whole body adipose tissue plus skeletal muscle LPL activity was about two times higher in runners than in control subjects. The adipose tissue LPL activity showed a significant positive correlation to the average weekly running mileage. In contrast to the long-distance runners, the sprinters with mainly non-endurance (power) training had tissue LPL activities no different from those of sedentary controls (75). In the whole group, there was a highly significant positive ($r = +0.72$) correlation between the plasma HDL cholesterol levels and the adipose tissue LPL activity (75). On the basis of these results, it was suggested that aerobic training induces the LPL activity (at least that fraction which is bound to capillary endothelium) of muscle and adipose tissue.

These findings have been amply confirmed in subsequent studies. In a cross-sectional examination of young healthy males, Marniemi et al. (76) found a significant linear positive correlation between the reported weekly physical activity and adipose tissue LPL activity. Lithell et al. (77,78) studied an unselected sample of middle-aged men from a Swedish population survey and showed that the heparin-releasable LPL activity level of the gastrocnemius muscle correlated positively with the capillary density, but inversely with the mean muscle fiber area and relative body weight. Unexpectedly, no relationship has been found between the muscle fiber composition and LPL activity (75,77).

Most convincingly, the effects of training become evident from longitudinal studies where the same subjects are assessed before and after either shorter periods of strenuous exercise, or less exhaustive but systematic long-term aerobic training. Costill et al. (79) trained normal healthy young males by a 10-week running program and could demonstrate a significant average 30% increase in the LPL activity of the gastrocnemius muscle. Peltonen et al. (80) subjected sedentary middle-aged men to a 15-week moderate endurance training and followed the response of postheparin plasma LPL activity, comparing it to respcctive assays made in a parallel untrained control group. A significant increase was already observed after one week of training and this change persisted throughout the exercise period. The adipose tissue LPL activity studied before and at the end of the program also increased by an average of 30% over that of the control group. However, the magnitude of the individual LPL responses to training did not correlate with the increase in physical fitness. In a similar follow-up study, Svedenhag et al. (81) found a 47% average increase in the skeletal muscle LPL activity during 8 weeks of regular cycle ergometer training of healthy young males. The capillary density of the exercising muscles was also increased, but there was no correlation between the individual changes of the capillary density and LPL activity. Simultaneous administration of a beta-adrenergic blocking drug did not abolish the enzyme or capillary response to training (81). Cessation of exercise for ten days in highly trained men resulted in a significant fall of postheparin plasma LPL activity (82). Simultaneously, the

HDL and HDL_2 cholesterol levels decreased progressively while no change was observed in HDL_3 cholesterol or apo A-I concentrations (82).

In persons with good basal physical fitness and a high muscular LPL activity level, an additional strenuous training (exercise) period increases the enzyme activity further. Lithell et al. (83) carried out serial muscle biopsies in soldiers during five-day field maneuvers and found a threefold increase in the LPL activity of the vastus lateralis muscle. The high levels persisted for at least five days after the end of the exercise period. Serum triglyceride concentration decreased concomitant with the rise of LPL activity (83). In another similar study, the same group of investigators followed well-trained soldiers during a heavy 10-day mountain march (84). The muscle LPL activity attained a maximal level by the second day, being higher in the afternoons than in the mornings. These very high activities (up to tenfold normal) were obviously caused by a combination of the effects of training and acute exercise. Interestingly, the afternoon muscle LPL activities were significantly correlated with urinary epinephrine excretion rates measured at the same time. In covariance analysis, the epinephrine accounted for 71% of the variation of the muscle LPL activity (84). These findings in man are consistent with the earlier observations in rats (47) and further support the view that the exercise-induced increase in muscle (including myocardium) LPL activity is mediated by catecholamines.

Only few studies have been published on the response of LPL to training or exercise in disease conditions. Costill et al. (79) found that male juvenile-onset (Type I) diabetic patients showed an increase in muscle LPL activity during systematic endurance training similar to that found in nondiabetic males. In contrast, Lithell et al. (85) failed to observe any change in the skeletal muscle LPL of Type I or Type II (adult-onset) diabetic patients, or of nondiabetic obese women during a 10-week training period. Since the capillary density also did not increase in the diabetic subjects, the absent response of LPL was accounted for by the failure of capillary density to change during training (85). This might also explain why strength athletes with mainly anaerobic training do not show any increase in the muscle LPL activity (75). Upon training, these subjects develop a muscle fiber hypertrophy without a parallel increase of capillarization, resulting in the decrease of capillary density (86). On the other hand, the reasons for the defective muscle capillarization during training in diabetics are not clear. No studies have been carried out on the possibility of increasing muscle or adipose tissue LPL by exercise in patients with hypertriglyceridemia and subnormal LPL activity.

Summary and Conclusions

The working muscles cover their extra fuel requirements either from intramuscular glycogen and triglyceride stores, or from blood glucose or FFA. According to current evidence, the plasma triglycerides transported as chylomicrons or VLDL, although a potential source of fatty acids, contribute little direct energy to contracting skeletal muscles, but may be utilized by heart muscle. However, skeletal muscles and myocardium possess a high activity of LPL which regulates the uptake of chylomicron and VLDL fatty acids in these tissues. Both acute exercise and endurance training influence the LPL activity of skeletal muscles, heart, and adipose tissue.

In both animals and man, the skeletal muscle LPL activity is increased by acute exercise. The effect persists for hours or even days after the exercise has come to end. It is, however, completely abolished by eating. The increase occurs primarily in the LPL located at muscle capillary endothelial cells and it is probably caused by an increased rate of translocation of the enzyme to capillaries from myocytes. Upon continued exercise, the intramuscular lipase activity will also increase. The mechanism of this adaptive change is so far unknown, but it might be mediated by the exercise-induced increase in muscle catecholamines. In adipose tissue of experimental animals, exercise causes a decrease of LPL activity. This effect may result from product inhibition by the FFA released in larger amounts from fat cells during exercise. Paradoxically, the adipose tissue LPL activity has been found to rise in man after acute exercise. However, this change is much less remarkable than the change which occurs in skeletal muscle.

Regular endurance training increases the LPL activity in both skeletal muscle and adipose tissue of man. The change is roughly proportional to the intensity of training. Good physical fitness is accompanied by high average LPL activity in muscle, adipose tissue, and postheparin plasma. Since the LPL influences both removal of triglycerides from the plasma and the synthesis of plasma high density lipoproteins (HDL), it is likely that both the low VLDL and high HDL concentrations characteristic for physically well-trained people are explained by the induction of LPL upon regular exercise. The mechanism of this adaptive change is not clear, but it might be related to the increase of capillary density of skeletal muscles during endurance training. In anaerobic power type training, the muscle capillaries do not proliferate and the LPL activity remains at the level of untrained muscle.

Training adapts the muscles to utilize fatty acids as fuel for exercise more readily than the untrained state, and thus to spare glycogen and produce less lactate. Whether the increase of LPL activity enables the skeletal muscles and heart to directly oxidize circulating triglyceride fatty acids during exercise is not known, but this would be a plausible possibility. Regardless, the increased rate of uptake of chylomicron and VLDL triglyceride fatty acids due to the high LPL activity provides the trained muscles an opportunity to rapidly replace the intramuscular triglyceride stores utilized during exercise. Because the size of the muscles' own triglyceride pool is thought to be the key determinant of total work performance, the rate of refilling of this pool may become the crucial factor deciding both the maximal working capacity and the length of time which an individual can exercise at submaximal work load. Thus, ultimately the LPL may have a key position in the determination of the individual fitness level reached by a given intensity of training.

The writing of this review has been generously supported by a grant from the Finnish Medical Research Council (Academy of Finland).

References

1. Wetzel, M. G., and R. O. Scow. 1984. *Am J. Physiol.* 246:C467–C485.
2. Severson, D. L. 1979. *J. Molec. Cell. Cardiol.* 11:569–583.
3. Chohan, P., and A. Cryer. 1979. *Biochem. J.* 181:83–93.
4. Palmer, W. K., R. A. Caruso, and L. B. Oscai. 1981. *Biochem. J.* 198:159–166.
5. Stam, H., and W. C. Hülsmann. 1983. *Biochem. Int.* 7:187–195.
6. Strohfeldt, P., and C. Heugel. 1984. *Biochem. Biophys. Res. Commun.* 121:87–94.
7. Hülsmann, W. C., H. Stam, and H. Jansen. 1984. *Basic Res. Cardiol.* 79:268–273.
8. Spitzer, J. J., and M. Gold. 1964. *Am. J. Physiol.* 206(I):159–163.
9. Havel, R. J., B. Pernow, and N. L. Jones. 1967. *J. Appl. Physiol.* 23(I):90–99.
10. Havel, R. J., L. -G. Ekelund, and A. Holmgren. 1967. *J. Lipid Res.* 8:366–373.
11. Issekutz, B. Jr., H. I. Miller, P. Paul, and K. Rodahl. 1964. *Am. J. Physiol.* 207(3):583–589.
12. Carlson, L. A., L. -G. Ekelund and S. O. Fröberg. 1971. *Europ. J. Clin. Invest.* 1:248–254.
13. Dagenais, G. R., R. G. Tancredi, and K. L. Zierler. 1976. *J. Clin. Invest.* 58:421–431.
14. Zierler, K. L. 1976. *Circulation Res.* 38:459–463.
15. Fröberg, S. O., and F. Mossfeldt. 1971. *Acta physiol. scand.* 82:167–171.
16. Baldwin, K. M., J. S. Reitman, R. L. Terjung, W. W. Winder, and J. O. Holloszy. 1973. *Am. J. Physiol.* 225(5):1045–1050.
17. Lithell, H., J. Örlander, R. Schéle, B. Sjödin, and J. Karlsson. 1979. *Acta Physiol. Scand.* 107:257–261.
18. Hurter, R., M. A. Peyman, J. Swale, and C. W. H. Barnett. 1972. *Lancet* II:671–675.
19. Taskinen, M. -R., E. A. Nikkilä, S. Rehunen, and A. Gordin. 1980. *Artery* 6(6):471–483.
20. Thompson, P. D., E. Cullinane, L. O. Henderson, and P. N. Herbert. 1980. *Metabolism* 29:662–665.
21. Dufaux, B., G. Assmann, U. Order, A. Hoederath, and W. Hollmann. 1981. *Int. J. Sports Med.* 2:256–260.
22. Cullinane, E., S. Siconolfi, A. Saritelli, and P. D. Thompson. 1982. *Metabolism* 31:844–847.
23. Carlson, L. A., and F. Mossfeldt. 1964. *Acta physiol. scand.* 62:51–59.
24. Young, D. R., J. Shapira, R. Forrest, R. R. Adachi, R. Lim, and R. Pelligra. 1967. *J. Appl. Physiol.* 23:716–725.
25. Enger, S. C., S. B. Strømme, and H. E. Refsum. 1980. *Scand. J. clin. Lab. Invest.* 40:341–345.
26. Nikkilä, E. A., and A. Konttinen. 1962. *Lancet* I:1151–1154.
27. Jones, M. L., and R. J. Havel. 1967. *Am. J. Physiol.* 213(4):824–828.
28. Terjung, R. L., L. Budohoski, K. Nazar, A. Kobryn, and H. Kaciuba-Uscilko. 1982. *J. Appl. Physiol.* 52(4):815–820.
29. Mackie, B. G., G. A. Dudley, H. Kaciuba-Uscilko, and R. L. Terjung. 1980. *J. Appl. Physiol.* 49(5):851–855.
30. Carlson, L. A., L. -G Ekelund, S. O. Fröberg, and D. Hallberg. 1967. *Acta Med. Scand. suppl.* 472:245–252.
31. Kantor, M. A., E. M. Cullinane, P. N. Herbert, and P. D. Thompson. 1984. *Metabolism* 33:454–457.

32. Holm, G., P. Björntorp, and R. Jagenburg. 1978. *J. Appl. Physiol.* 45(1):128–131.
33. Hagenfeldt, L., and J. Wahren. 1973. *Metabolism* 22:815–820.
34. Kaijser, L., and S. Rössner. 1975. *Acta med. scand.* 197:289–294.
35. Carlson, L. A., L. Kaijser, S. Rössner, and M. L. Wahlqvist. 1973. *Acta med. scand.* 193:233–245.
36. Linder, C., S. S. Chernick, T. R. Fleck, and R. O. Scow. 1976. *Am. J. Physiol.* 231(3):860–864.
37. Tan, M. H., T. Sata, and R. J. Havel. 1977. *J. Lipid Res.* 18:363–370.
38. Enser, M. B., F. Kunz, J. Borensztajn, L. H. Opie, and D. S. Robinson. 1967. *Biochem. J.* 104:306–317.
39. Borensztajn, J., and D. S. Robinson. 1970. *J. Lipid Res.* 11:111–117.
40. Ben-Zeev, O., H. Schwalb, and M.C. Schotz. 1981. *FEBS Lett.* 136:95–97.
41. Oscai, L. B., R. A. Caruso, and A. C. Wergeles. 1982. *J. Appl. Physiol.* 52(4):1059–1063.
42. Hülsmann, W. C., H. Stam, and W. A. P. Breeman. 1982. *Biochem. Biophys. Res. Commun.* 108:371–378.
43. Stam, H., and W. C. Hülsmann. 1984. *Biochim. Biophys Acta* 794:72–82.
44. Simpson, J. 1979. *Biochem. J.* 182:253–255.
45. Borensztajn, J., P. Keig, and A. H. Rubenstein. 1973. *Biochem. Biophys. Res. Commun.* 53:603–608.
46. Nikkilä, E. A., P. Torsti, and O. Penttilä. 1963. *Metabolism* 12:863–869.
47. Nikkilä, E. A., P. Torsti, and O. Penttilä. 1965. *Life Sci.* 4:27–35.
48. Askew, E. W., G. L. Dohm, R. L. Huston, T. W. Sneed, and R. P. Dowdy. 1972. *Proc. Soc. Exp. Biol. Med.* 141:123–129.
49. Kozlowski, S., L. Budohoski, E. Pokoska, and K. Nazar. 1979. *Pflügers Arch.* 382:105–107.
50. Budohoski, L., S. Kozlowski, R. L. Terjung, H. Kaciuba-Uscilko, K. Nazar, and I. Falecka-Wieczorek. 1982. *Pflügers Arch.* 394:191–193.
51. Budohoski, L. 1985. *Pflügers Arch.* 405:188–192.
52. Barakat, H. A., D. S. Kerr, E. B. Tapscott, and G. L. Dohm. 1981. *Proc. Soc. Exper. Biol. Med.* 166:162–166.
53. Goldberg, D. I., W. L. Rumsey, and Z. V. Kendrick. 1984. *Metabolism* 33:964–969.
54. Nikkilä, E. A., and P. Torsti. 1967. *In:* Physical Activity and the Heart. M. J. Karvonen, and A. J. Barry, editors. Chapter 19:216–224. Charles C Thomas Publisher/Springfield, 1967.
55. Nikkilä, E. A., and O. Pykälistö. 1968. *Life Sci* 7:1303–1309.
56. Patten, R. L. 1970. *J. Biol. Chem.* 245:5577–5584.
57. Lithell, H., K. Hellsing, G. Lundqvist, and P. Malmberg. 1979. *Acta Physiol. Scand.* 105:312–315.
58. Holloszy, J. O., and E. F. Coyle. 1984. *J. Appl. Physiol.* 56(4):831–838.
59. Björntorp, P., M. Fahlén, G. Grimby, A. Gustafson, J. Holm, P. Renström, and T. Schersten. 1972. *Metabolism* 21:1037–1044.
60. Askew, E. W., R. L. Huston, and G. L. Dohm. 1973. *Metabolism* 22:473–480.
61. Morgan, T. E., F. A. Short, and L. A. Cobb. 1969. *Amer. J. Physiol.* 216:82–86.
62. Fröberg, S. O. 1971. *Metabolism* 20:714–720.
63. Askew, A. W., C. G. Huston, C. G. Plopper, and A. L. Hecker. 1975. *J. Clin. Invest.* 56:521–529.
64. Fröberg, S. O., I. Östman, and N. O. Sjöstrand. 1972. *Acta Physiol. Scand.* 86:166–174.
65. Bukowiecki, L., J. Lupien, N. Follea, A. Paradis, D. Richard, and J. LeBlanc. 1980. *Am. J. Physiol.* 239:E422–E429.
66. Wood, P. D., and W. L. Haskell. 1979. *Lipids* 14:417–427.
67. Dufaux, B., G. Assmann, and W. Hollmann. 1982. *Int. J. Sports Med.* 3:123–136.
68. Simonelli, C., and R. P. Eaton. 1978. *Am. J. Physiol.* 234(3):E221–E227.
69. Mondon, C. E., C. B. Dolkas, T. Tobey, and G. M. Reaven. 1984. *J. Appl. Physiol.* 57(5):1466–1471.

70. Borensztajn, J., M. S. Rone, S. P. Babirak, J. A. McGarr, and L. B. Oscai. 1975. *Am. J. Physiol.* 229:394–397.
71. Zavaroni, I., Y. I. Chen, C. E. Mondon, and G. M. Reaven. 1981. *Metabolism* 30:476–480.
72. Tan, M. H., A. Bonen, J. B. Garner, and A. N. Belcastro. 1982. *J. Appl. Physiol.* 52(6):1514–1518.
73. Kimball, T. J., M. T. Childs, D. Applebaum-Bowden, and W. L. Sembrowich. 1983. *Metabolism* 32:497–503.
74. Walberg, J. L., M. R. C. Greenwood, and J. S. Stern. 1983. *Am. J. Physiol.* 245:R706–712.
75. Nikkilä, E. A., M. -R. Taskinen, S. Rehunen, and M. Härkönen. 1978. *Metabolism* 27:1661–1671.
76. Marniemi, J., P. Peltonen, I. Vuori, and E. Hietanen. 1980. *Acta Physiol. Scand.* 110:131–135.
77. Lithell, H., F. Lindgärde, K. Hellsing, G. Lundqvist, E. Nygaard, B. Vessby and B. Saltin. 1981. *Diabetes* 30:19–25.
78. Lithell, H., F. Lindgärde, E. Nygaard, and B. Saltin. 1981. *Acta Physiol. Scand.* 111:383–384.
79. Costill, D. L., P. Clearly, W. J. Fink, C. Foster, J. L. Ivy, and F. Witztum. 1979. *Diabetes* 28:818–822.
80. Peltonen, P., J. Marniemi, E. Hietanen, I. Vuori, and C. Ehnholm. 1981. *Metabolism* 30:518–525.
81. Svedenhag, J., H. Lithell, A. Juhlin-Dannfelt, and J. Henriksson. 1983. *Atherosclerosis* 49:203–207.
82. Thompson, P. D., E. M. Cullinane, R. Eshleman, S. P. Sady, and P. N. Herbert. 1984. *Metabolism* 33:943–950.
83. Lithell, H., R. Schéle, B. Vessby, and I. Jacobs. 1984. *J. Apply. Physiol.* 57:698–702.
84. Lithell, H., M. Cedermark, J. Fröberg, P. Tesch, and J. Karlsson. 1981. *Metabolism* 30:1130–1134.
85. Lithell, H., M. Krotkiewski, B. Kiens, Z. Wroblewski, G. Holm, G. Strömblad, G. Grimby, and P. Björntorp. 1985. *Diabetes Res.* 2:17–21.
86. Tesch, P. A., A. Thorsson, and P. Kaiser. 1984. *J. Appl. Physiol.* 56:35–38.

Chapter 8

LIPOPROTEIN LIPASE IN HYPERTRIGLYCERIDEMIAS

Marja-Riitta Taskinen

Hypertriglyceridemias are a heterogeneous group of lipid disorders which can be due to primary metabolic abnormalities or secondary to a variety of other diseases. In an individual, the concentration of plasma triglycerides depends on the balance between the rates of production and removal of triglyceride-rich particles. Because lipoprotein lipase (LPL) is the rate limiting enzyme in the removal process, the reduction of its activity can lead to hypertriglyceridemia—the best documented example being Type I hyperlipoproteinemia which occurs as a result of LPL deficiency. The role of LPL defects in the etiology of other genetic, as well as secondary, hypertriglyceridemias is largely inconclusive. The lack of adequate methodology to measure LPL activity in human subjects was for a long time a major limiting factor. However, methodological advances during the past ten years have allowed assays of LPL activity in postheparin plasma as well as small samples of human adipose tissue and skeletal muscle, and thus advanced our understanding of the role of LPL in hypertriglyceridemias. This overview examines recent data on LPL activity in primary hypertriglyceridemias and in specific secondary hypertriglyceridemias which can be causally related to alterations of LPL activity.

LPL Activity in Normolipidemic Subjects

In human subjects, heparin-releasable LPL activity has been measured in postheparin plasma and tissue specimens of adipose tissue and skeletal muscle taken by needle biopsy techniques. Table 1 shows reference values for the LPL activity in tissues and in postheparin plasma of healthy men and women. The enzyme activity in gluteal adipose tissue is higher in women than in men as documented in two previous studies (1,2). In contrast, no sex difference is apparent for muscle LPL activity. Huttunen et al. (3), have previously reported that LPL activity in postheparin plasma is higher in women than in men. However, this was not confirmed by the data in Table 1. The lack of sex difference has also been noted in several other studies (4–7). The values for LPL activity differ markedly amongst various studies. The difference for postheparin plasma has been reported to be 10-fold (7) and it is even greater for adipose tissue LPL activity (0.34 vs 6.63 micromol FFA/g/h) (8,9). Alterations seem to be less in muscle LPL than in adipose tissue LPL (9,10). The reference values shown in Table 1 are clearly lower than those reported previously (9). This was due to slight modifications in the preparation of the substrate used in the assays. Similar variations in reference values within the same laboratory has also been reported by Lithell et al. (11,12) for muscle LPL and is apparent from the data from other laboratories as well (13,14). These observations emphasize the need for adequate and actual reference material analyzed in parallel with experimental samples for each study. The normal range for both muscle and adipose tissue LPL activity is considerable (Table 1), indicating that the removal capacity varies considerably from person to person.

Figure 1 shows that in normal subjects, postheparin plasma LPL activity correlates positively with the enzyme activity in both adipose tissue and skeletal muscle. Thus, postheparin plasma LPL can be used as an indicator for tissue LPL activities in normal subjects. The role of LPL activity as a physiological determinant for the concentration of serum triglycerides is supported by observations that in nonobese normolipidemic men, the concentration of very low density lipoproteins (VLDL) triglycerides correlates inversely with adipose tissue LPL ($r = -0.32$, $P < 0.05$), skeletal muscle LPL ($r = -0.54$, $P < 0.01$) and with postheparin plasma LPL activity ($r = -0.56$, $P < 0.01$). The data suggest that muscle tissue is more important

TABLE I LPL activity in tissues and in postheparin plasma in non-obese healthy subjects

LPL Activity in	Men	Women
adipose tissue*	1.98 ± 0.30 (n = 26)	3.10 ± 0.35[xx] (n = 20)
skeletal muscle*	0.57 ± 0.04 (n = 19)	0.62 ± 0.06 (n = 20)
postheparin plasma†	23.3 ± 1.3 (n = 49)	22.8 ± 1.1 (n = 47)

*μmol FFA.g^{-1}.h^{-1}, †μmol FFA.ml^{-1}.h^{-1}
Figures in parenthesis represent the number of subjects.
[xx]$p < 0.01$ for the difference from men.

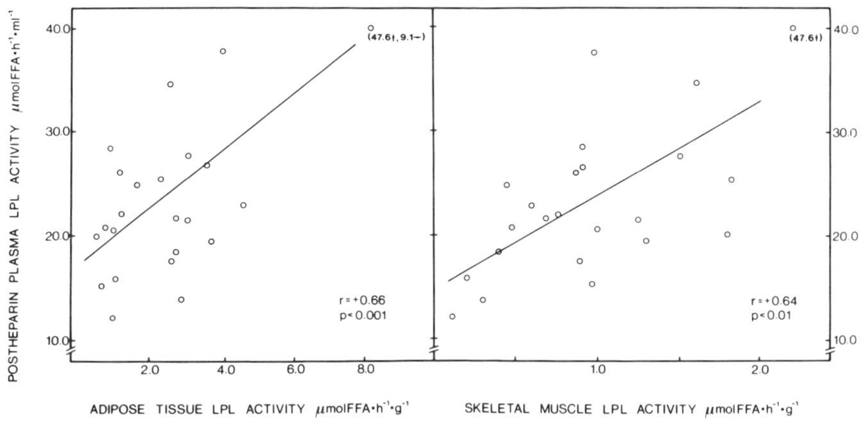

FIGURE 1 Simple (Pearson) correlations for postheparin plasma LPL activity with adipose tissue LPL activity (left) and skeletal muscle LPL activity (right) in nonobese normolipidemic men.

in the removal of circulating VLDL than adipose tissue. This concept is consistent with the data of Lithell (10) and with the results obtained from forearm studies (15).

LPL Activity in Familial Chylomicronemias

Type I hyperlipoproteinemia

Type I hyperlipoproteinemia has been defined as an inherited deficiency of LPL since the pioneer work of Havel and Gordon (16) who documented the absence of lipolytic activity as the cause of this disorder. More recently, however, it has been shown that Type I hyperlipoproteinemia is etiologically heterogeneous, and that several inborn defects can lead to the impairment of chylomicron removal and resultant hyperchylomicronemia (Table 2). In Type I, the plasma lipoprotein pattern is characterized by chylomicronemia, normal or marginally increased VLDL level, and by decreased low density (LDL) and high density lipoproteins (HDL) concentrations. The restriction of dietary fat is followed by a fall of serum triglycerides and the disappearance of chylomicrons; the disorder has also been defined as fat-induced hyperlipidemia. The clinical picture includes recurrent abdominal pains, pancreatitis, hepato- and splenomegaly, eruptive xanthoma, lipemia retinalis and, commonly, an onset in early childhood. On the basis of the clinical presentation alone, it is not possible to distinguish the different inborn errors behind the Type I phenotype (17). This requires the measurements of LPL activity in tissues (adipose tissue and skeletal muscle) and in postheparin plasma, the assay of plasma activator capacity for LPL, the measurements of apoprotein concentrations, and the verification of the presence or absence

TABLE II Etiology of hyperchylomicronemia syndromes

Type I hyperlipoproteinemia
• LPL deficiency
• Apo CII deficiency
• Other genetic defects
• Acquired disorder
Type V hyperlipoproteinemia
• Familial disorder
• Sporadic disorder
• Secondary to other diseases

of plasma inhibitors for LPL. An excellent review on familial LPL deficiency and related disorders of chylomicron metabolism was recently authored by Nikkilä (17).

LPL deficiency. LPL deficiency is a rare autosomal recessive disorder with an estimated frequency of less than one per million (17). In earlier studies, the diagnosis of LPL deficiency was based on the measurement of postheparin plasma lipolytic activity (16–23). In Type I patients, the postheparin plasma lipolytic activity (PHLA) is negligible when chylomicrons are used as substrate (16,18–21). The data were less consistent in assay systems using artificial fat emulsions as the substrate, and both low and low-normal values have been reported for patients with Type I hyperlipoproteinemia (16,18–21,23). As discussed by Nilsson-Ehle (see Chapter 3), the lipolytic activity in postheparin plasma contains LPL from different sources (adipose tissue, skeletal muscle, lungs) and other lipolytic enzymes (phospholipases and monoglyceride hydrolase). Hepatic lipase is another enzyme which, like LPL is released into circulation by heparin. Since the hepatic lipase activity in postheparin plasma of Type I patients is within normal range (4,5,24–28), the variation in their PHLA activity is explicable and the interpretation of earlier data ought to be reconsidered.

Specific methods which separate LPL and hepatic lipase activities in postheparin plasma, have been available since 1974. The absence or extremely low LPL activity (less than 10% of the mean levels in normolipidemic controls) characterize the probands with Type I hyperlipoproteinemia (4,5,24,26–30). This is consistent with absent or very low enzyme activity in adipose tissue (31). Interestingly, although the LPL activity has not yet been measured in the skeletal muscle of Type I patients, the markedly reduced LPL activity in postheparin plasma implies that the muscle LPL must be low. Brunzell et al. (32) have documented two unique cases: In one case, the LPL activity was absent in adipose tissue but the postheparin plasma LPL value was close to normal. In the second case, the enzyme activity in adipose tissue was normal but that in postheparin plasma was markedly reduced. These individual cases suggest that LPL deficiency can be selective at the tissue level. However, the majority of the diagnosed patients have presented "classical" LPL deficiency.

Havel and Gordon (16) were the first to demonstrate that the catabolic rate of chylomicrons is reduced in Type I patients. Further metabolic studies in LPL deficient subjects have confirmed these preliminary findings, and convincingly proved the central role of LPL in the catabolism of triglyceride-rich particles (20,27). LPL deficiency has also provided a model to study metabolic interrelations between different lipoproteins (26,33,34). A puzzling question has, however, remained unsolved: Why is the concentration of triglycerides increased only in chylomicrons but not in VLDL in Type I patients? Kinetic studies have demonstrated that the removal rate of large triglyceride-rich particles is slow in Type I patients (16,20,33) whereas the fractional catabolic rate as well as the synthetic rate of VLDL apoprotein B is nearly normal (26,35). Thus, patients with LPL deficiency appear able to clear VLDL particles from circulation. Consequently, VLDL particles must be removed by some alternative mechanisms which do not involve LPL.

Substantial evidence has been derived from family studies for an autosomal recessive trait in Type I hyperlipoproteinemia (21,28–31,36). Several investigators have documented low LPL activity in postheparin plasma or in adipose tissue together with an elevation of serum triglyceriides in at least one or two siblings of the proband (16,19–21,25,27,28,31,36). Parental consanguinity has been present in several (22,26,31) but not all families (16,20,21,27,28). Studies in pedigrees with several generations have indicated that a subnormal or intermediate LPL activity is a marker in heterozygotes (19,21,25,28,36). The majority of the heterozygotes have, however, normal fasting serum triglyceride levels (28,31), but they show an impaired clearance of chylomicrons during an oral fat tolerance test (31). In conclusion, an autosomal recessive pattern of inheritance seems to be valid for LPL deficiency. Wilson et al. (27) have recently questioned this concept and suggested that multiple-gene mechanisms could be involved at least in some kindreds with Type I hyperlipoproteinemia. They reported a large pedigree with Type I hyperlipoproteinemia coexisting with mixed-phenotype hyperlipidemia. This interesting data indicates the need for further genetic studies with more specific markers.

The molecular basis of LPL deficiency remains unknown. Theoretically, the synthesis of the enzyme may be defective or the enzyme may be a nonfunctional mutant. The development of specific immunoassays which measure the amount of the enzyme protein, as well as the use of monoclonal antibodies which identify different structural units within the enzyme, are needed to solve this problem.

Apoprotein CII deficiency. A prerequisite for the function of LPL is its interaction with apoprotein CII (apo CII), which is a specific activator of LPL-induced lipolysis (37). Apo CII is normally carried in triglyceride-rich particles and in HDL. Nascent VLDL particles pick up apo CII from HDL particles, but during lipolysis apo CII is transferred from chylomicrons and VLDL back to HDL (37). In 1978, Breckenridge and coworkers (38) described the first case of apo CII deficiency as the cause of Type I phenotype. Since the original report, at least twenty two new cases have been documented (39). The studies in patients with apo CII deficiency have established the functional role of this apoprotein in LPL-induced lipolysis (37).

The lipoprotein pattern in both apo CII deficiency and LPL deficiency is very similar (17,39) although the clinical presentation reveals some differences. In apo CII deficiency the age of onset of the clinical symptoms seems to be slightly later than in LPL deficiency. The hepato- and splenomegaly are less common, the occurrence of eruptive xanthoma is rare and episodes of recurrent abdominal pains and pancreatitis are frequent (17,38,39). The lipoprotein pattern is characterized by hyperchylomicronemia, normal or slightly increased VLDL level but low LDL and HDL levels (38–40). The cornerstone of the diagnosis is the absence of apo CII in the whole plasma and/or in triglyceride-rich particles. In patients with apo CII deficiency, postheparin plasma LPL activity is markedly reduced or undetectable if the patient's own plasma is the source of both the enzyme activity and its activator (38,41,42). In contrast, if the assay system for LPL includes normal plasma or purified apo CII as activator source, the enzyme activity may be increased (38,41,42) or normal (28,38). Brunzell et al. (43) reported very high LPL activity in the adipose tissue of a patient with apo CII deficiency and concluded that high LPL activity is a compensatory mechanism to counterbalance the defective catabolism of chylomicrons (43).

The infusion of normal plasma into patients with apo CII deficiency results in a rapid and dramatic decrease of serum triglyceride levels and in the disappearance of plasma chylomicrons (38,42,44,45). While it has been shown that these alterations are accompanied by increases in LDL (42,45), the data on HDL is less conclusive (42,45). Thus, patients with apo CII deficiency provide another excellent model with which to study the metabolic interrelations between different lipoproteins during lipolysis.

The family studies indicate that the absence of apo CII, like LPL deficiency, is an autosomal recessive disorder (28,41,42,46). The concentration of apo CII in obligate heterozygotes in different kindreds is low, averaging 30–50% from that in normal subjects (46). Interestingly, the heterozygotes have normal or only marginally increased levels of serum triglycerides when compared with age and sex-matched normolipidemic subjects (28,46). This implies that less than half the normal concentration of apo CII in plasma is sufficient to guarantee an adequate rate of lipolysis. For example, the concentration of apo CII in homozygotes after infusions of normal plasma remained low (less than 10–20% of normal levels) but, nevertheless, intravascular lipolysis occurred (38). Therefore, the concentration of apo CII cannot be a rate-limiting factor *in vivo* in the catabolism of triglyceride-rich particles under physiological conditions (37). Recent studies have shown that in one kindred both homozygotes and heterozygotes with apo CII deficiency have two non-functional mutant forms of apo CII; i.e. apo CII-X and apo CII-Y (47). In addition, four other types of molecular defects have been identified in apo CII deficient kindreds (H. B. Brewer, Jr., personal communication). It is evident that although many questions remain to be answered regarding apo CII deficiency, more is known about the genetic and molecular basis of this condition than LPL deficiency.

Other genetic Type I hyperlipoproteinemias. Stalenhoef et al. (48) have described two siblings with Type I phenotype resulting from the deficiency of LPL activity together with the absence of both apo CII and apo E-3. The lipoprotein pattern is characteristic for Type I phenotype and the family study suggested an autosomally recessive trait. The infusion of normal plasma into the patients could not restore the lipolytic activity and the fall of serum triglycerides was small. Brunzell and co-workers (43) reported another unique family with Type I phenotype, where the cause of hyperlipoproteinemia was the presence of LPL inhibitor in plasma. These studies demonstrate that Type I phenotype can be caused by several metabolic errors which prevent the removal of chylomicrons from circulation.

Acquired Type I hyperlipoproteinemias. Type I hyperlipoproteinemias can also be acquired i.e., secondary to other diseases. Glueck et al. (49) described three patients with Type I phenotype who had dysglobulinemias, and proposed that the observed low PHLA activity in these cases was due to an interaction between heparin and immunoglobulins. The gross hyperlipidemia in these patients suggests that immunoglobulins interact with LPL at the endothelial surface and prevent its physiological function.

Type V Hyperlipoproteinemia

Patients with Type V hyperlipoproteinemia show fasting chylomicronemia as well as elevation of VLDL triglyceride. Although this disorder is more common than Type I hyperlipoproteinemia, it is, nevertheless, a rare cause of hypertriglyceridemia with a highly diverse etiology. Common secondary causes for Type V hyperlipoproteinemia are diabetes, alcoholism, nephrotic syndrome and hypothyroidism (50–52). The clinical features of Type V share many similarities with Type I patients (50–52). In contrast to Type I, the onset of Type V appears later in adulthood. Typical clinical manifestations for Type V are frequent associations of impaired glucose tolerance, hyperuricemia and hyperinsulinism (17,50,53). It has been recently demonstrated that the rate of glucose metabolism *in vivo*, measured by using the euglycemic clamp technique, is markedly reduced in Type V patients with a normal glucose tolerance test (54). The data indicate that insulin resistance is a characteristic feature of Type V patients.

The existence of familial Type V has been well documented (36,52,53), but the lack of a specific genetic marker for Type V phenotype has impeded the detection of the pattern of inheritance which remains unresolved. The first degree relatives for the probands with Type V express either Type IV or Type V hyperlipoproteinemia (36,52,53). The clustering of the two disorders in the pedigrees is puzzling, and it is possible that familial Type V disorder is not a single entity but a heterogeneous group, one sub-group being clearly related to familial Type IV.

LPL activity in Type V hyperlipoproteinemia. The basic biochemical defect producing Type V phenotype has not been fully established. Kinetic studies in Type V patients have consistently shown a substantial increase in both VLDL-TG and VLDL-apo B transport rates (55–57). Thus, the overproduction of VLDL seems to be one basic defect in Type V hyperlipoproteinemia. However, the degree of VLDL overproduction in Type V is not clearly excessive in comparison to that of Type IV patients who do not demonstrate as severe hypertriglyceridemia or hyperchylomicronemia. Kesäniemi and Grundy (57) have documented the defective clearance of VLDL as a second abnormality in all their patients with Type V. The data are consistent with the low fractional catabolic rate of VLDL and VLDL apo-B observed in previous studies (55,56). Kesäniemi and Grundy (57) proposed that Type V hyperlipoproteinemia is characterized by a dual defect in the metabolism of triglyceride-rich particles i.e., an overproduction of VLDL and a defective clearance of triglyceride-rich particles.

The mechanisms underlying the impaired clearance of VLDL in Type V patients is not clear. In several studies, postheparin plasma LPL activity in Type V patients was within normal range (4,25,52,53). In contrast, Greten et al. (5) observed low postheparin plasma LPL activity in two of their four patients with Type V, and Huttunen et al. (3) also documented low LPL activity in postheparin plasma in three of their patients with Type V. We have recently studied heparin-releasable LPL activity in adipose tissue, skeletal muscle and postheparin plasma in fourteen patients with primary Type V hyperlipoproteinemia. The LPL activity in both adipose tissue and skeletal muscle was markedly reduced in comparison to values in normolipidemic control subjects (Table 3). Similarly, Persson (1) has also measured low LPL activity in adipose tissue of patients with Type V. Table 3 shows

TABLE III Lipoprotein lipase activity (mean ± SEM) in patients with Type V hyperlipoproteinemia

LPL activity	Type V (n = 14)	Controls (n = 28)
Adipose tissue*	0.91 ± 0.23^{xx}	2.16 ± 0.26
Skeletal muscle*	0.36 ± 0.08^{xx}	0.85 ± 0.10
Postheparin plasma†	15.67 ± 0.80^{x}	21.60 ± 1.02

* = μmol FFA.h^{-1}.g^{-1}, †μmol FFA.h^{-1}.ml^{-1}
The relative body weight of the patients averaged 126 ± 8%.
$^{x}p < 0.05$; $^{xx}p < 0.01$ for the difference from controls.

that the average enzyme activity in skeletal muscle was one third of that found in controls. This is consistent with earlier data from a smaller group of patients (17) where the decrease of LPL activity in postheparin plasma was less pronounced than that in tissues.

In our group of patients with Type V, no correlations existed between serum triglyceride levels and adipose tissue LPL or skeletal muscle LPL. Postheparin plasma LPL showed an inverse correlation, albeit not statistically significant, with serum triglycerides. The lack of any correlation between serum triglyceride levels and LPL activities indicates that the reduced LPL activity in Type V is not the only factor contributing to the elevation of serum triglycerides. Interestingly, the adipose tissue and muscle LPL activities in Type V patients were not markedly lower than in nonobese patients with Type IV (Table 6).

Five out of fourteen cases represented familial Type V, and all the probands had skeletal muscle LPL segregated clearly below the normal range. Tissue LPL activities have not yet been systematically assayed in the relatives of the patients with Type V. Table 4 displays the results of one family where all the siblings and the parents were available for the studies. The proband (M.P.) had low muscle LPL activity. Interestingly, the two brothers as well as the mother and father also had clearly reduced muscle LPL activity. The enzyme activity in adipose tissue and in postheparin plasma was within the normal range in all other family members except in the proband. These findings suggest that low muscle LPL activity can be an inherited abnormality in familial Type V hyperlipoproteinemia. Further, the data show that the postheparin plasma LPL activity does not clearly reflect the selective reduction of the enzyme at the tissue level.

Dunn et al. (58) recently described a family where the impaired catabolism of VLDL triglyceride seemed to be an inherited defect and responsible for hypertriglyceridemia. The expression of Type IV and Type V phenotypes in this family was related to the degree of VLDL production. The subjects with high VLDL production showed Type V, whereas those with only a moderate increase in VLDL production expressed Type IV. In our studies,

TABLE IV Serum lipids and LPL activities in family members for Type V proband (M.P.)

						LPL activity in		
		Age	TG mg/dl	LDL-chol. mg/dl	HDL-chol. mg/dl	adipose* tissue	skeletal* muscle	postheparin† plasma
Mother	(M.P.)	51	327	166	54	2.69	0.35	19.98
Father	(K.P.)	53	1391	66	35	0.99	0.21	15.39
Proband	(M.P.)	30	1340	50	15	0.40	0.39	12.86
Brother	(S.P.)	28	398	162	46	1.05	0.23	22.80
Brother	(J.P.)	24	336	186	39	1.00	0.38	16.56

*μmol FFA.h^{-1}.g^{-1}, †μmol FFA.h^{-1}.ml^{-1}.

the proband and his father had Type V phenotype, whereas the other affected family members had Type IV hyperlipoproteinemia. Unfortunately kinetic data from this family is not presently available to compare with that of the family described by Dunn et al. (58). In summary, the reduction of LPL activity in either adipose tissue and/or skeletal muscle in many patients with Type V suggests that low LPL activity can be a cause for reduced VLDL removal. Since some patients with Type V have LPL activities within the normal range, it is probable that other factors may also account for a slow VLDL removal; i.e., defective function of LPL, or the presence of enzyme inhibitors in the plasma. In conclusion, Type V is a heterogeneous disorder and more extended family studies are needed to define the prevalence of different defects in the removal system.

LPL Activity in Familial Hypertriglyceridemias

Genetic disorders with hypertriglyceridemia include familial hypertriglyceridemia (FHT), familial combined hyperlipidemia (FCHT) and dysbetalipoproteinemia. The familial nature of all three disorders is well established (59–61). The biochemical defects leading to dysbetalipoproteinemia are relatively well characterized (60,61). The disorder is characterized by defective catabolism of remnants (60,61) and recent evidence suggest that VLDL shows abnormal interaction with LPL (62–64). Apparently, VLDL particles have compositional changes which render them resistant to LPL action (63,64) whereas LPL activity is normal (4,5,65). In contrast, the underlying mechanism of FHT and FCHT is less well established. So far, no genetic or biochemical marker is available for the classification of individual cases without extensive family studies. The problem is most apparent in FCHT, where different phenotypes (Type IIa, IIb, IV and V) appear within the same kindred (59). In FHT, the phenotype is by definition Type IV although affected family members can have also Type V. Kinetic studies have consistently confirmed the overproduction of VLDL in most patients with both FHT and FCHT (55,56,66,67). The oversecretion of VLDL triglycerides and VLDL-apo B is typical for Type IV, whereas the increased synthesis of only VLDL-apo B is more characteristic for the combined hyperlipoproteinemia (66). However, VLDL kinetics do not distinguish well between Type IV patients with FHT and FCHT genotypes (68,69).

Circumstantial evidence suggests that a defective removal plays a role in the pathogenesis of familial hypertriglyceridemias. Several kinetic studies have indicated that a defect of VLDL clearance co-exists with VLDL overproduction and contributes to the elevation of serum triglycerides in Type IV (55,56,67,69). The fractional removal rate of VLDL-apo B correlates positively with LPL activity in adipose tissue (70) and in postheparin plasma (71) in patients with a wide range of serum triglyceride levels. Nevertheless, data on LPL activity in Type IV are inconsistent (Table 5). The discordance of available data needs careful consideration. Obesity and diabetes frequently co-exist with hypertriglyceridemia, and both influence LPL activity

TABLE V Lipoprotein lipase activity in adipose tissue, skeletal muscle and postheparin plasma in patient with primary familial hypertriglyceridemia (Type IV FHT)

		LPL activity		
		Postheparin plasma	Adipose tissue	Skeletal muscle
Persson	(1)		decreased	
Krauss et al.	(4)	normal		
Larsson et al.	(72)		decreased	
Huttunen et al.	(3)	decreased		
Greenberg et al.	(53)	normal		
Günther et al.	(73)		normal	
Goldberg et al.	(74)		normal	
Taylor et al.	(75)		decreased	
Taskinen et al.	(76)	decreased	decreased	decreased
Beil et al.	(67)	decreased		
Stalenhoef	(68)	normal		
Boberg et al.	(77)	decreased		

The table includes only studies where specific methods have been used to separate LPL and hepatic lipase activities in postheparin plasma.

as discussed elsewhere in this volume (Chapters 4 and 9). The impact of these confounding factors was not taken into consideration in all studies (1,4,53,74,75). Another methodological reason for variable results in postheparin plasma LPL may be attributed to differences in the heparin dose which has varied from 10 to 100 IU/kg, and the use of different substrates for LPL. Moreover, the lack of an accurate classification of the patients without family studies can contribute to the inconsistency of the data since in most studies the patients have not had a definite genetic diagnosis (1,4,67,72,73,75–77).

Table 5 shows that in the majority of the studies, the LPL activity is reduced in Type IV patients. Taskinen et al. (76) recently studied the heparin-releasable LPL activity of adipose tissue, skeletal muscle and postheparin plasma in men with primary hypertriglyceridemia (Type IIb and IV phenotypes), and compared the values of those in normolipidemic men with a comparable degree of obesity. Because the relatives of the patients were not studied, the group is heterogeneous, including both familial and sporadic cases of hypertriglyceridemia. Table 6 shows that the mean activity of adipose tissue LPL was significantly lower in nonobese men with Type IIb and IV, regardless of whether expressed per tissue weight, per fat cell or per estimated total body fat. The range of LPL values in both patient groups overlapped with that of normolipidemic control subjects. However, in most men with Type IIb and IV, LPL activity in the adipose tissue segregated below the mean value for men in the control group (Figure 2). In contrast, most obese men with Type IIb and IV had adipose tissue LPL values within the reference limits for obese normolipidemic men, and the mean enzyme

TABLE VI Lipoprotein lipase activities in adipose tissue, skeletal muscle and in postheparin plasma of Type IIb and Type IV men in comparison to normolipidemic control subjects

Group	No	Adipose tissue per weight	Adipose tissue per cell	Adipose tissue per total fat mass	Skeletal muscle per weight	Postheparin plasma	
		μmol FFA.h^{-1}.g^{-1}	pmol FFA.h^{-1}.cell^{-1}	mmol FFA.h^{-1}	μmol FFA.h^{-1}.g^{-1}	μmol.h^{-1}.ml^{-1}	
Nonobese							
Normolipidemic	42	2.45 ± 0.19	1.46 ± 0.11	45 ± 4	0.84 ± 0.07	23.5 ± 1.7	(23)
Type IIb	10	1.33 ± 0.26[b]	0.83 ± 0.21[b]	25 ± 4[b]	0.91 ± 0.12	18.8 ± 1.4[a]	(8)
Type IV	10	1.01 ± 0.11[c]	0.70 ± 0.08[c]	24 ± 3[c]	0.46 ± 0.06[b,i]	17.6 ± 1.5[a]	(9)
Obese							
Normolipidemic	28	2.16 ± 0.26	1.93 ± 0.26	84 ± 9[c]	0.85 ± 0.10	21.6 ± 1.0	(26)
Type IIb	10	1.46 ± 0.24	1.05 ± 0.18[e]	49 ± 8[e]	0.64 ± 0.13	19.5 ± 2.1	(9)
Type IV	23	1.63 ± 0.18[h]	1.29 ± 0.18[d]	65 ± 10	0.70 ± 0.10[g]	21.6 ± 1.2	(21)

[a]$p < 0.05$, [b]$p < 0.01$, [c]$p < 0.001$ for difference from nonobese normolipidemic subjects
[d]$p < 0.05$, [e]$p < 0.01$, [f]$p < 0.001$ for difference from obese normolipidemic subjects
[g]$p < 0.05$, [h]$p < 0.01$ for difference from nonobese patients with Type IV
[i]$p < 0.01$ for difference from patients with Type IIb.
The figures in parentheses give number for subjects who had a heparin test.
The data are reproduced with the permission from Blackwell Scientific Publications, limited, Oxford (76).

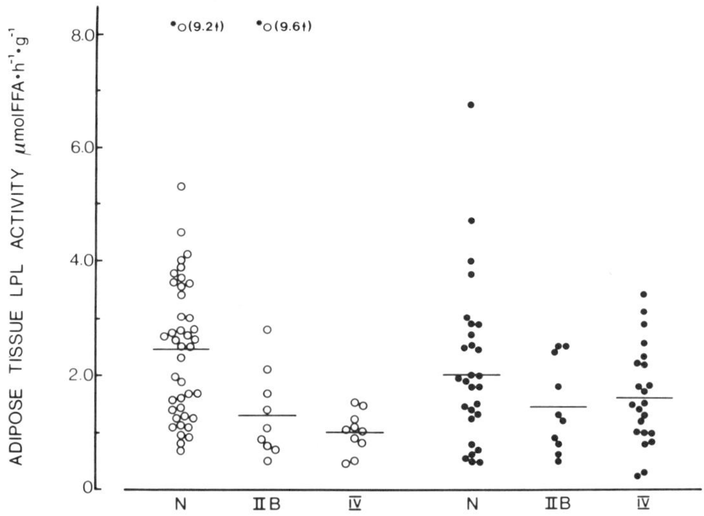

FIGURE 2 Individual values of adipose tissue LPL activity in nonobese (○) and obese (●) normolipidemic subjects (N) and patients with Type IIb and IV hyperlipoproteinemia. The solid lines present the mean values in each group (* subjects excluded from calculations). The data are reproduced with the permission from Blackwell Scientific Publications limited, Oxford (76).

activity was marginally reduced when expressed per fat cell (Table 6). In obese groups, LPL activity per total fat mass is similar or higher than in nonobese controls (Table 6). This rules out an overall removal defect of VLDL as a cause of hypertriglyceridemia if the VLDL production rate is normal.

The mean LPL activity in skeletal muscle was clearly lower in nonobese men with Type IV than in the respective control group (average change = −45%). Figure 3 shows that all Type IV patients had muscle enzyme values within the low normal range of the respective control men. Interestingly, the reduction of skeletal muscle LPL in nonobese Type IV men was only slightly less than in Type V men (see Table 3). In contrast, nonobese and obese men with Type IIb, and obese men with Type IV, had skeletal muscle LPL activity similar to their respective control groups.

Postheparin plasma LPL activity in nonobese men with Type IIb and IV was lower than in corresponding control groups. Relative reduction of postheparin plasma LPL was, however, less than that in adipose tissue LPL (20 vs. 46% in Type IIb and 25 vs. 59% in Type IV). Consequently, postheparin plasma LPL activity was not related to the LPL activity in either adipose tissue or skeletal muscle. In conclusion, postheparin plasma LPL does not reflect the enzyme activities at the tissue level in hypertriglyceridemic patients, as it does in normolipidemic subjects (see Figure 1). The reasons for this discordance are not clear.

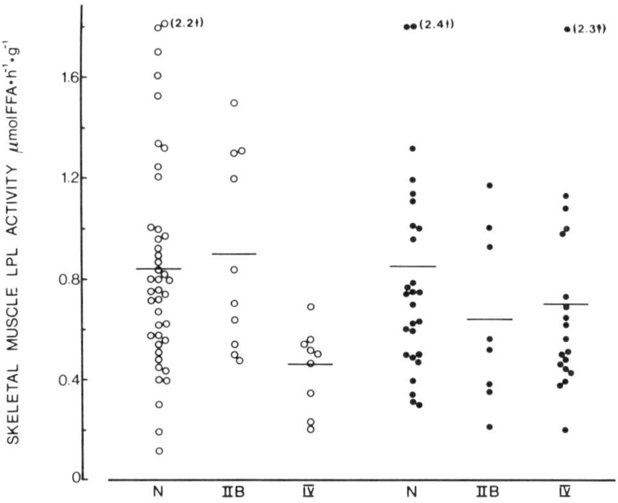

FIGURE 3 Individual values of skeletal muscle LPL activity in nonobese (○) and obese (●) normolipidemic men (N) and patients with Type IIb and IV hyperlipoproteinemia. Solid lines present the mean value in each group. The data are reproduced with the permission from Blackwell Scientific Publications limited, Oxford (76).

In order to address the possible familial nature of the changes in LPL activity, Sane (69) recently studied nine kindreds with familial hypertriglyceridemia (FHT) and six kindreds with combined hyperlipidemia (FCHT). The criteria used for the classification of the families were as follows: a) A family which included at least three subjects (proband included) with Type IV and V represented FHT. b) A family which included the proband, at least one member with Type IIb, and at least two members with Type IIa, IV or V represented FCHT. Table 7 shows the LPL activity in the adipose tissue, skeletal muscle and postheparin plasma of normotriglyceridemic and hypertriglyceridemic family members. The mean values of the LPL activity in both tissues and postheparin plasma were reduced in hypertriglyceridemic subjects of FHT families. In contrast, LPL activities in normolipidemic members of FHT families, as well as in both non-affected and affected subjects of the families with FCHT, were no different from those in the members of control families. The individual values in FHT families for adipose tissue and skeletal muscle LPL showed a wide range which overlapped with the distribution of the values in control families. The data suggest that Type IV hyperlipidemia is often associated with mild to moderate reduction of LPL activity, but it is not a distinct genetic marker. Several subjects with Type IV had quite normal LPL activities in adipose tissue and skeletal muscle LPL. This data supports the findings of previous studies which have shown that postheparin plasma and adipose tissue LPL activities are normal in combined hyperlipidemia (3,67).

TABLE VII LPL activities of adipose tissue, skeletal muscle and postheparin plasma in pedigrees with familial hypertriglyceridemia (FHT) and combined hyperlipidemia (FCHT)

	FHT		FCHT		NTC
	NT (n = 45)	HT (n = 33)	NT (n = 27)	HT (n = 12)	(n = 20)
LPL activity in					
adipose tissue*	1.73 ± 0.25	1.29 ± 0.16[x]	1.96 ± 0.25	1.78 ± 0.46	1.91 ± 0.35
skeletal* muscle	0.57 ± 0.04	0.48 ± 0.04[x]	0.55 ± 0.05	0.53 ± 0.06	0.61 ± 0.07
postheparin† plasma	19.53 ± 0.84	19.13 ± 0.90[x]	18.97 ± 1.08	20.71 ± 1.57	23.5 ± 1.74

NT = normotriglyceridemic subject
HT = hypertriglyceridemic subject
NTC = normolipidemic control families
* = μmol FFA.g^{-1}.h^{-1}, † = μmol FFA.ml^{-1}.h^{-1}
The numbers in parenthesis indicate first degree relatives who were studied.
[x] = $p < 0.05$ for difference from values in normolipidemic subjects of control families.
The number of families with FHT, FCHT and NTC were 9, 6 and 6 respectively. Source: Sane (69).

LPL Activity in Secondary Hypertriglyceridemias

Several exogenous factors can cause the elevation of serum triglycerides in the absence of genetic disorders. This overview will focus on those acquired hypertriglyceridemias where the pathogenesis is related to LPL activity. Such disorders are diabetes, obesity, alcohol, hypothyroidism and renal disease. Diabetes and obesity are covered in Chapters 4 and 9. Carbohydrate-induced hypertriglyceridemia, as well as the elevation of serum triglycerides in connection with the use of estrogens and oral contraceptives, are not discussed because the underlying mechanisms are not related to changes in LPL.

Alcohol-induced hypertriglyceridemia

Effects of alcohol on serum triglycerides. The intake of alcohol has varied and complex effects on serum lipids and lipoproteins. Alcohol-induced changes depend on the mode and amount of alcohol consumption, and the acute and chronic effects of alcohol are markedly different. Alcohol-induced hypertriglyceridemia is probably the most common form amongst secondary hyperlipidemias. Hypertriglyceridemia occurs in about 25–30% of all alcoholics (78–81). In some population studies, the amount and frequency of alcohol intake shows a weak positive correlation with the concentration of serum triglycerides (82,83). The hypertriglyceridemic effect of both acute and short term ethanol intake is well documented in several studies (84–90). It has been shown that a moderate intake of alcohol in the evening increases the fasting serum triglyceride levels on the following morning (86).

In one fourth of normolipidemic subjects, serum triglyceride levels exceeded the upper limit of normal and exposed these subjects to an incorrect classification as Type IV cases (86). The response to alcohol was clearly exaggerated in hyperlipidemic subjects (86). Further, acute alcohol intake aggravates and prolongs the post-prandial hyperlipidemia in normal subjects (85,89–92).

The regular intake of alcohol in doses exceeding 60 g/day is associated with a rise of serum triglycerides in healthy volunteers (89,93–95). Again, the response of serum triglycerides to regular alcohol consumption is exacerbated in patients with primary hypertriglyceridemia (93). The lipoprotein profile in chronic alcoholics without liver disease is characterized by either normal or marginally elevated VLDL triglyceride levels (96–101). In contrast, alcoholic patients with liver disease generally show hypertriglyceridemia (97,99). These studies suggest that alcohol-induced hypertriglyceridemia is not the result of a single entity, but is due instead, to several different effects of alcohol on VLDL metabolism.

Effects of alcohol on LPL activity.

Acute effects. Several years ago Nikkilä et al. (102) showed that three hours of ethanol infusion in normal subjects is followed by a significant decrease in postheparin plasma LPL activity as well as a rise in serum triglyceride levels. The reduction of LPL activity is also evident five hours after the oral ethanol load (92). Further, ethanol ingestion decreases fasting LPL activity in adipose tissue and prevents the glucose-induced rise in adipose tissue enzyme activity (87). The suppression of LPL activity is still apparent ten hours after ethanol intake (89). The inhibitory effect of ethanol on LPL activity is, however, transitory. If the enzyme activity in postheparin plasma is measured on the morning following an evening of ethanol intake, postheparin plasma LPL activity is normal (86).

Recently, Taskinen et al. (90) carried out a study where healthy volunteers were served 5.5 grams of ethanol per kg body weight over two and a half days, together with their normal meals. The actual amount of alcohol per day corresponded to five drinks of whisky, within four hours, twice a day. Adipose tissue LPL activity increased 2.3-fold in contrast to no change in LPL activity in the absence of any alcohol intake. However, the postheparin plasma enzyme activity remained constant despite the changes in the adipose tissue enzyme. Alcohol intake was followed by a progressive rise in VLDL triglyceride concentration in the fasting serum, and by an exaggerated postprandial response of VLDL triglyceride.

Chronic effects. Two studies have shown that long-term intake of alcohol increases adipose tissue LPL activity in normolipidemic volunteers (89,103), but one group observed no change in LPL activity (95). Schneider and coworkers (89) followed postheparin plasma LPL activity during the regular daily intake of alcohol (70–80 g/day) for four weeks. Postheparin plasma

LPL activity increased significantly on alcohol intake within one week and the rise of LPL activity averaged 86% after four weeks. These findings support the observations that in chronic alcoholics, postheparin plasma LPL activity is consistently high in comparison to non-alcoholic control subjects (96,100,104). The cessation of drinking is followed by a rapid fall of postheparin plasma LPL activity (Figure 4) (104). The average LPL activity declined by 34% during the first two days. The time course of LPL changes during the alcohol withdrawal is consistent with that observed during short-term alcohol intake (90). Thus, the action of alcohol on LPL activity seems to be bi-phasic; the acute intake of ethanol inhibits the enzyme activity, whereas chronic exposure to ethanol induces LPL activity. The mechanisms behind the alcohol-induced changes in LPL are not clear. Hansson and Nilsson-Ehle (91) have shown that the acute inhibitory effect of ethanol is not mediated by acetate in humans. Further, acetate and acetaldehyde *in vitro* have no effect on adipose tissue LPL activity (91). These findings suggest that ethanol itself might be the active factor.

Interrelations between serum lipoproteins and LPL activity. It appears that the rise of VLDL triglycerides after a single or short term intake of ethanol is due to the impaired removal of VLDL which results from the reduction of LPL activity (101). This is consistent with the observation that the clearance of chylomicrons is markedly delayed (five hours) after the ethanol load (92). On the other hand, the rise of VLDL triglycerides upon

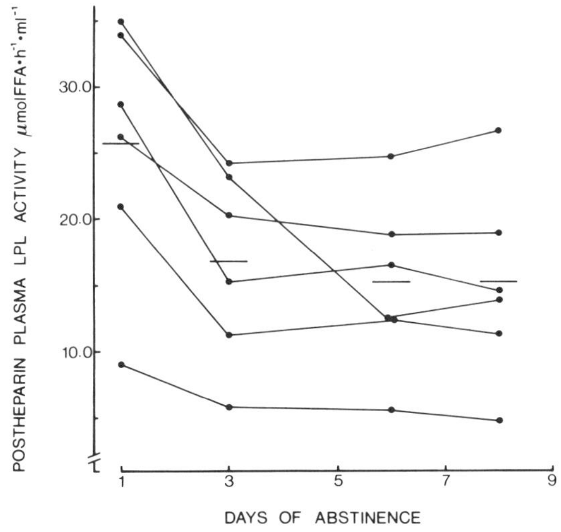

FIGURE 4 Individual responses of postheparin plasma LPL activity in 6 alcoholic men during alcohol abstinence. The solid lines present the mean values on admission and 2, 5 and 7 days after the cessation of drinking.
The data are reproduced with the permission from Elsevier Science Publishers BV. Amsterdam (104).

the continuance of alcohol intake for weeks cannot be attributed to a defect of VLDL catabolism because the LPL activity is high. It has been observed that whereas there is an increase in the fractional catabolic rate of VLDL in chronic alcohol users, the rate declines to normal during abstinence (105). Because in chronic alcoholics the VLDL production rate is also increased, the total VLDL turnover rate is enhanced although this enhancement diminishes after cessation of drinking (105). Thus, in chronic alcoholics, VLDL triglyceride increases if the enhancement of the clearance capacity is not high enough to compensate for the increase in VLDL production. In normal subjects, moderate daily intake of alcohol for four weeks clearly increases VLDL production without any concomitant change in postheparin plasma LPL activity (95). In this situation, the elevation of serum triglycerides reflects primarily VLDL overproduction induced by alcohol (95). Thus, the effect on VLDL may also be dependent on the dose of alcohol.

The major effects of alcohol on lipoproteins are not restricted to VLDL, but are also reflected in LDL and HDL. It is well established that alcohol induces changes in HDL (101). In chronic alcoholics the concentration of HDL is usually elevated, a change caused mainly by a rise of the HDL_2 (81,96–101). Further habitual alcohol intake is related to HDL levels (83,106,107). According to current thinking, HDL_2 particles are partly derived from LPL-induced hydrolysis of triglyceride-rich particles (108). Therefore, the rise of HDL (HDL_2) in chronic alcoholics can be explained by the increase in the VLDL turnover rate due to high LPL activity (105). This explanation is supported by the observations that the fall of LPL and HDL_2 occurs in parallel after the cessation of drinking in chronic alcoholics (100,104). In contrast, the small or moderate intake of alcohol is associated with a rise of HDL_3, without changes in HDL_2 (109,110). Apparently, alcohol also influences HDL levels through mechanisms other than LPL.

Hypertriglyceridemias Secondary to Renal Disease

LPL activity in chronic renal failure. Hypertriglyceridemia is a common abnormality in both dialyzed and undialyzed patients with chronic renal failure and is present in 40–60% of all patients studied (111–115). The lipoprotein pattern is characterized by an increase in serum total- and VLDL triglycerides, normal or even sub-normal serum total- and LDL cholesterol, and by a reduction in plasma HDL (113,116–120). The picture is essentially similar in both untreated patients and in patients on maintenance dialysis (112–118). The mechanisms behind these changes have been addressed in several studies but the picture is as yet not well defined.

Bagdade et al. (111) reported low postheparin plasma lipolytic activity in patients with chronic renal disease and proposed that defective triglyceride removal contributes to the elevation of serum triglycerides. This initial finding was confirmed in subsequent studies (118,121). Selective measurements of LPL and hepatic lipase activities in postheparin plasma have revealed that both enzyme activities are reduced in undialyzed patients with chronic renal failure (119,122–124). The start of hemodialysis does not affect the enzyme activities which are lower in those patients than in control subjects (115,119,122,125). Fasting LPL activity in adipose tissue is also low in uremic patients compared to control subjects (126,127). Further, the response of adipose tissue LPL to feeding is blunted i.e., adipose tissue LPL activity in the fed state is clearly sub-normal (127). These data are contrasted by two studies where only hepatic lipase activity, but not LPL activity, was found to be reduced in uremic patients (113,128). These seemingly contrasting results may be explained by the differences in sex distribution and by the small size of the study cohorts. Recent evidence suggests that the reduction of LPL activity is related to the impairment of renal function, being most pronounced in patients with severe renal failure (122,124).

The biochemical defect responsible for the reduction of LPL activity in chronic renal failure is unclear. Murase et al. (129) suggested that uremic plasma contains an inhibitor of LPL activity. However, attempts to confirm the inhibition of LPL by uremic plasma failed in two other assay systems which used diluted plasma samples (113,119). The hemodialysis procedure requires repeated administration of heparin and, therefore, it is possible that this may deplete the tissue pools of LPL. Apparently, this concept is not valid in undialyzed patients. Further, LPL activity remains unchanged after the initiation of hemodialysis (119). Finally, in normal subjects, intermittent administration of heparin is not followed by a reduction in the LPL activity (119). One possible intriguing explanation is that low LPL activity in uremia is related to insulin resistance (124), a common finding in chronic renal failure (130).

The relevance of low LPL activity to the elevation of serum triglycerides is supported by substantial evidence. Chan et al. (115) observed that logarithms of serum triglyceride values correlated inversely with postheparin plasma LPL activity. Kinetic studies have shown that the fractional removal rate of VLDL triglyceride is clearly reduced in both undialyzed and dialyzed patients with chronic renal failure (112,123,131,132). Consistently, the fractional clearance rate of Intralipid is markedly delayed in uremic subjects and correlates inversely with the levels of serum triglycerides (114,121,133). In turn, postheparin plasma LPL activity correlates positively with *in vivo* measured postheparin clearance rate of Intralipid (115). Further evidence is provided by the observation that in hemodialysis patients, clofibrate treatment is associated with a fall of serum triglycerides accompanied by a rise in LPL (134). In addition, low LPL activity provides an appropriate explanation for the reduction of HDL in uremic patients because LPL activity is one determinant of plasma HDL level (108). Indeed, Chan et al. (115) showed that in hemodialysis patients, HDL cholesterol is related positively to LPL activity.

It should be pointed out that the elevation of VLDL triglyceride in uremic patients occurs at an early stage of renal failure and is apparent before any change occurs in LPL activity (124). Further, compared to normal subjects, patients with chronic renal failure often have higher serum triglyceride levels for any given removal rate of Intalipid (114). This indicates that increased VLDL production contributes to the elevation of serum triglycerides. Kinetic studies have consistently confirmed that the total VLDL turnover rate is increased in many patients with uremia and contributes to the pathogenesis of uremic hypertriglyceridemia (131,132).

LPL activity in post-transplantation patients. It is well documented that hyperlipidemia is also very common in transplant recipients with stable graft function (116,117,121,122,135–137). The lipoprotein patterns are more variable than in the uremic state, showing increases in both VLDL and LDL (116,117,136). The pathogenetic mechanisms also seem to be different from those seen in chronic renal failure. It has been shown in several studies that LPL activity in postheparin plasma is normal in patients with successful transplantation (122–124). Data from kinetic studies suggest that post-transplantation VLDL production is clearly increased (137). This is thought to be due to the administration of corticosteroids as part of immunosuppressive therapy (136,137).

LPL activity in nephrotic syndrome. By definition, nephrotic syndrome is characterized by increases in both serum triglycerides and cholesterol i.e., VLDL and LDL levels. The data on plasma HDL have been less definitive; low (138,139), normal (140,141) and even high HDL values (142,143) have been reported for patients with nephrotic syndrome. Kinetic studies have demonstrated that VLDL triglyceride production is increased in nephrotic syndrome, but at the same time the fractional catabolic rate of VLDL is decreased (144,145). Chan et al. (140) have observed a marginally reduced removal rate of Intralipid during fat tolerance test. The data on LPL activity is so far limited in patients with nephrotic syndrome. Kashyap et al. (146) measured postheparin plasma LPL activity in nine patients with nephrotic syndrome. Two of the patients showed subnormal enzyme activity, whereas the others had LPL activity within normal range. Oetliker et al. (142) assayed postheparin plasma LPL activity in nine children with proteinuric nephrotic syndrome. The enzyme activity was clearly reduced compared to that in control children. Further, there was a significant inverse correlation between serum triglycerides and postheparin plasma LPL activity (142). In nephrotic syndrome, apo CII is lost in the urine and consequently VLDL may have decreased LPL activator potency (146). It is possible that this altered VLDL composition is related to its defective clearance. In summary, hyperlipidemia in nephrotic syndrome appears to be due to a combination of both the overproduction and the defective clearance of VLDL. However, metabolic interrelations between different lipoproteins have not yet been established.

LPL in hypothyroidism

In overt hypothyroidism, the lipoprotein pattern is characterized by an increase in serum total- and LDL cholesterol, whereas HDL cholesterol is within the upper normal range or slightly elevated (147,148). Alterations in serum triglyceride levels are less consistent; the values have been reported to be normal or moderately elevated in comparison to euthyroid subjects (147,148). Hypothyroidism is also associated with an accumulation of triglyceride-rich particles within the intermediate density (IDL) range (149). Nevertheless, serum triglyceride levels decrease after the substitution therapy (150–154).

The mechanisms behind the hypertriglyceridemia of hypothyroidism have been addressed in several studies. Substantial evidence indicates that the changes in serum triglyceride levels in hypothyroidism are due to a clearance defect. Data from kinetic studies show that the fractional removal rate of VLDL triglycerides is clearly reduced (150) or within the low normal range (152), but that it increases during thyroxine substitution therapy (150,152). These observations suggest that thyroxine can enhance the elimination rate of VLDL triglyceride. Accordingly, the removal rate of exogenous triglycerides during an Intralipid tolerance test, as well as chylomicron clearance, is clearly improved upon replacement therapy (150,152,153,155). In contrast, the elimination rate of both exogenous and endogenous triglycerides is markedly accelerated in hyperthyroidism but decreases during anti-thyroid therapy (147).

The data strongly suggest that thyroid hormones influence LPL activity. Several studies have demonstrated that this concept is valid although the molecular basis has remained unclear. First, low levels of postheparin plasma lipolytic activity (PHLA) have been reported in earlier studies for hypothyroid patients (150,151,156,157). Pykalisto et al. (151) first demonstrated that LPL activity in adipose tissue is reduced in hypothyroidism and that the enzyme activity increases during replacement therapy with thyroxine. This observation was confirmed by Lithell et al. (155) who, in addition, documented low LPL activity in the skeletal muscle of hypothyroid patients. The substitution of thyroxine was accompanied by a concomitant increase of LPL activity in tissues and in postheparin plasma (155). Therefore, it seemed reasonable to conclude that the low PHLA activity was due to the reduction of tissue LPL activity. However, selective measurements of both LPL and hepatic lipase activity revealed that both enzyme activities are reduced in hypothyroidism and thus contribute to low PHLA (152,153). Further, it is now evident that hepatic lipase is actually more sensitive to the effects of thyroid hormones than LPL (147). The reduction of LPL is apparent only in severe hypothyroidism, whereas the enzyme activity remains normal in subclinical disease (155,158). This observation may explain why some studies have not confirmed the low LPL activity in hypothyroidism (152). In summary, the reduction of LPL activity in hypothyroidism may well explain the defective clearance of triglyceride-rich particles and also the elevation of serum triglycerides.

LPL in endocrinological disorders

Active acromegaly is commonly associated with mild or moderate hypertriglyceridemia (159,160). Murase et al. (160) reported that LPL activity in postheparin plasma is decreased in active acromegaly. Recent data by Asayama et al. (161) have demonstrated that the administration of growth hormone in idiopathic pituitary dwarfism is followed by a decline in postheparin plasma LPL activity. Although these studies indicate that growth hormone influences LPL activity, the mechanism behind the observed changes remain unknown.

Another interesting observation is that postheparin plasma LPL activity also seems to be reduced in patients with prolactinoma who have mild hypertriglyceridemia (162). The exact mechanisms linking prolactin and LPL activity are unclear, but an intriguing possibility is that low LPL activity may be related to insulin resistance (162).

Endogenous hypercortisolism is another endocrinological abnormality which is associated with mild to moderate hypertriglyceridemia (163). However, in patients with Cushing's disease, the LPL activity of adipose tissue, skeletal muscle, and postheparin plasma is similar to that in control subjects (163). Thus, the LPL system is not involved in the pathogenesis of hyperlipidemia in Cushing's disease (163).

Conclusions

The importance of LPL in the pathogenesis of hypertriglyceridemias has been underestimated in past studies due to the inadequate methodology for the assay of LPL activity. Recent research has provided a strong body of evidence to support the assertion that changes in LPL activity are involved in the pathogenesis of both primary hypertriglyceridemias and in secondary hypertriglyceridemias due to acute alcohol intake, renal disease and hypothyroidism. A complete deficiency of LPL is characteristic for Type I hyperlipoproteinemia. LPL activity is often low or subnormal in patients with familial Type IV and V hyperlipoproteinemias. The reduction of LPL activity in both disorders seems more pronounced in the skeletal muscle than in the adipose tissue. Since postheparin LPL does not appear to be a sensitive parameter for mild to moderate changes in LPL activity in hypertriglyceridemic patients, further metabolic and family studies are needed to define the prevalence of changes in tissue LPL activities in patients with familial hypertriglyceridemias. Other areas for future studies include: 1) Recognition of those factors which affect the function of LPL in hypertriglyceridemic patients with a known removal defect but normal enzyme activity. 2) The genetic and molecular basis behind the changes of LPL activity in both primary and secondary hypertriglyceridemias. 3) The development of methods which measure the amount of enzyme protein, as well as methods to relate changes in the structure of LPL to its function.

The author appreciates greatly the collaborative work and discussions with the members of the research group in the Third Department of Medicine, University of Helsinki; Drs. Esko A. Nikkilä, Timo Kuusi, Timo Sane, Matti Välimäki and Reino Ylikahri. The studies by the author and coworkers have been supported by grants from the Sigrid Juselius Foundation and

Finnish State Alcohol Monopoly (Alko) Helsinki, Finland. This review was written during the research fellowship provided by Finnish State Medical Research Council (Academy of Finland) and Paavo Nurmi Foundation, Helsinki, Finland. The author is indebted to Miss Heli Vainio and Raija Selivuo for their assistance in the preparation of this manuscript.

References

1. Persson, B. 1973. *Acta Med. Scand.* 193:447–456.
2. Björntorp, P., G. Enzi, R. Ohlson, B. Persson, P. Sponbergs, and U. Smith. 1975. *Horm. Metabl. Res.* 7:230˜37.
3. Huttunen, J. K., C. Ehnholm, M. Kekki, and E. A. Nikkilä. 1976. *Clin. Sci. Molec. Med.* 50:249–260.
4. Krauss, R. M., R. I. Levy, and D. S. Fredrickson, 1974. *J. Clin. Invest.* 54:1107–1124.
5. Greten, H., R. DeGrella, G. Klose, W. Rascher, J. L. de Gennes, and E. Gjone. 1976. *J. Lipid Res.* 17:203–210.
6. Boberg, J., M. Boberg, R. Gross, J. D. Turner, J. Augustin, and W. V. Brown. 1979. *Upsala J. Med. Sci* 84:215–227.
7. Applebaum-Bowden, D., S. M. Haffner, P. W. Wahl, J. J. Hoover, G. R. Warnick, J. J. Albers, and W. R. Hazzard. 1985. *Arteriosclerosis* 5:273–282.
8. Pykälistö, O. J., P. H. Smith, and J. D. Brunzell. 1975. *J. Clin. Invest* 56:1108–1117.
9. Taskinen, M. -R., E. A. Nikkilä, J. K. Huttunen, and H. Hilden. 1980. *Clin. Chim. Acta* 104:107–117.
10. Lithell, H. 1977. *Acta Universitatis Upsaliensis* No. 272.
11. Lithell, H., J. Boberg, K. Hellsing, G. Lundqvist, and B. Vessby. 1978. *Atherosclerosis* 30:89–94.
12. Lithell, H., F. Lindgärde, K. Hellsing, G. Lundqvist, E. Nygaard, B. Vessby, and B. Saltin. 1981. *Diabetes* 30:19–25.
13. Sadur, C. N., and R. H. Eckel. 1982. *J. Clin. Invest.* 69:1119–1125.
14. Sadur, C. N., T. J. Yost, and R. H. Eckel. 1984. *J. Clin. Endocrinol. Metab.* 59:1176–1182.
15. Rössner, S., B. Eklund, L. Kaijser, A. G. Olsson, and G. Walldius. 1976. *Eur. J. Clin. Invest.* 6:299–305.
16. Havel, R. J., and R. S. Gordon, Jr. 1960. *J. Clin. Invest.* 39:1777–1790.
17. Nikkilä, E. A. 1983. *In*: The Metabolic Basis of Inherited Disease. 5th ed. J. B. Stanbury, J. B. Wyngaarden, D. S. Fredrickson, J. L. Goldstein and M. S. Brown, editors. McGraw-Hill, New York. 622–642.
18. Steiner, G. 1968. *N. Engl. J. Med.* 279:70–74.
19. Bradford, R. H., and R. H. Furman. 1968. *Biochim. Biophys. Acta* 164:172–184.
20. Ford, S. Jr., W. K. Schubert, C. J. Glueck, R. C. Bozian. 1971. *Am. J. Med.* 50:536–541.
21. Schreibman, P. H., D. L. Arons, C. D. Saudek, and R. A. Arky. 1973. *J. Clin. Invest.* 52:2075–2082.
22. Berger, G. M. B., and F. Bonnici. 1977. *S. Afr. Med. J.* 51:623–628.
23. Fredrickson, D. S., K. Ono, and L. L. Davis. 1963. *J. Lipid Res.* 4:24–33.
24. Berger, G. M. B., and P. R. Abraham. 1977. *Clin. Chim. Acta* 81:219–228.
25. Potter, J. M., and W. B. Macdonald. 1979. *Aust. N. Z. J. Med.* 9:688–693.
26. Nicoll, A., and B. Lewis. 1980. *Eur. J. Clin. Invest.* 10:487–495.
27. Wilson, D. E., C. Q. Edwards, and I. -F. Chan. 1983. *Metabolism* 32:1107–1114.
28. Fellin, R., G. Baggio, A. Poli, J. Augustin, M. R. Baiocchi, G. Baldo, M. Sinigaglia, H. Greten, and G. Crepaldi. 1983. *Atherosclerosis* 49:55–68.
29. Kashyap, M. L., L. S. Srivastava, R. C. Tsang, M.-R. Taskinen, B. A. Hynd, G. Perisutti, D. W. Brady, C. J. Glueck, C. A. Ahumada, J. A. McCarthy, R. A. Sosa, and T. O. Reeds. 1980. *J. Lab. Clin. Med.* 95:180–187.

30. Go, T., H. Ohkubo, Y. Mochizuki, T. Murase, and N. Yamada. 1983. *J. Pediatr.* 102:405–407.
31. Harlan, W. R. Jr., P. S. Winesett, and A. J. Wasserman. 1967. *J. Clin. Invest.* 46:239–247.
32. Brunzell, J. D., A. Chait, E. A. Nikkilä, C. Ehnholm, J. K. Huttunen, and G. Steiner. 1980. *Metabolism* 29:624–629.
33. Stalenhoef, A. F. H., M. J. Malloy, J. P. Kane, and R. J. Havel. 1984. *Proc. Natl. Acad. Sci. USA* 81:1839–1843.
34. Rubinstein, A., J. C. Gibson, J. R. Paterniti, Jr., G. Kakis, A. Little, H. N. Ginsberg, and W. V. Brown. 1985. *J. Clin. Invest.* 75:710–721.
35. Berman, M., M. III Hall, R. I. Levy, S. Eisenberg, D. W. Bilheimer, R. D. Phair, and R. H. Goebel. 1978. *J. Lipid. Res.* 19:38–56.
36. Fredrickson, D. S. and R. J. Levy. 1972. *In*: The Metabolic Basis of Inherited Disease. 3rd ed. J. B. Stanbury, J. B. Wyngaarden, and D. S. Fredrickson, editors. McGraw-Hill, New York. 545–614.
37. Quinn, D., K. Shirai, and R. L. Jackson. 1982. *Prog. Lipid Res.* 22:35–78.
38. Breckenridge, W. C., J. A. Little, G. Steiner, A. Chow, and M. Poapst. 1978. *N. Engl. J. Med.* 298:1265–1273.
39. Saku, K., C. Cedres, B. McDonald, B. A. Hynd, B. W. Liu, L. S. Srivastava, and M. L. Kashyap. 1984. *Am. J. Med.* 77:457–462.
40. Breckenridge, W. C., P. Alaupovic, D. W. Cox, and J. A. Little. 1982. *Atherosclerosis* 44:223–235.
41. Yamamura, T., H. Sudo, K. Ishikawa, and A. Yamamoto. 1979. *Atherosclerosis* 34:53–65.
42. Miller, N. E., S. N. Rao, P. Alaupovic, N. Noble, J. Slack, J. D. Brunzell, and B. Lewis. 1981. *Eur. J. Clin. Invest.* 11:69–76.
43. Brunzell, J D., N. E. Miller, P. Alaupovic, R. J. St. Hilaire, C. S. Wang, D. L. Sarson, S. R. Bloom, and B. Lewis. 1983. *J. Lipid Res.* 24:12–19.
44. Catapano, A. L., G. L. Mills, P. Roma, M. La Rosa, and A. Capurso. 1983. *Clin. Chim. Acta* 130:317–327.
45. Manzato, E., G. Baggio, G. Gabelli, S. Zambon, R. Marin, and G. Crepaldi. 1985. *Giornale dell'arteriosclerosi suppl.* 1:138.
46. Cox, D. W., W. C. Breckenridge, and J. A. Little. 1978. *N. Engl. J. Med.* 299:1421–1424.
47. Maguire, G. F., J. A. Little, G. Kakis, and W. C. Breckenridge. 1984. *Can. J. Biochem. Cell Biol.* 62:847–852.
48. Stalenhoef, A. F. H., A. F. Casparie, P. N. M. Demacker, J. T. J. Stouten, J. A. Lutterman, and A. van 't Laar. 1981. *Metabolism* 30:919–926.
49. Glueck, C. J., A. P. Kaplan, R. I. Levy, H. Greten, H. Gralnick, and D. S. Fredrickson. 1969. *Ann. Intern. Med.* 71:1051–1062.
50. Gotto, A. M. Jr. 1973. *Clin. Endocrinol. Metab.* 2:11–39.
51. Kwiterovich, P. O. Jr., J. R. Farah, W. V. Brown, P. S. Bachorik, S. B. Baylin, and C. A. Neill. 1977. *Pediatrics* 59:513–525.
52. Fallat, R. W., and C. J. Glueck. 1976. *Atherosclerosis* 23:41–62.
53. Greenberg, B. H., W. C. Blackwelder, and R. I. Levy. 1977. *Ann. Intern. Med.* 87:526–534.
54. Yki-Järvinen, H., M.-R. Taskinen, and E. A. Nikkilä. 1986. *Clin. Res.* 34:67A.
55. Sigurdsson, G., A. Nicoll, and B. Lewis. 1976. *Eur. J. Clin. Invest.* 6:167–177.
56. Packard, C. H., J. Shepherd, S. Joerns, A. M. Gotto, and O. D. Taunton. 1980. *Metabolism* 29:213–222.
57. Kesäniemi, Y. A., and S. M. Grundy. 1984. *JAMA* 251:2542–2547.
58. Dunn, F. L., S. M. Grundy, D. W. Bilheimer, R. J. Havel, and P. Raskin. 1985. *Metabolism* 34:316–324.
59. Fredrickson, D. S., J. L. Goldstein, and M. S. Brown. 1978. *In*: The Metabolic Basis of Inherited Disease. 4th ed. J. B. Stanbury, J. B. Wyngaarden, D. S. Fredrickson, editors. McGraw-Hill, New York, 604–655.

60. Brown, M. S., J. L. Goldstein, and D. S. Fredrickson. 1983. *In*: The Metabolic Basis of Inherited Disease. 5th ed. J. B. Stanbury, J. B. Wyngaarden, D. S. Fredrickson, J. L. Goldstein, M. S. Brown, editors. McGraw- Hill, New York. 655–671.
61. Mahley, R. W., and B. Angelin. 1984. *Adv. Intern. Med.* 29:385–411.
62. Chait, A., W. R. Hazzard, J. J. Albers, R. P. Kushwaha, and J. D. Brunzell. 1978. *Metabolism* 27:1055–1066.
63. Chung, B. H., and J. P. Segrest, 1983. *J. Lipid Res.* 24:1148–1159.
64. Kushwaha, R. S., S. M. Haffner, D. M. Foster, and W. R. Hazzard. 1985. *Metabolism* 34:1029–1038.
65. Goldberg, A. P., D. M. Applebaum-Bowden, and W. R. Hazzard. 1979. *Metabolism* 28:1122–1126.
66. Chait, A., J. J. Albers, and J. D. Brunzell. 1980. *Eur. J. Clin. Invest.* 10:17–22.
67. Beil, U., S. M. Grundy, J. R. Crouse, and L. Zech. 1982. *Arteriosclerosis* 2:44–57.
68. Stalenhoef, A. F. H., P. N. M. Demacker, J. A. Lutterman, and A. van 't Laar. 1982. *In*: Metabolic Studies in Various Forms of Hypertriglyceridemia in Man. A. F. H. Stanlenhoef, editor. Drukkerij Dukenburch-Wijchen. 43–61.
69. Sane, T. 1983. *Academic Dissertation, Helsinki.*
70. Magill, P., S. N. Rao, N. E. Miller, A. Nicoll, J. Brunzell, J. St. Hilaire, and B. Lewis. 1982. *Eur. J. Clin. Invest.* 12:113–120.
71. Reardon, M. F., H. Sakai, and G. Steiner. 1982. *Arteriosclerosis* 2:396–402.
72. Larsson, B., P. Björntorp, J. Holm, T. Schersten, L. Sjöström, and U. Smith. 1975. *Metabolism* 24:1375–1389.
73. Günther, W., W. Leonhardt, M. Hanefeld, and H. Haller. 1977. *Endokrinologie* 70:176–181.
74. Goldberg, A. P., A. Chait, and J. D. Brunzell. 1980. *Metabolism*, 29:223–229.
75. Taylor, K. G., G. Holdsworth, and D. J. Galton. 1980. *Eur. J. Clin. Invest.* 10:133–138.
76. Taskinen, M. -R., E. A. Nikkilä, and T. Kuusi. 1982. *Eur. J. Clin. Invest.* 12:433–438.
77. Boberg, J. 1972. *Acta Med. Scand.* 191:97–102.
78. Johansson, B. G., and A. Medhus. 1974. *Acta Med. Scand.* 195:273–277.
79. Böttiger, L. E., L. A. Carlson, E. Hultman, and V. Romanus. 1976. *Acta Med. Scand.* 199:357–361.
80. Baumgartner, H. P., and L. Filippini. 1977. *Schweiz. Med. Wochenschr.* 107:1406–1411.
82. Avogaro, P., G. Cazzolato, and G. B. Bittolo. 1979. *In*: Metabolic Effects of Alcohol. P. Avogaro, C. R. Sirtori and E. Tremoli, editors. Elsevier/North-Holland Biomedical Press. 157–164.
82. Ostrander, L. D. Jr., D. E. Lamphiear, W. D. Block, B. C. Johnson, C. Ravenscroft, and F. H. Epstein. 1974. *Arch. Intern. Med.* 134:451–456.
83. Castelli, W. P., T. Gordon, M. C. Hjortland, A. Kagan, J. T. Doyle, C. G. Hames, S. B. Hulley, and W. J. Zukel. 1977. *Lancet II*: 153–155.
84. Avogaro, P., and G. Cazzolato. 1975. *Metabolism* 24:1231–1242.
85. Barboriak, J. J., and W. J. Hogan. 1976. *Atherosclerosis* 24:323–325.
86. Taskinen, M. -R., and E. A. Nikkilä. 1977. *Acta Med. Scand.* 202:173–177.
87. Nilsson-Ehle, P., S. Carlström, and P. Belfrage. 1978. *Lipids* 13:433–437.
88. Kaffarnik, H., J. Schneider, R. Schubotz, L. Hausmann, G. Mühlfellner, O. Mühlfellner, and P. Zöfel. 1978. *Atherosclerosis* 29:1–7.
89. Schneider, J., A. Liesenfeld, R. Mordasini, R. Schubotz, P. Zöfel, F. Kubel, C. Vandre-Plozzitzka and H. Kaffarnik. 1985. *Atherosclerosis* 57:281–291.
90. Taskinen, M. -R., M. Välimäki, E. A. Nikkilä, T. Kuusi, and R. Ylikahri. 1985. *Metabolism* 34:112–119.
91. Hansson, P., and P. Nilsson-Ehle. 1983. *Ann. Nutr. Metab.* 27:328–337.
92. Schneider, J., E. Panne, H. Braun, R. Mordasini, and H. Kaffarnik. 1983. *J. Lab. Clin. Med.* 101:114–122.
93. Ginsberg, H., J. Olefsky, J. W. Farquhar, and G. M. Reaven. 1974. *Ann. Intern. Med.* 80:143–149.

94. Belfrage, P., B. Berg, I. Hägerstrand, P. Nilsson- Ehle, H. Törnqvist, and T. Wiebe. 1977. *Eur. J. Clin. Invest.* 7:127–131.
95. Crouse, J. R., and S. M. Grundy. 1984. *J. Lipid Res.* 25:486–496.
96. Ekman, R., G. Fex, B. G. Johansson, P. Nilsson-Ehle, and J. Wadstein. 1981. *Scand. J. Clin. Lab. Invest.* 41:709–715.
97. Devenyi, P., G. M. Robinson, B. M. Kapur, and D. A. K. Roncari. 1981. *Am. J. Med.* 71:589–594.
98. Barboriak, J. J., P. Alaupovic, and P. Cushman. 1981. *Drug Alcohol Depend.* 8:337–343.
99. Peynet, J., A. Legrand, P. Techenet, J. P. Isal, P. J. Guillausseau, and F. Rousselet. 1982. *Nouv. Presse. Med.* 11:3179–3183.
100. Taskinen, M. -R., M. Välimäki, E. A. Nikkilä, T. Kuusi, C. Ehnholm, and R. Ylikahri. 1982. *Metabolism* 31:1168–1174.
101. Nikkilä, E. A., M. -R. Taskinen, M. Välimäki, and R. Ylikahri. 1984. *In*: Diet, Diabetes and Atherosclerosis. G. Pozza, P. Micossi, A. L. Catapano and R. Pasletti, editors. Raven Press, New York. 167–175.
102. Nikkilä, E. A., M. -R. Taskinen, and J. K. Huttunen. 1978. *Horm. Metab. Res.* 10:220–223.
103. Belfrage, P., P. Nilsson-Ehle, and T. Wiebe. 1973. *Acta Med. Scand. suppl.* 552:19–26.
104. Välimäki, M., E. A. Nikkilä, M. -R. Taskinen, and R. Ylikahri. 1986. *Atherosclerosis* 59:147–153.
105. Sane, T., E. A. Nikkilä, M. -R. Taskinen, M. Välimäki, and R. Ylikahri. 1984. *Atherosclerosis* 53:185–193.
106. Angelico, F., A. Bucci, R. Capocaccia, G. Morisi, M. Terzino, and G. Ricci. 1982. *Ann. Nutr. Metab.* 26:73–76.
107. Gruchow, H. W., R. G. Hoffmann, A. J. Anderson, and J. J. Barboriak. 1982. *Atherosclerosis* 43:393–404.
108. Nikkilä, E. A., T. Kuusi, M. -R. Taskinen, and M. J. Tikkanen. 1984. *In*: Treatment of Hyperlipoproteinemia. L. A. Carlson and A. G. Olsson, editors. Raven Press, New York. 77–84.
109. Camargo, C. A. Jr., P. T. Williams, K. M. Vranizan, J. J. Albers, and P. D. Wood. 1985. *JAMA* 253:2854–2857.
110. Williams, P. T., R. M. Krauss, P. D. Wood, J. J. Albers, D. Dreon, and N. Ellsworth. 1985. *Metabolism* 34:524–530.
111. Bagdade, J. D., D. Porte, Jr., and E. L. Bierman. 1968. *N. Engl. J. Med.* 279:181–185.
112. Cattran, D. C., S. S. A. Fenton, D. R. Wilson, and G. Steiner. 1976. *Ann. Intern. Med.* 85:29–33.
113. Mordasini, R., F. Frey, W. Flury, G. Klose, and H. Greten. 1977. *N. Engl. J. Med* 297:1362–1366.
114. Chan, M. K., Z. Varghese, J. W. Persaud, R. A. Baillod, and J. F. Moorhead. 1982. *Clin. Nephrol.* 17:183–190.
115. Chan, M. K., J. Persaud, Z. Varghese, and J. F. Moorhead. 1984. *Kidney Int.* 25:812–818.
116. Ibels, L. S., L. A. Simons, J. O. King, P. F. Williams, F. C. Neale, and J. H. Stewart. 1975. *Q. J. Med.* 176:601–614.
117. Bagdade, J., A. Casarltto, and J. Albers. 1976. *J. Lab. Clin. Med.* 87:37–48.
118. Daubresse, J. C., G. Lerson, G. Plomteux, G. Rorive, A. S. Luyckx, and P. J. Lefebvre. 1976. *Eur. J. Clin. Invest.* 6:159–166.
119. Huttunen, J. K., A. Pasternack, T. Vänttinen, C. Ehnholm, and E. A. Nikkilä. 1978. *Acta Med. Scand.* 204:211–218.
120. Norbeck, H. E., and L. A. Carlson. 1981. *Acta Med. Scand.* 209:489–503.
121. Ibels, L. S., M. F. Reardon, and P. J. Nestel. 1976. *J. Lab. Clin. Med.* 87:648–658.
122. Crawford, G. A., E. Savdie, and J. H. Stewart. 1979. *Clin. Sci.* 57:155–165.
123. Savdie, E., J. C. Gibson, G. A. Crawford, L. A. Simons, and J. F. Mahony. 1980. *Kidney Int.* 18:774–782.

124. Asayama, K., H. Ito, C. Nakahara, A. Hasegawa, and K. Kato. 1984. *Pediatr. Res.* 18:783–788.
125. Applebaum-Bowden, D., A. P. Goldberg, W. R. Hazzard, D. J. Sherrard, J. D. Brunzell, J. K. Huttunen, E. A. Nikkilä, and C. Ehnholm. 1979. *Metabolism* 28:917–924.
126. Persson, B. 1973. *Acta Med. Scand.* 193:457–462.
127. Goldberg, A., D. J. Sherrard, and J. D. Brunzell. 1978. *J. Clin. Endocrinol. Metab.* 47:1173–1182.
128. Bolzano, K., F. Krempler, and F. Sandhofer. 1978. *Eur. J. Clin. Invest.* 8:289–293.
129. Murase, T., D. C. Cattran, B. Rubenstein, and G. Steiner. 1975. *Metabolism* 24:1279–1286.
130. DeFronzo, R. A., and A. Alvestrand. 1980. *Am. J. Clin. Nutr.* 33:1438–1445.
131. Verschoor, L. R., R. Lammers, and J. C. Birkenhäger. 1978. *Metabolism* 27:879–883.
132. Reaven, G. M., R. S. Swenson, and M. L. Sanfelippo. 1980. *Am. J. Clin. Nutr.* 33:1476–1484.
133. Norbeck, H. E., and S. Rössner. 1982. *Acta Med. Scand.* 211:69–74.
134. Goldberg, A. P., D. M. Applebaum-Bowden, E. L. Bierman, W. R. Hazzard, L. B. Haas, D. J. Sherrard, J. D. Brunzell, J. K. Huttunen, C. Ehnholm, and E. A. Nikkilä. 1979. *N. Engl. J. Med.* 301:1073–1076.
135. Casaretto, A., R. Goldsmith, T. L. Marchioro, and J. D. Bagdade. 1974. *Lancet I*:481–484.
136. Ibels, L. S., A. C. Alfrey, and R. Weil, III. 1978. *Am. J. Med.* 64:634–642.
137. Cattran, D. C., G. Steiner, D. R. Wilson, and S. S. A. Fenton. 1979. *Ann. Intern. Med.* 91:554–559.
138. Baxter, J. H., H. C. Goodman, and R. J. Havel. 1960. *J. Clin. Invest.* 39:455–465.
139. Gherardi, E., E. Rota, S. Calandra, R. Genova, and A. Tamborino. 1977. *Eur. J. Clin. Invest.* 7:563–570.
140. Chan, M. K., J. W. Persaud, L. Ramdial, Z. Varghese, P. Sweny, and J. F. Moorhead. 1981. *Clin. Chim. Acta.* 117:317–323.
141. Appel, G. B., C. B. Blum, S. Chien, C. L. Kunis, and A. S. Appel. 1985. *N. J. Engl. Med.* 312:1544–1548.
142. Oetliker, O. H., R. Mordasini, J. Lütschg, and W. Riesen. 1980. *Pediatr. Res.* 14:64–66.
143. Michaeli, J., H. Bar-on, and E. Shafrir. 1981. *Isr. J. Med. Sci.* 17:1001–1008.
144. McKenzie, I. F. C., and P. J. Nestel. 1968. *J. Clin. Invest.* 47:1685–1695.
145. Kekki, M., and E. A. Nikkilä. 1971. *Eur. J. Clin. Invest.* 1:345–351.
146. Kashyap, M. L., L. S. Srivastava, B. A. Hynd, D. Brady, G. Perisutti, C. J. Glueck, and P. S. Gartside. 1980. *Atherosclerosis* 35:29–40.
147. Valdemarsson, S. 1983. *Acta Endocrinol.* 103: suppl 255, 1–52.
148. Heimberg, M., J. O. Olubadewo, and H. G. Wilcox. 1985. *Endocrin. Rev.* 6:590–607.
149. Ballantyne, F. C., A. A. Epenetos, M. Caslake, S. Forsythe, and D. Ballantyne. 1979. *Clin. Sci.* 57:83–88.
150. Nikkilä, E. A., and M. Kekki. 1972. *J. Clin. Invest.* 51:2103–2114.
151. Pykälistö, O., A. P. Goldberg, and J. D. Brunzell. 1976. *J. Clin. Endocrinol. Metab.* 43:591–600.
152. Abrams, J. J., S. M. Grundy, and H. Ginsberg. 1981. *J. Lipid Res.* 22:307–322.
153. Valdemarsson, S., P. Hedner, and P. Nilsson-Ehle. 1982. *Eur. J. Clin. Invest.* 12:423–428.
154. Muls, E., M. Rosseneu, G. Lamberigts, and P. De Moor. 1985. *Metabolism* 34:345–353.
155. Lithell, H., J. Boberg, K. Hellsing, S. Ljunghall, G. Lundqvist, B. Vessby, and L. Wide. 1981. *Eur. J. Clin. Invest.* 11:3–10.
156. Porte, D. Jr., D. D. O'Hara, and R. H. Williams. 1966. *Metabolism* 15:107–113.
157. Lisch, H. -J., M. Ogriseg, Ch. Breier, H. Drexel, H. Fill, und S. Sailer. 1982. *Klin. Wochenschr.* 60:337–342.
158. Valdemarsson, S., P. Hansson, P. Hedner, and P. Nilsson-Ehle. 1983. *Acta Endocrinol.* 104:50–56.
159. Nikkilä, E. A., and R. Pelkonen. 1975. *Metabolism* 24:829–838.

160. Murase, T., N. Yamada, N. Ohsawa, K. Kosaka, S. Morita, and S. Yoshida. 1980. *Metabolism* 29:666–672.
161. Asayama, K., S. Amemiya, S. Kusano, and K. Kato. 1984. *Metabolism* 33:129–131.
162. Pelkonen, R., E. A. Nikkilä, and B. Grahne. 1982. *Clin. Endocrinol.* 16:383–390.
163. Taskinen, M. -R., E. A. Nikkilä, R. Pelkonen, and T. Sane. 1983. *J. Clin. Endocrinol. Metab.* 57:619–626.

Chapter 9

DIABETES AND LIPOPROTEIN LIPASE ACTIVITY

Patricia A. O'Looney and George V. Vahouny

In 1967 Bagdade et al. (1) described the syndrome called diabetic lipemia. Untreated diabetic individuals with marked hypertriglyceridemia, showed a decrease in their triglyceride levels towards normal when treated with insulin. It was also demonstrated that these subjects had low postheparin plasma lipolytic activity, which was used as an indirect measure of lipoprotein lipase (LPL), and suggested that the hypertriglyceridemia was due to a defect in LPL (1,2). Furthermore, insulin treatment normalized the heparin-releasable enzymatic activity in plasma (1,2).

In the present chapter, we will summarize the status of the knowledge regarding the activity of LPL in both human and experimental diabetes. This will include a discussion of lipolytic activities in postheparin plasma and of LPL activity in adipose and muscle tissue. Where appropriate, the differences between the insulin-dependent diabetes (IDD) and the non-insulin dependent diabetes (NIDD) will be indicated.

Human Diabetes

Postheparin Lipolytic Activity

Adults with mild diabetes (IDD) exhibit a disproportionate prevalence of hypertriglyceridemia (3,4), with elevated levels of both the very low density lipoprotein (VLDL) fraction and of chylomicrons. Severe uncontrolled diabetes is always associated with hypertriglyceridemia, and treatment of the diabetes has been shown to be associated with a decrease in plasma triglyceride levels (5).

These changes in blood triglycerides appear to be due, at least in part, to insulin-dependent alterations in LPL activity, which has been suggested to account for the removal of as much as 90% of chylomicron triglycerides from blood (6). LPL can be released from the capillary endothelia into plasma by small intravenous doses of heparin (7), and this activity is referred to as postheparin lipolytic activity, or PHLA (7). Postheparin lipolytic activity is now known to consist of multiple enzymatic activities that emanate from different tissue sources (8–11). LPL release, induced by heparin, has been demonstrated to be multiphasic in rat hearts (12), as has the PHLA release in man (13). PHLA levels have been measured during the early phase [10–30 minutes following a single low dose (10 units/kg) of intravenous heparin] and during the late phase [prolonged 3–6 hour infusion of a high dose (60 units/kg) of heparin]. Despite the apparent problems in assays of PHLA, which are described below, there is evidence relating the degree of diabetic hypertriglyceridemia with levels of plasma PHLA.

In the studies measuring the early phase release of PHLA in untreated diabetic patients, low (1,2,14), high (15) and normal activities (16,17) have been reported. Low PHLA levels have been reported in several patients with untreated overt diabetes and hypertriglyceridemia (1). In the studies of Bagdade et al. (1), PHLA was only 44% of control (45 minutes after heparin) while plasma triglycerides remained markedly elevated ($>$ 5450 mg/dl). PHLA remained severely depressed (28%) of control) after only 4 hours of insulin therapy. However, both the elevated plasma triglyceride levels and the low PHLA levels returned toward normal (PHLA was 89% of controls) after a 24 hour insulin therapy. Bagdade et al. (2) also reported that when insulin was withdrawn for 48 hours from insulin-dependent juvenile diabetics, there was an increase in triglyceride levels and a fall in PHLA. This inverse correlation between the degree of hypertriglyceridemia and PHLA levels was further substantiated by the findings of Shigeta et al. (17). Although PHLA was found to be normal in IDD after only 10 minutes postheparin, there was a significant decrease in lipase activity at 20 minutes after heparin. PHLA was shown to be inversely correlated with the degree of hypertriglyceridemia, i.e. with plasma triglyceride levels of 80–119 mg/dl, the lipase activity was 69% of control; at levels of 120–149 mg/dl, activity was 45% of control; and at levels greater than 150 mg/dl, the activity was only 8% of control levels. Similar variability in PHLA levels was observed based on the degree of hyperglycemia. Those diabetic patients with the highest fasting glucose levels had the lowest PHLA levels during the early phase of PHLA release (15) and during the late phase of heparin infusion (16). Impaired clearance of intravenously-injected, labeled VLDL from the plasma following 48 hours insulin withdrawal in IDD patients suggested that PHLA might reflect a measure of the functionally important activity in triglyceride removal (2).

In contrast, elevated levels of PHLA were reported in thirteen diabetics who were studied 24 hours after their last dose of insulin, or 48 hours after their last dose of oral hypoglycemic agents (15). When the study was initiatcd, the triglyceride levels were slightly elevated at 110 mg/dl. At 15 minutes postheparin, the lipolytic activity measured with an olive oil emulsion was 162% of the mean of normal male and female patients. With this marked increase in PHLA in diabetic patients, it is questionable as to whether a 24 hour insulin withdrawal is sufficient for marked alterations in blood components to occur. There is, however, no mention of the basal insulin levels at the time of the heparin injection, the duration of insulin therapy prior to study, or the blood glucose levels before and after heparin injection. It should be noted that a 48 hour withdrawal of insulin was reported in the studies by Bagdade et al. (1,2), in which a decrease in PHLA in insulin-deficient diabetes was reported.

To assess the differences between effects of short and long term insulin therapy on the multiphasic responses of PHLA, Brunzell et al. (16) designed an extensive study to determine whether abnormalities in multiphasic release of LPL were associated with hypertriglyceridemia in diabetes mellitus. In 12 diabetic patients with hypertriglyceridemia, 25 nondiabetic hypertriglyceridemic patients and 7 normal patients, PHLA was measured during a standard low heparin dose and a high dose constant heparin infusion to study the early and late phase of PHLA release, respectively. The standard low dose PHLA response (10 minutes) was in the normal range in both groups of hypertriglyceridemic patients. It appeared to be lower in the untreated diabetic patients (0.369 ± 0.104 units) than in the nondiabetic hypertriglyceridemic patients (0.466 ± 0.163 units), but the difference was not significant. During the constant infusion of heparin for 3–5 hours, the peak PHLA was reached at 60 minutes and, there was found to be no difference between these three groups. The equilibrium PHLA resulting from constant infusion of heparin was defined as the mean of three values during the last hour of the heparin infusion (the late phase of release), and this produced different results. Although there was no difference between the normal and nondiabetic hypertriglyceridemic patients, the equilibrium PHLA was significantly lower in the untreated diabetic patients (0.388 ± 0.133 units) than the nondiabetic patients (0.495 ± 0.167 units). This difference in PHLA value during the late phase of release was not improved after 2 months of insulin treatment, but was significantly improved after 6 months of insulin therapy.

These contrasting early studies are typical of the variability in data during attempts to directly relate PHLA with diabetic hypertriglyceridemia. It is now clear that there are several explanations for this high degree of variability in studies on PHLA. Among these are: the cause(s) and levels of hypertriglyceridemia (and hyperglycemia); the method of enzyme assay; and the dose of intravenous heparin employed and the time of plasma collection after the administration of heparin. In many studies, it is not possible to compare data or evaluate the reasons for differences in results. However, it does seem, based on the discussions above, that the last of the variables mentioned above, namely, the heparin dose and the timing of blood collection, has a major influence on the data.

The fact that PHLA is composed of several lipolytic enzymes, which originate from different tissues (18,19) and have different functions in the triglyceride-removal process, may provide a possible explanation for discrepancies in the studies of PHLA levels. Huttunen et al. (20) reported that the appearance of these lipolytic enzymes into plasma after heparin injection was dependent on the dose of heparin and time of blood collection. The release into plasma of LPL and a second lipolytic activity, referred to as hepatic lipase (HL), occurred at different heparin dose levels. At 10 units/kg, heparin released approximately 75% of the maximal activity of HL but only about 30% of the activity of LPL. A dose of 100–200 units/kg of heparin was needed for the release of maximal LPL activity but only about 50 units/kg was required for maximal release of HL (20). Furthermore, the activity of HL reached a peak at 2–5 minutes after a 100 units/kg dose of heparin, whereas the peak activity of LPL occurred 15–20 minutes later (20). In addition, there appear to be other variables that require consideration. These are briefly described below.

The inconsistencies reported on the levels of PHLA during the early phase in insulin-deficient diabetics, particularly after a low dose of heparin, may partly be due to the duration and severity of the diabetic condition. It would appear that hyperglycemia in the presence of hypertriglyceridemia significantly affects PHLA in diabetic patients. These two clinical symptoms should be considered when comparisons are made. For example, in the study by Perry (15), in which a higher than normal level of PHLA was found in diabetics, the patients had undergone treatment (either oral hypoglycemic agents or insulin) to control the diabetes, and they did not display hypertriglyceridemia either before (110 mg/dl) or 15 minutes after heparin injection (90 mg/dl). In that report, the insulin or oral hypoglycemic agents were withheld for only 24 hours prior to study and as a result, may have obscured the effect on PHLA levels. This is also reflected in the finding that even after 60 minutes, the plasma triglyceride levels in the diabetic patients was only 100 mg/dl. There was no data on the plasma glucose levels either before of after insulin withdrawal, as a reflection of the severity of the diabetic state.

To compare the use of different substrates in PHLA assay, similar rates of hydrolysis for chylomicrons and for artificially prepared fat emulsions have been found in early studies with LPL (21,22). Therefore, the variability which has been reported in PHLA studies is not a reflection of the different substrates used in the assay. This has recently been supported by the work of Wilson et al. (14) who showed the normal rates of hydrolysis with either soybean oil substrate or chylomicrons substrate from a normolipemic or a hyperlipemic donor.

The method used to assay PHLA in diabetic patients is critical when evaluating and comparing various reports. To illustrate this point, Wilson et al. (14) measured the PHLA in diabetic patients with hyperlipemia, using the methods of Datta (23) and Muir (24). The basic difference between these two methods is in the use of calcium chloride as the fatty acid acceptor in the method by Datta (23), and albumin as the fatty acid acceptor in the procedure by Muir (24). It was reported by Datta (23) that the use of calcium chloride as the sole fatty acid acceptor improved the extraction of fatty acids, and thus, led to a higher postheparin LPL activity. Of the five patients studied, four were non-insulin dependent diabetes and one was an insulin-dependent diabetic. In some patients, there appeared to be a decrease in PHLA when compared to normal values using the Datta procedure, i.e. the lipolytic activity was only 24% to 44% of normal. However, when PHLA was assayed in the same samples according to the method of Muir, the lipolytic activity was in the normal range, and in one patient, the activity was 160% of normal.

Other methods employed to measure postheparin lipolytic activity have been described by Fredrickson et al. (7), in which albumin was used as the sole fatty acid acceptor, and by Korn (21), in which both calcium chloride and albumin were used as the acceptor of fatty acids. The Fredrickson's procedure was employed in the studies by Bagdade et al. (1,2), Brunzell et al. (16) and Porte et al. (25) while Shigeta et al. (17) used the method of Korn.

An additional variable may involve the tissue sites of lipolytic enzyme-release following heparin injection. The late phase of heparin-releasable PHLA may relate to adipose tissue storage or synthesis of the enzyme or enzyme precursors (26) and, thus could be the site of the abnormality produced by insulin deficiency. Decreased protein synthesis is known to occur secondary to insulin deficiency.

The assumption that the late phase of lipolytic activity is derived from adipose tissue has been supported by the study of Pfeifer et al. (27), who demonstrated a biphasic release of LPL activity in postheparin plasma of noninsulin dependent diabetic patients. Pfeifer et al. (27) postulated that the first phase originates from muscle, while the second phase is derived from adipose tissue (28,29).

The variety of problems relating to measurements of PHLA as a reflection of LPL activity strongly indicates that this procedure is of little value in assessing triglyceride clearance defects in diabetes. In addition, the lipolytic enzymes of different tissues are apparently not equally sensitive to insulin deficiency (30–32). Based on the availability of a specific immunochemical method (20), LPL and HL can now be assayed separately in postheparin plasma, and these methods should be employed for a reexamination of the effects of diabetes on these individual enzymes. Some studies of this nature are described below.

Postheparin Lipoprotein Lipase and Hepatic Lipase

LPL is defined as the triglyceride lipase of postheparin plasma that is inhibited by high salt concentration and activated by addition of serum (apo

C-II). HL, in contrast, is resistant to high salt concentrations and is active in the absence of added serum. The selective assay of LPL and HL in postheparin plasma (29) is based on the inactivation of HL by a specific antiserum to allow specific assay of LPL, and on the use of a high salt concentration and omission of additional serum for the specific assay of HL.

A lower level of specific postheparin LPL has been reported in a variety of patients with untreated diabetes. The postheparin plasma LPL activity was found to be lower in patients with untreated ketotic diabetes (56% of controls), and in patients with untreated mild to moderate nonketotic early-onset diabetes (80% of controls) (33). In these studies, postheparin plasma was obtained at 5 minutes and 15 minutes after an injection of heparin (100 units/kg body weight). Insulin-treatment of ketotic diabetes resulted in a rapid increase in the activity of serum LPL, and a decreases in serum triglyceride levels. These results are in total agreement with the earlier demonstration of low PHLA in human insulin-deficient diabetes (2), and support the view that hypertriglyceridemia accompanying severe insulin deficiency is due, at least in part, to a decreased activity of LPL (2,3,4) and concomitant impairment of triglyceride removal (34).

Insulin-treated juvenile diabetics, who have had diabetes up to 18 years and have been on continuous insulin treatment, have been reported to have either normal or elevated postheparin LPL activity (33,35). The activity of LPL in postheparin plasma is significantly higher in both male and female diabetic patients with good diabetic control, in comparison to normal values. In these studies, control of diabetes was defined as good, if fasting blood glucose was 100 mg/dl or less. Diabetic men with poor control of diabetes (blood glucose > 250 mg/dl) had slightly lower LPL activity than did men with good control (26.6 units versus 32.9 units, respectively).

In untreated NIDD patients who also had hypertriglyceridemia, the postheparin LPL activity was only 74% of control values (33). However, in non-insulin dependent diabetic subjects without concomitant hypertriglyceridemia, it is unclear whether or not plasma postheparin lipolytic activity is decreasesd (24), or normal (33) after only 15–60 minutes of heparin treatment. Since these lipase levels were determined from plasma withdrawn relatively early after heparin injection, Pfeifer et al. (24) extended their study to include the late phase (210–240 minutes postheparin) activity of LPL from NIDD patients. Analysis of the two phases (early and late) of the postheparin LPL activity in plasma showed that the abnormal early phase in untreated NIDD was corrected to normal values in less than one month of therapy, while the late phase activity was not corrected until 3 months of therapy. These results are in good agreement with those previously reported by Brunzell et al. (16), where the late phase abnormality of PHLA in untreated diabetic patients was not corrected until after 6 months of antihyperglycemic therapy.

The HL activity of postheparin plasma appears to be similar to control values in both IDD (33) and NIDD patients (24,33). The only reported exception has been in hypertriglyceridemic NIDD, where there was a higher HL activity than in the corresponding control group (33).

Lipoprotein Lipase of Adipose Tissue and Skeletal Muscle

Adipose Tissue. Various methods have been devised to measure the LPL, specifically dervied from adipose tissue, due to the discrepancies in determining LPL activity based only on measurements of PHLA. The principal approaches have been either to elute extracellular enzyme from intact tissues by incubation with heparin at 37° C (36) or at 4° C (37), or to extract intra- and extracellular enzyme from either fresh tissue homogenates (38), or from tissues defatted with acetone-ether (39). The recovery of total LPL eluted from adipose tissue with heparin has been improved by the inclusion of serum activator in the medium to provide a protein carrier and to further stabilize the lipase (40). By including a detergent (e.g. sodium deoxycholate) in the extraction medium, the yield of recovered enzyme is increased markedly (40). Iverius and Brunzell (40) have suggested that elution of LPL from tissue homogenates at 4° C represents only the extracellular enzyme activity, and therefore correlates directly with the physiologically active LPL on the endothelial surface. In addition, elution at 37° C may also reflect some intracellular enzyme secreted during the incubation period (40).

It has been reported that heparin-releasable LPL activity from biopsies of subcutaneous adipose tissue from insulin-deficient, untreated diabetic patients was 37% of control values (41,42). The acetone-ether powder preparation of adipose tissue from IDD also exhibited a statistically lower LPL activity when compared to controls (41). After two weeks of insulin treatment, the mean LPL activity of adipose tissue of diabetic patients increased significantly, but still was subnormal (56 and 65% of controls when expressed as μmol FFA/h per gram or pmol FFA/h per cell, respectively) (42). A 36% increase in the activity of LPL of adipose tissue was shown in insulin-treated diabetic patients who were deprived of insulin for only 12 hours prior to LPL assay and were given an 8 hour intravenous infusion of insulin (43). Pykalisto et al. (41) reported no change in the activity of heparin-releasable LPL of fresh adipose tissue or of acetone-ether powders of the tissue from diabetic patients after a one week treatment of the hyperglycemia. However, the diabetic patients were treated with oral sulphonylurea and not with insulin. This unaltered LPL activity after sulphonylurea treatment is not surprising, since insulin has been found to be essential for the maintenance of normal adipose tissue LPL activity, and can promote the *in vitro* synthesis of LPL in rat adipose tissue (44,45).

The finding of low heparin-releasable LPL activity in adipose tissue of insulin-deficient diabetics is in agreement with earlier data demonstrating the presence of an LPL defect in postheparin plasma of untreated ketotic diabetics, and its correction with insulin treatment (33). A similar defect has also been found in adipose tissue of patients who have non-insulin dependent diabetes combined with hypertriglyceridemia (41,46,47). The close dependence of the adipose tissue LPL on insulin levels is further documented by the decline of the activity during total starvation or restriction of caloric intake (42). On the other hand, the activity is rapidly increased by a high carbohydrate diet, and by oral or intravenous glucose loads (48). However, in untreated insulin-dependent diabetic patients, in the absence of adequate insulin response, even high carbohydrate feeding will not cause an increase in adipose LPL activity (41).

Skeletal Muscle. There is less information on insulin regulation of human skeletal muscle LPL. Muscle LPL activity decreases slowly during low caloric diets (49) and can be increased by glucose infusion (42). These data suggest that human skeletal muscle LPL behaves differently than it does in the rat since, in this latter species, muscle LPL is either not influenced or only mildly affected (50) by insulin.

The LPL activity has been determined from biopsy samples of skeletal muscles in patients with newly-detected, untreated insulin-deficient diabetes and non-insulin dependent diabetes (42,47). The skeletal muscle of NIDD men showed an insignificantly lower level of heparin-releasable LPL activity than in controls (42). In the skeletal muscle of IDD patients, the LPL activity averaged 46% of the mean value of controls. After initiation of insulin treatment, LPL activity increased significantly in skeletal muscle, but as in the case of the adipose tissue, the activity was still subnormal after 2 weeks (78% of control values). These results (42) suggest that human skeletal muscle LPL is also dependent on insulin, although it appears less sensitive than the adipose tissue enzyme. This conclusion is supported by recent findings (43), in which insulin-treated diabetic patients, who were deprived of insulin for only 12 hours prior to LPL assay, were studied. In spite of development of hyperglycemia during the insulin deprivation, the LPL activity of adipose and skeletal muscle remained within the normal range. This is most likely due to residual insulin still present only after 12 hours of withdrawal (43). During subsequent insulin administration, the skeletal muscle LPL remained unchanged, whereas the LPL activity of adipose tissue was significantly increased (by 36%). These additional observations by Taskinen et al. (43) are compatible with the concept that human adipose tissue LPL is more sensitive to insulin than is muscle LPL, although skeletal muscle LPL may also retain limited insulin sensitivity.

Experimental Diabetes

Lipoprotein Lipase Activity in Adipose Tissue

In tissues such as adipose tissue and heart, LPL exists in both functional and nonfunctional forms (51,52). The functional form appears to be largely associated with the endothelial surface of tissue capillaries and is readily released by heparin (52). This LPL activity is responsible for the degradation of lipoprotein triglyceride during tissue assimilation of the triglyceride fatty acids. The nonfunctional form of LPL which is not readily releasable by heparin, appears to be associated with the tissue parenchymal cells (52). This activity has also been termed "residual" and may represent the ultimate source of the vascular endothelial activity (23,53).

Although most studies show that rat adipose tissue LPL is an insulin-dependent enzyme (54,55), conflicting results have been reported on the adipose tissue LPL activity of diabetic rats (30,32,56–60). Adipose tissue LPL activity in diabetic rats has been reported to be high (61), low (30,32,56,58–60,62), only moderately decreased (58), or even normal (57). As in the case of the human studies, these conflicting reports may be a result of a number of variables including the method chosen for the expression of enzyme activity, and the methods of tissue preparation. Since diabetic rats exhibit a marked loss of adipose tissue weight, it has been suggested that the enzyme activity should be expressed per total tissue and not per gram tissue weight (60). Ishikawa et al. (60) demonstrated that epididymal adipose tissue weight is closely related to its LPL activity and as such, the LPL activity in whole adipose tissue may reflect, more adequately, the functional state of the tissue. Interestingly, in their study, diabetes caused a marked reduction (15–41% of control values) in the total activity of LPL in the whole adipose tissue in rats, but there was no change when expressed per gram of tissue weight.

The level of enzyme activity measured may also be a reflection of the dependency of LPL on heparin concentration (63), presence of serum, pH of buffer (64), the concentration of the diabetogenic agent used to induce diabetes, and the duration and severity of the diabetes. Additional variables in enzyme activity have reported utilizing homogenates of acetone-ether powder, sliced tissue, or homogenates of epididymal fat tissue.

Although there is variability in the reported activity of adipose LPL in experimental diabetes, the existing evidence suggests a significant reduction of the activity released from epididymal adipose tissue (Table 1). The changes in the lipolytic activity are parallel in the heparin-releasable fraction of fresh tissue and in the activity of the acetone-dried preparations. The results suggest that the regulation of the LPL activity in rat adipose tissue is sensitive to acute changes in serum insulin concentrations, resulting from administration of either streptozotocin or alloxan. Administration of insulin, in doses sufficient to control the diabetes, appears to restore the lipolytic activity of adipose tissue to normal (30). The low activity of LPL in untreated diabetes occurs concomitantly with a rise in plasma triglycerides, suggesting that a deficiency of LPL activity may contribute significantly to the elevated plasma triglycerides of uncontrolled diabetes in rats (56,59). On the other hand, the closest relationship noted by Chen et al. (58) was between the magnitude of hyperglycemia and the decline in adipose tissue LPL activity. When streptozotocin-induced diabetic rats were divided into two groups on the basis of their plasma triglyceride levels (those with triglyceride concentration above or below 150 mg/dl), there were no differences between adipose tissue LPL activity of the two diabetic groups, in spite of

TABLE I Adipose Tissue Lipolytic Activity of Normal and Diabetic Rats

Lipoprotein Lipase Activity Control	Diabetic	Percent of Control	Reference
**Units/mg*			
3.0	0.8	27	(56)
Units/g			
5.0	1.6	32	(20)
10.7	5.8	54	(58)
9.4	3.1	33	(59)
9.8	2.4	25	
12.1	5.0	41	(60)
20.1	3.0	15	
21.2	5.4	26	
37.0	13.3	36	(30)

*μeq FFA/h

the fact that their plasma triglyceride levels were significantly different. However, when the animals were divided into two groups on the basis of their plasma glucose concentrations (above and below 275 mg/dl), the lowest levels of LPL activity was found in the rats with the most severe degree of hyperglycemia (58). Although the lower levels of adipose tissue LPL activity in insulin-deficient rats may play a role in determining the degree of hypertriglyceridemia, it remains uncertain whether other factors may also participate in the defect in triglyceride removal from plasma that could lead to hypertriglyceridemia.

Lipoprotein Lipase Activity in Muscle

Heart Muscle. As discussed in the previous section, the measurement of LPL activity in adipose tissue of diabetic rats indicates a reduction associated with insulin deficiency and a restoration by treatment with insulin. The increased LPL activity induced by insulin appears to be related to increased protein synthesis (55,65), and also to enzyme secretion from the adipocyte to the endothelial site of activity (51,55,66).

Studies with heart LPL in response to insulin deficiency have not been consistent. It has been reported that during experimental diabetes, heart LPL activity remains unchanged (32,58,61), is decreased (12,30,64,67) or is increased (30,59,62) with various experimental approaches (Table 2). A lack of change or an increase in myocardial LPL during experimental diabetes is inconsistent with the observed defect in lipoprotein clearance by this organ (30,67,68), if, in fact, LPL activity represents the "rate-limiting" step in lipoprotein triglyceride metabolism.

The reason for the conflicting reports concerning the effect of diabetes on myocardial LPL activity is not clear. One possible explanation might be the methods employed for the assay of LPL activity in heart muscle, and

TABLE II Lipolytic Activity in Myocardial Muscle of Experimental Diabetes

Diabetogenic Agent & Concentration	Source of Enzyme	LPL Activity percent of normal	Reference
Alloxan, (50 mg/kg)	Acetone-dried preparation	253	(30)
Streptozotocin (225 mg/kg)	Post-mitochondrial supernatant	215	(59)
Streptozotocin (65 mg/kg)	Tissue homogenate	252	(62)
Alloxan (50 mg/kg)	Heart Perfusion, 65 min	32	(12)
	Tissue Homogenate	61	
	Tissue Slices	51	
Streptozotocin (65 mg/kg)	Heart Perfusion, 45 min	47	(67)
	Tissue Homogenate	63	
Streptozotocin (65 mg/kg)	Tissue Homogenate at 3 days diabetes	15	(64)
	Tissue Homogenate at 4 weeks diabetes	38	
Alloxan (200 mg/kg)	Acetone-dried preparation	110	(32)
Pancreatectomy	Tissue Homogenate	116	(61)

to the different states of diabetes. Acetone-ether preparations, a post-mitochondrial supernatant of cardiac muscle homogenates, and cardiac homogenates were used by Kessler (30), Rauramaa et al. (59) and Nomura et al. (62), respectively, and all demonstrated a 230–250% increase in heart LPL activity in the diabetic rats when compared to controls. However, Aktin and Meng (12) have reported lower activity of LPL in the hearts of diabetic rats, using three different systems (heart slices, heart homogenates and perfusion of the heart.)

As in the earlier studies in which adipose tissue LPL was determined in diabetic rats, the diabetogenic agent used to induce diabetes has differed among these studies of muscle LPL. Diabetic states were induced either by intravenous injection of alloxan, 50 mg/kg body weight (12,30) and 200 mg/kg (32), or of streptozotocin at 45 mg/kg body weight (58), 65 mg/kg (62,64,67) and 225 mg/kg (59), or by pancreatectomizing the rats (61). It has also been shown that the activity of this enzyme in heart is greatly influenced by the nutritional state of the animal, and as such, Kotlar and Borensztajn (69) have emphasized the importance of the actual time of sacrifice when reporting results on myocardial LPL activity. It is well-established (54,70,71) that animals with free access to food show oscillations in muscle LPL activity which coincide with their feeding habits. Moreover, Nakai et al. (64) have reported an increase of heart muscle LPL activity after a 12-hour fast, with a significant decrease in LPL activities after 48 and 72-hours of fasting. However, these rhythmic variations in LPL activity in normal rats have been shown to be markedly altered in the diabetic animals (72). Whether the assay procedures of LPL activity in heart muscle, the drugs used for the induction of diabetes, the different levels of blood glucose, or the nutritional state of the animal can partly explain the different results of insulin deficiency on myocardial LPL activity is uncertain.

As mentioned previously, Aktin and Meng (12) have clearly demonstrated lower enzyme activity in the hearts of diabetic rats using different tissue systems. Although there was no difference in the heparin-releasable LPL from hearts of normal and diabetic rats during the first 5 minutes of heparin perfusion, the enzyme released from diabetic rat heart was significantly lower than controls after a 45 minute perfusion with heparin. The greatest difference occurred after 65 minutes of perfusion, when the LPL activity was only 32% of control values. These findings have been supported by studies in our laboratory (67) in which we reported a lower level of heparin-releasable LPL activity from hearts of diabetic rats after a 45 minute perfusion (47% of controls). This decrease in heart muscle LPL in untreated diabetic rats correlated with the findings of defective clearance of VLDL-triglyceride both *in vivo* (73) and by the isolated heart in recirculating perfusion (67,74). Our studies on the recirculating perfusion of VLDL clearly demonstrated a defective triglyceride clearance associated with insulin deficiency within 48 hours of a single dose of 65 mg/kg of streptozotocin. These data (56% reduction in clearance of 0.32 mM triglyceride) were entirely consistent with those of Kreisberg (68), who earlier had shown a 70% reduction in chylomicron triglyceride (0.3–0.5 mM triglyceride) clearance by perfused hearts from rats rendered insulin-deficient by a single injection of 45 mg/kg of alloxan 3–5 days earlier. The reduced removal rate of VLDL triglyceride by hearts from streptozotocin-induced diabetic rats was further substantiated by *in vivo* studies (73). Several laboratories (75–77) have shown that VLDL isolated from the plasma of diabetic rats have a considerably slower disappearance rate than VLDL of non-diabetic rats when injected into normal animals. The disappearance rate of VLDL-triglyceride isolated from diabetic rats, and reinjected into normal or diabetic recipient rats, was about half that of VLDL-triglycerides from non-diabetic rats (73,76). This reduced clearance of VLDL triglycerides both *in vivo* and by perfused hearts from diabetic rats, and the measurable decrease in functional myocardial LPL, are difficult to reconcile with earlier reports of unchanged or even increased levels of myocardial LPL associated with insulin deficiency (30,32,58,59,61,62).

Contrasting results have been reported regarding the reversability of LPL activity with the addition of insulin to the heart perfusion. Aktin and Meng (12) were unable to reverse the low LPL activity with insulin, and

Borensztajn et al. (78) postulated that the heart lipase activity might be regulated by mechanisms independent of insulin. We (67), on the other hand, were able to show a direct effect of insulin on myocardial LPL activity. Administration of a pharmacological dose of insulin (5 units) to diabetic rats resulted in a normalization of VLDL triglyceride lipolysis by perfused hearts and significantly increased the functional LPL activity of hearts from diabetic rats over that in animals not given insulin, and the activity was comparable to that in control hearts. In addition, to assess the direct effect of insulin on myocardial VLDL-triglyceride clearance, insulin was included in the recirculating perfusion media of isolated hearts. With the high levels of insulin (100 milliunits/ml) present during the entire perfusion period, the lipolysis of VLDL triglyceride by diabetic hearts was markedly improved (by 3.3-fold) and the activities of both functional and tissue LPL were significantly increased to levels comparable to those in control hearts.

A reduction of total protein synthesis has been demonstrated in perfused hearts from rats following alloxan-induced diabetes (79). This reduciton can be largely restored to normal levels by the perfusion of insulin for 1 hour. Furthermore, Morgan et al. (80) have reported the stimulation of protein synthesis by insulin and its inhibition by cycloheximide during short-term perfusions of rat hearts. Evidence for the involvement of protein synthesis during insulin-induced increases in myocardial triglyceride utilization was reported by our laboratory (67). The increased LPL activities in response to insulin *in vitro* under optimized conditions, were completely blocked by pretreatment of hearts with cycloheximide (Figure 1). However, using the more physiological measurement of VLDL triglyceride lipolysis during organ perfusion, cycloheximide only partially prevented the insulin-stimulated improvement in lipolysis (Figure 2). Nevertheless, these studies collectively imply that protein synthesis is at least in part involved in the effect of insulin on LPL activity.

Skeletal Muscle. The activity of LPL was found to be greater in red skeletal muscle that in white (61,71); however, the activity varied among the different types of red muscle (61). In diabetic rats, there are conflicting reports regarding the LPL activity of white and red skeletal muscle. In pancreatectomized rats, Linder et al. (61) have reported a 60% decrease in LPL activity of white skeletal muscle, 74% decrease in red soleus muscle and a 75% reduction in the LPL activity of the diaphragm. However, in streptozotocin-induced diabetic rats, the LPL activity of red soleus muscle has been shown to be either normal (58,59), or to exhibit a marked increase (166% of control values) at 4 days post-streptozotocin (59). It should be noted that the concentration of the diabetogenic drug, streptozotocin, used to induce diabetes in these 2 studies differed. An intravenous dose of 45 mg/kg body weight of streptozotocin was employed by Chen et al. (58), whereas Rauramaa et al. (59) used a 225 mg/kg dose of the agent.

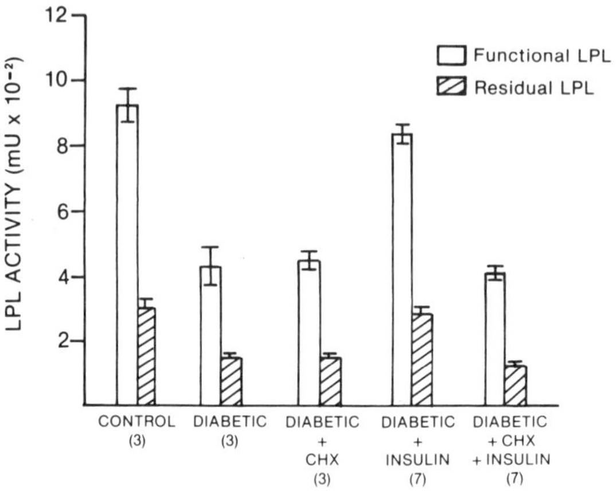

FIGURE 1 *Effects of Insulin and Cycloheximide (CHX) on Functional and Residual Activities of Perfused Rat Hearts.* All perfusions were for 40 minutes, and heparin (5 units/ml) was included during the final 10 minutes. Control and diabetic hearts were perfused with buffer for 40 minutes. Diabetic hearts were also perfused with buffer or buffer plus 20 μM cycloheximide for 10 minutes prior to addition of insulin and continued perfusion for 30 minutes.

Hepatic Lipase

Although numerous studies have been reported regarding the postheparin and tissue LPL activity in both human and experimental diabetes, the relationship between HL activity and diabetes is less clear. In animal models of insulin deficiency (streptozotocin-treated rats), low tissue and postheparin plasma HL activity have been documented (64,81,82), returning toward normal or even higher than control levels with diet modification or with insulin treatment. In contrast to these results in diabetic rats, postheparin plasma HL activity was increased in severely hyperglycemic insulin-requiring diabetic dogs (83). It was suggested (83) that the marked difference in HL activity between the rat and dog models of diabetes may be related to the differences in the means of inducing diabetes (streptozotocin vs. pancreatectomy).

Summary

The hypertriglyceridemia encountered in human and experimental insulin-deficiency diabetes has been attributed to a defect in the removal of triglyceride-containing lipoprotein particles from the circulation. Data attempting to relate the defective clearance of lipoprotein triglycerides during diabetes and the activity of LPL have not been entirely consistent.

In humans, the original observations by Bagdade et al. (1,2) suggested a decrease in PHLA in insulin-deficient diabetic patients. Both the elevated plasma triglyceride levels and the low PHLA levels returned toward normal

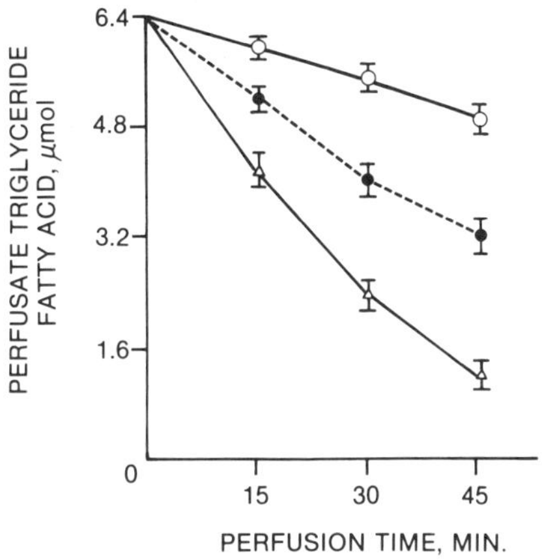

FIGURE 2 *Effects of Insulin and Cycloheximide on VLDL Triglyceride Utilization by Perfused Hearts from Diabetic Rats.* Hearts were pre-perfused for 10 minutes with buffer, 100 millunits/ml of insulin, or insulin and 20 μM cycloheximide, prior to addition of VLDL glyceryl tri [1-^{14}C] oleate and determination of lipolysis. Data represent means ± S.E. for three perfusions in each group. ○———○, buffer pre-perfusion; △———△, insulin pre-perfusion; •———•, insulin plus cycloheximide.

after a 24 hour insulin therapy. These data, however, have been questioned in part, on the basis that PHLA represents multiple enzyme activities derived from various tissues. More direct measurements of lipolytic activity, however, have supported these earlier findings in which low LPL activity was reported in adipose and muscle tissues from untreated insulin-deficient diabetic patients.

Similar to the studies of LPL activity in human diabetes, conflicting reports have been reported on the lipolytic activity in experimental diabetes. These inconsistencies reported on the levels of LPL in experimental diabetes may be due to the diabetogenic drug used and its concentration, the duration and severity of the diabetic condition, the nutritional state of the animal, and the presence of associated hyperglycemia. The majority of studies assaying LPL activity in adipose and muscle tissues of diabetic rats have indicated a reduction associated with insulin-deficiency and a restoration of activity following treatment with insulin. The low activity of myocardial LPL in insulin-deficient diabetic rats is compatible with the observations that perfused hearts from diabetic rats show a defective clearance of lipoprotein triglycerides. Hypertriglyceridemia accompanying severe insulin deficiency has been shown to be at least partly caused by a decrease of LPL activity and concomitant impairment of triglyceride removal.

In human diabetes, hyperglycemia associated with hypertriglyceridemia significantly affects PHLA. An inverse correlation exists between the degree of hypertriglyceridemia and PHLA levels in IDD (17). A similar correlation between PHLA levels and hyperglycemia has been reported (17).

It should be noted that the delayed removal of triglyceride-rich lipoproteins, observed in studies with diabetic animals and human diabetics, may not be solely due to changes in LPL activity. The diabetes-induced alterations in the composition and/or properties of the apolipoproteins of triglyceride-rich particle may also play a role in defective triglyceride removal and metabolism (74,77). Further studies will clarify these relationships.

References

1. Bagdade, J. D., D. Porte, Jr. and E. L. Bierman. 1967. *N. Eng. J. Med.* 276:427–433.
2. Bagdade, J. D., D. Porte, Jr. and E. L. Bierman. 1968. *Diabetes* 17:127–132.
3. Man, E. B. and J. P. Peters. 1935. *J. Clin. Invest.* 14:579.
4. New, M. I., T. N. Roberts, E. L. Bierman and G. G. Reader. 1963. *Diabetes* 12:208–12.
5. Chance, G. W., E. C. Albutt and S. M. Edkins. 1969. *Lancet* 1:1126.
6. Bergman, E. N., R. J. Havel, B. M. Wolfe and T. Bohmer. 1971. *J. Clin. Invest.* 50:1831–1839.
7. Fredrickson, D. A., K. Ono and L. L. Davis. 1963. *J. Lipid Res.* 4:24–33.
8. Biale, Y. and E. Shafrir. 1969. *Clin. Chim. Acta* 23:413–19.
9. Greten, H., R. I. Levy and D. S. Fredrickson. 1969. *J. Lipid Res.* 10:326–30.
10. Vogel, W. C., J. D. Brunzell and E. L. Bierman. 1971. *Lipids* 6:805–814.
11. Zieve, F. J. and L. Zieve. 1972. *Biochem. Biophys. Res. Commun.* 47:1480–1485.
12. Aktin, E. and H. C. Meng. 1972. *Diabetes* 21:149–56.
13. Brunzell, J. D., N. D. Smith, D. Porte, Jr. and E. L. Bierman. 1972. *J. Clin. Invest.* 51:16a.
14. Wilson, D. E., P. H. Schreibman and R. A. Arky. 1969. *Diabetes* 18:562–66.
15. Perry, W. F. 1967. *Clin. Chim. Acta* 16:189–194.
16. Brunzell, J. D., D. Porte and E. L. Bierman. 1975. *Metabolism* 24:1123–1136.
17. Shigeta, Y., K. Nakamura, M. Hoshi, M. Kim and H. Abe. 1967. *Diabetes* 16:238–41.
18. Krauss, R. M., H. G. Windmueller, R. I. Levy and D. S. Fredrickson. 1973. *J. Lipid Res.* 14:286–95.
19. Fielding, C. J. 1972. *Biochim. Biophys. Acta* 280:569–78.
20. Huttunen, J. K., C. Ehnholm, P. K. J. Kinnunen and E. A. Nikkilä. 1975. *Clin. Chim. Acta* 63:335–47.
21. Korn, E. D. 1955. *J. Biol. Chem.* 215:15–26.
22. Havel, R. J. and R. S. Gordon. 1960. *J. Clin. Invest.* 39:1777–1790.
23. Datta, D. V. 1963. *Proc. Soc. Exp. Biol. Med.* 112:1006–1008.
24. Muir, J. R. 1967. *Clin. Chim. Acta* 17:312–314.
25. Porte, D. Jr. and E. L. Bierman. 1969. *J. Lab. Clin. Med.* 73:631–48.
26. Schotz, M. C. and A. S. Garfinkel. 1972. *Biochim. Biophys. Acta* 270:472–78.
27. Pfeifer, M. M., J. D. Brunzell, J. D. Best, R. G. Judzewitsch, J. B. Halter and D. Porter, Jr. 1983. *Diabetes* 32:525–31.
28. Brunzell, J. D., W. R. Hazzard, A. G. Mobulsky, E. L. Bierman. 1975. *Metabolism* 24:115–22.
29. Brunzell, J. D., A. Chait, E. A. Nikkilä, C. Ehnholm, J. K. Huttunen and G. Steiner. 1980. *Metabolism* 29:624–29.
30. Kessler, J. I. 1963. *J. Clin. Invest.* 42:362–67.
31. Gries, F. A., S. Potthof and K. Jahnke. 1967. *Diabetologia* 3:311–17.
32. Elkeles, R. S. and E. Williams. 1974. *Clin. Sci. Mol. Med.* 46:661–64.
33. Nikkilä, E. A., J. K. Huttunen and C. Ehnholm. 1977. *Diabetes* 26:11–21.
34. Lewis, B., M. Mancini, M. Mattock, A. Chait and T. R. Fraser. *Eur. J. Clin. Invest.* 2:445–53.

35. Jones, D. P., G. R. Plotkin and R. A. Arky. 1966. *Diabetes* 15:565–70.
36. Persson, B. and B. Hood. 1970. *Atherosclerosis* 12:241–251.
37. Nilsson-Ehle, P., A. S. Garfinkel and M. C. Schotz. 1980. *Annu. Rev. Biochem.* 49:667–693.
38. Hietanen, E. and M. R. C. Greenwood. 1977. *J. Lipid Res.* 18:480–490.
39. Nilsson-Ehle, P., H. Torngvist and P. Belfrage. 1972. *Clin. Chim. Acta* 42:383–390.
40. Iverius, P. H. and J. D. Brunzell. 1985. *Am. J. Physiol.* 249:E107–E114.
41. Pykalisto, O. J., P. H. Smith and J. D. Brunzell. 1975. *J. Clin. Invest.* 56:1108–17.
42. Taskinen, M. R. and E. A. Nikkilä. 1979. *Diabetologia* 17:351–56.
43. Taskinen, M. R., Nikkilä, E. A., Nousiainen, R. and Gordin, A. 1981. *Scand. J. Clin. Lab Invest.* 41:263–68.
44. Wing, D. R., M. R. Salaman and D. S. Robinson. 1966. *Biochem. J.* 99:648–56.
45. Patten, R. L. 1970. *J. Biol. Chem.* 245:5577–84.
46. Taylor, K. G., D. J. Galton and G. Holdsworth. 1979. *Diabetologia* 16:313–17.
47. Taskinen, M. R., E. A. Nikkilä, R. Kuusi and K. Harno. 1982. *Diabetologia* 22:46–50.
48. Nilsson-Ehle, P. S. Carlstrom and P. Belfrage. 1975. *Scand. J. Clin. Lat. Invest.* 35:373–78.
49. Taskinen, M. R. and E. A. Nikkilä. 1979. *Atherosclerosis* 32:289–99.
50. Cryer, A., S. E. Riley, E. R. Williams and D. S. Robinson. 1976. *Clin. Sci. Mol. Med.* 50:213–21.
51. Wing, D. R. and D. S. Robinson. 1968. *Biochem. J.* 106:667–76.
52. Borensztajn, J. and D. S. Robinson. 1970. *J. Lipid Res.* 11:111–17.
53. Davies, P., A. Cryer and D. S. Robinson. 1974. *FEBS Lett.* 45:271–75.
54. Borensztajn, J., D. M. Samols and A. H. Rubenstein. 1972. *Am. J. Physiol.* 223:1271–75.
55. Garfinkel, A. S., P. Nilsson-Ehle and M. C. Schotz. 1976. *Biochim. Biophys. Acta* 424:264–73.
56. Schnatz, J. D. and R. H. Williams. 1963. *Diabetes* 12:174–78.
57. Redgrave, T. G. and D. A. Snibson. 1977. *Metabolism* 26:493–503.
58. Chen, Y. I., J. Howard, V. Huang, F. B. Kraemer and G. M. Reaven. 1980. *Diabetes* 29:643–47.
59. Rauramaa, R., P. Kuusela and E. Hietanen. 1980. *Horm. Metab. Res.* 12:591–95.
60. Ishikawa, A., T. Murase, N. Yamada, K. Tanaka, Y. Iwamoto, U. Akanuma and N. Ohsawa. 1982. *Endocrinol. Japan* 29:379–381.
61. Linder, C., S. S. Chernick, T. R. Fleck and R. O. Scow. 1976. *Am. J. Physiol.* 231:860–64.
62. Nomura, T., U. Hagino, M. Gotoh, A. Iguchi and N. Sakamoto. 1984. *Lipids* 19:594–599.
63. Elkeles, R. S. 1974. *Horm. Metab. Res.* 6:151–154.
64. Nakai, T., K. Oida, T. Tamai, S. Yamada, T. Kobayashi, T. Hayashi, Y. Kutsumi and R. Takeda. 1984. *Horm. Metab. Res.* 16:67–70.
65. Parkin, S. M., K. Walker, P. Ashby and D. S. Robinson. 1980. *Biochem. J.* 188:193–199.
66. Eckel, R. H., W. U. Fujimoto and J. D. Brunzell. 1978. *Biochim. Biophys. Res. Commun.* 84:1069–1975.
67. O'Looney, P., M. Vander Maten and G. V. Vahouny. 1983. *J. Biol. Chem.* 258:12994–13001.
68. Kriesberg, R. A. 1966. *Am. J. Physiol.* 210:379–384.
69. Kotlar, T. J. and J. Borensztajn. 1977. *Am. J. Physiol.* 233:E316–E319.
70. DeGasquet, P. and E. Pequignot. 1973. *Horm. Metab. Res.* 5:440–443.
71. Borensztajn, J., M. S. Rone, S. P. Babirak, J. A. McGarr, and L. G. Oscai. 1975. *Am. J. Physiol.* 229:394–397.
72. Borensztajn, J., S. Otway and D. S. Robinson. 1970. *J. Lipid Res.* 11:102–110.
73. O'Looney, P., T. Le and G. V. Vahouny. 1985. *Fed. Proc.* 44, 1762.
74. O'Looney, P., D. Irwin, P. Briscoe and G. V. Vahouny. 1985. *J. Biol. Chem.* 260:428–432.
75. Van Tol, A. 1977. *Atherosclerosis* 26:117–128.
76. Bar-On, H., E. Levy, Y. Oschry, E. Ziv and E. Shafrir. 1984. *Biochim. Biophys. Acta* 793:115–118.

77. Levy, E., E. Shafrir, E. Ziv and H. Bar-On. 1985. *Biochim. Biophys. Acta* 834:376–385.
78. Borensztajn, J., D. R. Samols and A. H. Rubenstein. 1972. *Am. J. Physiol.* 223:1271–1275.
79. Williams, I. H., B. H. L. Chua, R. H. Shams, D. Siehl and H. E. Morgan. 1980. *Am. J. Physiol.* 239:E178–E185.
80. Morgan, H. E., L. S. Jefferson, E. B. Wolpert and D. E. Rannels. 1971. *Biol. Chem.* 246:2163–2170.
81. Elkeles, R. S. and J. Hambley. 1977. *Diabetes* 26:58–60.
82. Knauer, T. E., J. A. Woods, R. G. Lamb and H. J. Fallon. 1982. *J. Lipid Res.* 23:631–637.
83. Muller, D. L., C. D. Saudek and D. Applebaum-Bowden, D. 1985. *Metabolism* 34:251–254.

Chapter 10

LIPROPROTEIN LIPASE IN TRAUMA AND SEPSIS

Gregory J. Bagby and Phillip H. Pekala

Various forms of trauma, especially when complicated by shock or sepsis, induce an array of changes in lipid metabolism which are potentially important in an individual's response to these insults. Lipids in the form of adipose tissue triglyceride (TG) constitute the major expendable fuel reserve in normal man. Consequently, their use is desirable when an individual must rely on an endogenous fuel to satisfy his energy requirements. Other fuel reserves are either limited in amount, carbohydrate stored as glycogen, or as in the case of proteins, required to perform other duties necessary for maintenance of homeostasis.

Fat as a fuel is supplied to cells primarily in the form of fatty acids. These fatty acids are delivered to tissues via the circulation as either albumin-bound free fatty acids (FFA) or triglyceride-fatty acids (TGFA) in chylomicra or very low density lipoproteins (VLDL). Typically, FFA quantitatively represent the major fatty acid form transported in the circulation to tissues in the postabsorptive state. Because of their central role in energy metabolism, extensive research has been conducted to elucidate the regulatory processes involved in FFA mobilization from adipose tissue and their flux through the vascular compartment. Plasma TG have not been viewed as important with regard to energy substrate transport. Nevertheless, conditions that influence plasma concentration and metabolism have been investigated because hypertriglyceridemia and other aspects of lipoprotein metabolism represent major risk factors in the development of atherosclerosis. However, there are two reasons why the importance of plasma TGFA as an energy substrate should not be overlooked. First, plasma TGFA can be regarded as a reservoir for plasma FFA in that the number of fatty acid equivalents in plasma TG normally outnumber FFA bound to albumin. Second, TGFA can be directed to extrahepatic tissues based on the prevalence of the enzyme lipoprotein lipase (LPL) within different tissues. This enzyme is responsible for the liberation of fatty acids from TG prior to their uptake by extrahepatic tissues. Once liberated, this fatty acid can not be distinguished from that transported to a tissue as FFA.

In line with the purpose of this book, we will focus our attention on the changes that take place in tissue LPL during various forms of shock, trauma and sepsis. To this end, we will consider other aspects of lipid metabolism only as they are influenced by changes in LPL. For those interested, several articles or chapters have been published in recent years which deal with more general aspects of lipid metabolism in this area (1,2,3,4).

Two rationales have been used to justify studies dealing with trauma or sepsis induced changes in LPL. Most investigators have looked for changes in LPL activity after trauma or shock in hopes of explaining apparent alterations in plasma TG metabolism. More recently, interest has been generated because of the increased use of artificial fat emulsions during intravenous nutritional support of critically ill patients who are either malnourished or incapable of enteral support.

Effects of Stress on Lipoprotein Lipase

Conceptually, trauma and sepsis can be viewed as specific types of stress. By stress we simply mean any external or internal environmental change that must be adapted to or compensated for in order to maintain the body in homeostasis. Stress can be local or general and include physical injury, exposure, deprivation, disease, and psychological categories which are not mutually exclusive.

Although the body does not respond to all stress challenges identically, many elicit a predictable endocrine response. Potentially, these endocrine changes can influence the prevailing level of LPL activity within various tissues. Acute stress states often result in decreased plasma insulin and increased plasma catecholamines, glucagon and glucocorticoids (5,6,7,8). Thus, to understand stress-induced changes in LPL activity in heart, skeletal muscle, and adipose tissue, it is necessary to know the role performed by these respective hormones in regulating this enzyme in these tissues.

As described in previous Chapters, insulin is thought to be an important positive modulator of adipose tissue LPL activity whereas catecholamines may exert a negative influence (Chapter 4). Briefly, an increase in plasma insulin levels increases adipose tissue LPL activity by eliciting a rapid release of enzyme from adipocytes and stimulating synthesis of LPL protein within these cells (9,10,11,12,13,14). Conversely, catecholamines can be regarded as negative modulators of adipose tissue LPL activity for two reasons. First, adrenergic stimulation of the pancreas decreases insulin secretion which would potentially suppress adipose tissue LPL activity. Second, and more directly, catecholamines and other adipose tissue modulators that increase cAMP levels decrease LPL activity by accelerating inactivation or degradation of the enzyme within the adipocyte (15,16,17,18).

Regulation of LPL activity in muscle was extensively covered in Chapter 5 and will only be summarized here. Although insulin may perform a permissive role in determining heart and skeletal muscle LPL activity, it is clearly not a primary regulator. Instead, several hormones have been implicated as regulators of LPL activity in these tissues including catecholamines, glucocorticoids, glucagon and thyroid hormones. Of this group, glucocorticoids and catecholamines are most likely to exert the greatest influences on LPL activity in heart and possibly skeletal muscle (12,19,20,21,22,23). An increase in the presence of either hormone class can typically be expected to increase LPL activity in heart. In skeletal muscle the picture is less clear.

Under many circumstances LPL activity in adipose tissue and muscle changes during stress states in a manner consistent with endocrine adjustments. The effect of stress induced by food deprivation, cold exposure, and exercise has been covered in previous Chapters and will thus only be briefly summarized at this time.

Figure 1 summarizes this response by illustrating adjustments taking place when an animal goes from a fed unstressed state to a fasted or stressed state. During stress conditions adipose tissue LPL activity decreases because plasma insulin levels decrease and catecholamine concentrations increase (not shown). Conversely, muscle LPL activity increases in response to either elevated glucocorticoids or catecholamines, or a combination of both modulators. Collectively these changes shift TGFA flux away from adipose tissue and toward muscle. In the unstressed animal, FFA output from adipose is relatively low. This is optimized when TG are being absorbed from the small intestines. Because adipose tissue LPL activity is high, most newly absorbed TGFA are directed toward this tissue for storage. As stress develops, FFA are mobilized from adipose tissue. Whereas a portion goes to muscle and other extrahepatic tissues where it is used primarily as an energy substrate, some is directed to the liver where it is either oxidized or incorporated into TG for subsequent secretion in VLDL complexes. Under these conditions, circulating TG are directed to muscle because of its relatively high level of LPL activity. This change is again consistent with our current understanding of humoral regulation of LPL activity within various tissues. From this, one would expect trauma and sepsis to result in similar changes in the tissue enzyme if endocrine responses to these challenges parallel those of other stress states and if other factors do not circumvent such a response.

Effects of Trauma and Sepsis on Lipoprotein Lipase

In the previous section, we summarized information available on the basic regulation of tissue LPL activity and demonstrated that a number of stressful challenges induce changes in the adipose tissue and skeletal muscle enzymes commensurate with their respective regulatory processes. In this

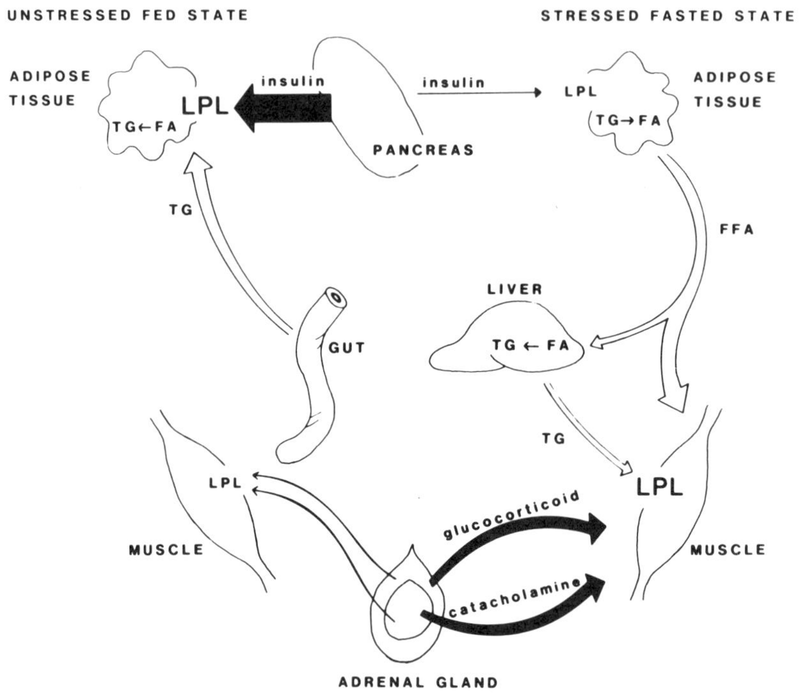

FIGURE 1 The basic regulation of adipose tissue and muscle lipoprotein lipase and how this regulation modulates the tissue distribution of lipoprotein triglyceride.

section we deal with the question: Do trauma and sepsis produce changes in tissue LPL activity that are consistent with these tissue specific regulatory processes?

To answer the above question, we must first consider the endocrine responses to traumatic and septic insults. Kinney and Felig (2) reviewed the metabolic and endocrine responses to injury and infection by dividing challenges into two phases based on the pioneering work of Cuthbertson (24). The early phase, called the "ebb" phase, is usually of short duration (less than 24 hours) and would include all forms of shock. The second phase, termed the "flow" or catabolic phase, is often a period of hypermetabolism and may be sustained for many days.

In discussing endocrine responses to trauma and sepsis, Kinney and Felig (2) point out that the type and severity of trauma or sepsis determines in part the endocrine response. In addition, a number of other variables can have an impact on these responses including species differences, and the nutritional and endocrine status of an animal or person prior to being challenged. Nevertheless, it is worthwhile to identify the endocrine changes that generally occur in response to trauma and sepsis.

The endocrine changes during the early phases of trauma and sepsis which may include shock consist of hypoinsulinemia, increased plasma glucocorticoid concentrations, and enhanced sympathetic and adrenal medullary activity (2). Under some conditions, e.g. bacterial endotoxin administration, transient hyperinsulinemia may occur if the insult induces a rapid onset of hyperglycemia, but this is usually followed by a shift to hypoinsulinemia (25). Indeed, decreased insulin concentrations have been observed despite hyperglycemia (26). This lack of pancreatic response to increased circulating glucose is likely due to the trauma-induced increase in norepinephrine or epinephrine and their inhibitory effect on the beta cell. In this regard, plasma concentration and urinary excretion of catecholamines are generally elevated in response to trauma, sepsis and shock (27,28,29,30,31), and blocking this reponse prevents hypoinsulinemia (32). Elevated catecholamines, as well as glucocorticoids, undoubtedly play modulating roles in other metabolic adjustments to these insults. However, the relative importance of these early endocrine changes to the concomitant metabolic alterations has yet to be established. Indeed, the multiple adjustments in endocrine status are likely to work in concert to produce the wide range of metabolic changes (33).

Increased plasma glucocorticoids and increased sympathetic-adrenal medullary activity along with hypergluconemia are typically observed during the sustained hypermetabolic phase of trauma and sepsis (30,34,35,36,37,38). The degree of elevation is positively related to the severity of injury. Because alpha- and beta-adrenergic blockades reduce the hypermetabolic response to thermal injury (30), catecholamines are thought to be determinants of hypermetabolism seen in these and other trauma patients.

Plasma insulin concentrations during the hypermetabolic phase are variable. Patients with extensive thermal injury can remain hypoinsulinemic during the flow phase (35), as can hypermetabolic septic rats (36). In contrast, hyperinsulinemia has been observed in a number of trauma states, but at times is accompanied by insulin resistance (39,40,41). Sustained elevation of catecholamines are thought to be, in part, responsible for this insulin resistance (33,41).

The general metabolic events taking place during either the ebb or flow phase following trauma or infection can not be attributed to a single hormonal change as the primary modulator (2,33,42). Therefore, these humoral changes either act synergistically and/or other modulators may be involved. In this regard, several secretory products from leukocytes have recently been implicated as important determinants of the metabolic response to trauma or sepsis (43). The interaction of these newly discovered hormone-like modulators and the more classic endocrine system has yet to be evaluated.

The response of LPL activity in tissues during the course of trauma and infection is predictable if the enzyme continues to be regulated during these states by a respective tissue's basic regulatory processes. Adipose tissue LPL activity should be low during these insults owing to reduced insulin concentrations (ebb phase) or reduced insulin responsiveness (flow phase). In contrast, heart and skeletal muscle LPL activity should be increased due to elevated levels of plasma glucocorticoids and increased activity of the sympatho-adrenal medullary system. Because trauma states and sepsis produce divergent effects on tissue LPL activity, they will be discussed separately.

Trauma. Hypertriglyceridemia develops in rabbits after various forms of shock and trauma. For example, repeated episodes of bleeding produces lipemia in rabbits. This phenomenon was primarily studied before the development of specific assays for LPL. Spitzer and Spitzer (44) attempted to learn about the genesis of hemorrhagic lipemia in rabbits by studying clearing-factor activities of postheparin plasma collected before and after removal of lipoproteins. In their studies, they found that the ability of postheparin plasma to clear added fat emulsions from lipemic rabbits was depressed. They were unable to determine if the decreased clearing ability was due to an actual decreased heparin-releasable clearing-factor lipase, or some other defect in the clearing reaction such as a decrease in an essential activator or a decreased capacity of albumin to accept liberated fatty acids. Their findings actually suggested that multiple etiologies lead to the development of the lipemic state in the rabbit. Although techniques are now available to resolve the cause or causes of hypertriglyceridemia in the hemorrhagic rabbit, we are not aware of any subsequent research on this phenomenon.

Hyperlipidemia has also been observed in rabbits exposed to lethal levels of whole body ionizing radiation (45,46). Feliste et al. (47) found that irradiation induced an accumulation of VLDL. This increase occurred at a time when postheparin plasma lipase activity was decreased (46). In subsequent studies, they demonstrated that postheparin plasma LPL, eluting from a heparin sepharose column with 1.5 M NaCl, was markedly reduced 16 to 24 hours after irradiation (48). Furthermore, when VLDL radiolabeled in the TG moiety with [^{14}C] palmitate was injected into irradiated rabbits, 100% of the label was retained in the VLDL fraction of plasma collected up to 60 min after injection. These findings are compatible with the postulate that suppression of LPL activity is responsible for hypertriglyceridemia in the irradiate rabbit. However, they also measured adipose tissue LPL activity and found it to be increased 3-fold in irradiated rabbits compared to control animals. From this finding, they suggested that adipocytes were still capable of producing LPL but that there was a defect in transport to its functional position on the luminal surface of capillary endothelial surface. However, their assay conditions may not have reflected the true adipocyte LPL activity since they measured lipase released from small pieces of adipose tissue after prolonged exposure to heparin. In this regard, the earlier work of Wooles (45) indicates that LPL activity in delipidated powders of rabbit adipose tissue is decreased 16 hours post-irradiation. Treatment of irradiated rabbits with hydrocortisone abolished the decrease in postheparin plasma lipase activity, but injection of an ACTH analog, synacthene, was ineffective (49). This indicates that pharmacological doses of a glucocorticoid were effective but that either endogenous corticosteroids were not produced in response to synacthene, or the amount produced was insufficient to overcome the effect of irradiation.

Oehler and associates (50) observed that hypertriglyceridemia developed in rabbits after experimental fracture of the femur. Concomitant with an increased plasma TG concentration was a pronounced decrease in postheparin plasma LPL activity. Lehr et al. (51) also studied the effect of bone fracture on postheparin plasma LPL activity in the dog. They were primarily investigating lung LPL activity because of their interest in elucidating the mechanism responsible for reducing pulmonary surfactant levels following trauma. Their results suggest that 5 hours after bone fracture heparin-releasable LPL activity from the lung was decreased and residual lipase activity was increased. An inappropriate sampling schedule after heparin injection makes a definitive interpretation of their data difficult. However, in agreement with findings in rabbits subjected to bone fracture, whole body heparin-releasable LPL activity was decreased in bone fracture traumatized dogs compared to control animals. Definitive studies on LPL activity in other tissues after bone fracture are missing making it difficult to determine which tissues are responsible for the suppression of postheparin plasma LPL activity. Oehler et al. (50) did find that catecholamine excretion into urine increased after bone fracture. If LPL activity in tissues is under normal humoral control, this would imply that the principal decrease would occur in adipose tissue due to the negative effect of catecholamines on pancreatic insulin release (7) and its enhancement of LPL degradation within this tissue (18). Increased catecholamines should also result in an increased heparin-releasable LPL activity from heart and possibly skeletal muscle (21). Since such a change would have the opposite effect on postheparin plasma lipase activity, this implies that the greatest changes were likely to take place in adipose tissue.

Although rabbits develop hyperlipidemia in response to a number of trauma states, this condition is not a typical response for all species. Elevated plasma TG concentrations have not been observed in dogs subjected to hemorrhagic shock (52), rats after surgical trauma (53), guinea pigs challenged by thermal injury (54), or in man after various forms of trauma including surgery and thermal injury (55,56). Adequate comparative studies to delineate the species dependent differences in plasma TG metabolism have not been performed. Two potential explanations are feasible. First, differences may exist among species in the ability of their livers to synthesize and secrete TG. Little or no information is available on this aspect of TG metabolism in animals or man following a traumatic insult. Second, the distribution or regulation of LPL activity may vary among species. In animals studied to date, most LPL activity is present in muscle and adipose tissue. One would expect trauma to increase heart and skeletal muscle LPL activities and decrease the adipose tissue enzyme. This reciprocal change would be consistent with our understanding of basic LPL regulation and is in line with changes that take place in other forms of stress. If these reciprocal changes take place during trauma, one would expect to see plasma TGFA directed toward muscle to increase as its LPL activity increases and directed away from adipose tissue as its LPL activity decreases. The composite clearance rate of plasma TG would depend on the degree that muscle LPL activity increases in comparison to a decrease in the adipose tissue enzyme activity. In an animal where trauma induces a marked decrease in adipose tissue LPL activity without producing a reciprocal increase in the muscle enzyme, one would expect to see a decrease in the overall TG clearance rate and a predisposition to hypertriglyceridemia. The rabbit may fit this pattern. In other species, increased muscle LPL activity may counterbalance a trauma induced decrease in the adipose tissue enzyme and preserve or even increase TG clearance and prevent the development of hypertriglyceridemia. Nonetheless, if the tissue distribution of LPL activity shifts following trauma, one would expect parallel changes to occur in the distribution of plasma TGFA.

Borbola and coworkers (57) found heart LPL activity to be increased in rats 6 hours after releasing tourniquets applied to hindlimbs for 3 hours. Heart and skeletal muscle LPL activity are increased in guinea pigs subjected to a 30% surface area full skin thickness thermal injury (54). However, skeletal muscle under the burned skin did not respond in the same way as muscle at sites distant from the injury. Consequently, significant increases in LPL activity were observed 24 hours after injury in all tissues except muscle obtained from beneath the site of thermal injury. The inability of this tissue to respond like other tissues may have been a direct consequence of the applied burn, although the muscle chosen was located adjacent to the femur and was thus somewhat insulated by overlying muscle. Interestingly, adipose tissue LPL activity was also increased. It is difficult to say whether muscle and adipose tissue LPL activity are both elevated after thermal injury in all species or if this represents a trauma induced change unique to the guinea pig. Guinea pigs have a distinct apolipoprotein profile and seem to lack apo CII (58). Because of this, few studies have been conducted on the regulation of LPL in this species.

Certain forms of surgical trauma also result in increased heart LPL activity. Bagby and Spitzer (53) found heart LPL activity to be increased in rats 24 hours after surgically implanting arterial and venous catheters. However in a separate study, laparotomy did not produce the same result (59). Carpentier and associates (60) also have reported an increased LPL activity in muscle and heart and a decreased activity in adipose tissue in traumatized rats but experimental details were not provided.

Robin et al. (56) did not observe changes in skeletal muscle LPL activity in various trauma patients; however, samples were not obtained until 3–7 days after the initial insult. Whether or not changes took place at a time more immediate to the initial insult was not determined. In this regard, the effect of prolonged stress on LPL activity in different tissues has not been extensively studied. In one study, stress produced by food deprivation resulted in a marked increase in heart LPL activity that was transient in nature (61). By the 72*nd* hour of starvation heart enzyme activity returned to unstressed levels. In contrast, Robin and associates (56) did observe an apparent difference in adipose tissue LPL activity of trauma patients given 5% dextrose intravenously. In these patients, adipose tissue LPL activity was elevated compared to normal subjects restricted to 5% dextrose for 4 days. The difference was coincident with significantly elevated plasma insulin concentrations and suggests that adipose tissue of traumatized patients retains its ability to respond to the prevailing plasma insulin level by maintaining an elevated LPL activity. Collectively, the sustained change in adipose tissue LPL activity and lack of increase in the muscle enzyme in trauma patients may imply that stress-induced changes in muscle LPL activity are short-lived while the adipose tissue enzyme can continue to respond to an insulin signal.

In another study, Heller and coworkers (62) found suppressed post-heparin plasma LPL activity in critically ill patients with multiple organ failure and in postoperative patients. Measurements were made within 24 hours of surgery or admittance to the Intensive Care Unit. Although information on the tissue distribution of LPL during this stage of trauma is not available in man, the endocrine balance at this time would be consistent with the primary decrease occurring in adipose tissue. These results suggest that composite tissue LPL activity is decreased early in the course of trauma, but this response may subside with time.

Although information regarding alterations in LPL activity in heart and adipose tissue in response to traumatic challenges is incomplete, existing evidence indicates that these changes are consistent with basic regulatory processes for this enzyme in each tissue. Trauma induced increases in heart and skeletal muscle LPL activity are compatible with increased catecholamine or glucocorticoid concentrations also present in such conditions (2). Studies are lacking on how long this response lasts.

Changes in the enzyme activity in adipose tissue also seem to follow changes in plasma insulin levels. Two groups have studied the effect of intravenous nutritional support of trauma and post-surgical patients on adipose tissue LPL activity. Taskinen and coworkers (63) found glucose alone, or Intralipid plus glucose, increased adipose tissue LPL activity in post-surgical patients. Although plasma insulin levels were not monitored, it is likely that elevated insulin concentrations in response to nutritive support was at least in part responsible for such increases in the adipose tissue enzyme. In this regard, Robin et al. (64) reported that trauma patients given glucose and Intralipid possessed increased enzyme activity in adipose tissue that paralleled increases in plasma insulin concentration.

In summary, in acute trauma states adipose tissue LPL activity is decreased whereas heart and skeletal muscle activity is often increased. This response is highly consistent with expected endocrine changes induced by the trauma state. The duration of this response has not been systematically studied. It is possible that muscle LPL activity may return to pretrauma levels. Finally, existing evidence indicates that adipose tissue LPL activity continues to respond to prevailing plasma insulin concentrations.

Sepsis. Although trauma produces variable responses in plasma TG concentrations, hypertriglyceridemia is a common feature of bacterial infections and particular gram-negative sepsis in human beings and animals (65,66,67,68). It is also observed in animals administered endotoxin, a lipopolysaccharide component of the cell wall of gram-negative organisms (59,69,70). In some circumstances, sepsis results in increased plasma FFA concentrations and turnover which may promote hepatic production and secretion of TG during infection (71,72); however, hypertriglyceridemia can occur during sepsis and endotoxemia in the absence of elevated FFA concentrations (53,56,73,74). Kaufmann and coworkers (70,75) observed that clearance of an injected artificial lipid emulsion was suppressed in monkeys given live *E. coli* or endotoxin from *E. coli.* They also observed a reduction in postheparin plasma lipase activity which led them to suggest that gram-negative sepsis and endotoxin induced elevated plasma TG concentrations by impairing the LPL mechanism of its disposal or clearance. Oehler et al. (76) also reported a decrease in postheparin plasma lipase activity following endotoxin administration to rabbits. However, neither study verified that the decrease in postheparin plasma lipase was specifically due to a decrease in LPL activity or resulted from a decrease in hepatic TG lipase activity. Kaufman et al. (75) commented on this limitation, arguing that suppression of LPL activity was probably responsible for the decrease in postheparin lipase activity since lipid clearance was imparied. However, additional studies were required to verify that gram-negative sepsis and endotoxemia result in suppression of LPL activity.

Bagby and Spitzer (77,78) reported decreases in heart LPL activity in endotoxin-treated rats. Endotoxin-treatment suppressed enzyme activity in heart to 20% of control levels in 7 hours and occurred even when sublethal doses of endotoxin were administered (79). The progressive decline in the myocardial enzyme activity resembled the decay curve seen in animals administered protein synthesis inhibitors. With suppression of this magnitude, one would expect LPL activity in the extracellular compartment to be substantially decreased. These investigators verified that heparin-releasable LPL activity was greatly decreased in hearts obtained from endotoxin-treated rats (80). Such a decrease is consistent with the hypothesis that endotoxin-induced hypertriglycerdemia results from suppression of LPL activity.

LPL activity in other extra hepatic tissues including both skeletal muscle and adipose tissue is reduced in response to endotoxin (59,79,81). In the rat, the decrease in the adipose tissue enzyme after endotoxin administration occurred in some but not all experiments (59,79,80). This variable response may be due to the fasted state of animals used in these experiments which would in itself suppress LPL activity in this tissue. In contrast to the response in rats, mice given endotoxin exhibit a pronounced reduction of adipose tissue LPL activity but not a decrease in the heart enzyme unless high doses are administered (81,82). Thus, some species differences may exist in the response of tissue LPL activity to endotoxin.

Suppression of adipose tissue and muscle LPL activity has also been observed in animals administered gram-negative organisms and in septic patients. Lanza-Jacoby et al. (83) found that rats injected intravenously with live *E. coli* developed hypertriglyceridemia and possessed reduced adipose tissue LPL activity 24 hours after initiation of sepsis. They also found the activity of the hepatic lipogenic enzyme, fatty acid synthase, to be increased in septic animals. This prompted these investigators to suggest that both hepatic TG synthesis and secretion, and impaired clearance may act in combination to elevate plasma TG concentrations.

Whereas Robin et al. (56) found trauma patients to possess increased adipose tissue LPL activity commensurate with elevated plasma insulin levels, their septic patients had decreased skeletal muscle and adipose tissue LPL activity. Plasma insulin levels during sepsis were also elevated in these patients; thus a drop in insulin concentration could not explain the suppression of the adipose tissue enzyme. Decreased skeletal muscle and adipose tissue LPL activity was particularly evident in septic patients having plasma TG levels higher than 1.5 mM.

Scholl and coworkers (59) examined the effect of endotoxin and sepsis in the rat on plasma TG concentrations and LPL activity in several tissues. Injection of *E. coli* endotoxin or live *E. coli* either intravenously or intraperitoneally resulted in hypertriglyceridemia and suppression of myocardial, skeletal muscle, and adipose tissue LPL activity. In contrast, rats subjected to peritonitis produced by cecal ligation and puncture or innoculation with rat feces did not exhibit hypertriglyceridemia or consistent decreases in tissue LPL activity. In response to peritonitis, adipose tissue LPL activity decreased but enzyme activity in heart and skeletal muscle increased. This divergent pattern between rats treated with endotoxin or live *E. coli,* and peritonitis occurred despite the presence of gram-negative organisms in rats subjected to either type of treatment (84,85). The fact that increases in plasma TG levels occurred only during conditions in which both skeletal muscle and adipose tissue LPL activity were suppressed implicates the importance of this enzyme in sepsis and endotoxin-induced hypertriglyceridemia.

Why does such a difference exist between animals treated with endotoxin or live *E. coli* and those subjected to peritoneal sepsis? The latter condition resembles changes in tissue LPL activity that take place during the early stages of stressful insults and trauma. Furthermore, these changes are consistent with expected endocrine changes (2). That is, rats challenged with peritonitis have elevated plasma glucocorticoid and catecholamine concentrations and decreased insulin levels which, in turn, should increase muscle and decrease adipose tissue LPL activity. Thus, the changes in tissue LPL activity during peritoneal sepsis are consistent with normal regulatory mechanisms for this enzyme. Although administration of endotoxin and live *E. coli* to rats produce a similar endocrine response (25), muscle LPL activity fails to increase but instead decreases. Furthermore, septic patients, who have low adipose tissue LPL activity, fail to increase that activity in response to nutritional intervention sufficient to elevate plasma insulin concentrations (64). Thus, neither muscle nor adipose tissue in septic animals or patients appear able to respond to normal endocrine signals. One possibility is that endotoxin in some forms of sepsis produces changes that circumvent the normal regulatory mechanisms controlling tissue LPL activity. Since sepsis often accompanies trauma, two opposing influences may be called into play. Whereas trauma increased myocardial LPL activity, endotoxin injection into surgically traumatized rats caused a decrease in the heart enzyme (53). Perhaps, the opposite takes place in rats subjected to peritonitis. That is, trauma associated with peritonitis or the symbiotic relationship among the mixed population of microorganisms present during peritoneal infections was sufficient to override any endotoxin or gram-negative bacterial effect on tissue LPL activities. In this regard, bacterial number or endotoxin concentration may not have reached sufficient levels to evoke their effect on this enzyme. In any event, the divergent response between trauma and endotoxin or gram-negative sepsis, despite similar endocrine responses, indicate that endotoxin or gram-negative organisms either directly interfere with mechanisms which normally regulate tissue levels of LPL or lead to the production of a modulator that circumvents "normal" regulation of the enzyme in tissues.

The Search for a Monokine Mediator(s) of Lipoprotein Lipase Activity

In 1980, Rouzer and Cerami (86) reported that rabbits became hypertriglyceridemic following infection with the protozoan parasite *Trypanosoma brucci* and attributed the condition to a deficiency of LPL activity. Since this change was consistent with alterations observed in animals after endotoxin administration or during sepsis, Kawakami and Cerami (82) further characterized this disorder using endotoxemia as an experimental model. Their results suggested that tissue suppression of LPL activity was due to a mediator that appeared in the serum in response to endotoxin. In these studies, two genetically similar strains of mice, one sensitive (C3H/HeN) and the other insensitive (C3H/HeJ) to bacterial endotoxin, were innoculated with *E. coli* endotoxin. In the endotoxin sensitive C3H/HeN mice, serum TG were elevated 2.6 times above control values 16 hours after injection with endotoxin. This increase correlated with a near total suppression of adipose tissue LPL activity. The endotoxin resistant C3H/HeJ mice did not exhibit as dramatic a response to similar concentrations of endotoxin. A 25-fold increase in endotoxin concentration was required to achieve the same degree of lipase activity suppression in these mice compared to the endotoxin sensitive murine strain. Further studies demonstrated that serum from endotoxin-treated C3H/HeJ mice could suppress adipose tissue LPL activity when administered to C3H/HeJ mice. Moreover, when adherent peritoneal exudate cells (primarily macrophages), obtained from endotoxin sensitive mice 6 days after intraperitoneal injection of thioglycollate broth, were cultured in the presence of endotoxin, the conditioned medium contained a mediator which, when administered to C3H/HeJ mice, resulted in the suppression of adipose tissue LPL activity. From these studies, it was concluded that the effects of bacterial endotoxin on lipase activity were mediated by a humoral factor synthesized by elicited peritoneal exudate cells (82). In separate experiments, it was observed that resident peritoneal exudate cells were not capable of producing such a mediator in response to endotoxin. (M. Kawakami and P. H. Pekala, unpublished observation).

Studies in the C3H/HeJ mouse suggested that endotoxin-induced suppression of adipose tissue LPL activity is due to the action of mediator(s) secreted by macrophages; however, confirmatory evidence was necessary because a portion of intravenously injected endotoxin remains in plasma for several hours in association with lipoproteins (87,88), and C3H/HeJ mice did exhibit some suppression of LPL activity after endotoxin. In addition, although adherent exudate cell preparations are predominantly macrophages, these cell preparations are usually contaminated with other leukocytic cells that may also respond to endotoxin.

To further investigate the actions of the mediator present in the conditioned medium, the well-defined 3T3-L1 preadipocyte system was employed (89,90,91,92). These cells, cloned from mouse embryo fibroblasts, differentiate in monolayer culture into cells having the biochemical and morphological characteristics of adipocytes (89,90,91). During adipocyte conversion, 3T3-L1 cells exhibit a coordinate rise in the enzymes of *de novo* fatty acid synthesis (93,94) and TG synthesis (95). Similarly, the activity of LPL rises 80- to 200-fold during differentiation (96). The activity of this enzyme appears to be identical to that of LPL of adipose tissue (97).

Incubation of differentiated 3T3-L1 (fatty) fibroblasts in the presence of conditioned medium from endotoxin-stimulated C3H/HeN mouse peritoneal exudate cells, resulted in both a dose and time dependent suppression of LPL activity to less than 10% of control values (98). In contrast, neither medium from untreated cells nor unconditioned medium containing endotoxin had a significant effect on lipase activity. Sonicates of the peritoneal exudate cells did not contain the mediator, suggesting that it was not constituitively synthesized and sequestered intracellularly in the absence of endotoxin. Moreover, partial characterization indicated the mediator was a protein.

The study of this endotoxin-induced macrophage secretory protein or monokine was greatly aided by the utilization of the RAW 264.7 mouse monocyte-macrophage cell line. These cells can be grown in large quantities and secrete a LPL suppressive activity in response in *E. coli* endotoxin that is identical to that described for the mouse exudate cells (99). This cell line was established from the ascites of a tumor induced in a male mouse by the intraperitoneal injection of Abelson leukemia virus. Utilizing the RAW 264.7 cell culture system in conjunction with the 3T3-L1 cells, two laboratories have reported purification schemes for a mediator protein that suppresses LPL activity (100,101,102). Because this protein suppresses LPL activity, a key anabolic enzyme, and may play a role in the stimulation of the catabolic state observed during certain chronic illnesses, the protein was termed cachectin. The purified protein exhibits an isoelectric point of 4.7 and a molecular weight of approximately 17,000 daltons under reducing and denaturing conditions (100,101,102). Molecular weight determinations under native conditions suggest that the protein aggregates to tri- and pentameric complexes. Specific receptors for cachectin appear to be present on a variety of cell types including the 3T3-L1 fatty fibroblasts which exhibit a K_d of approximately 3×10^{-10}M (102).

Recently, a high degree of homology between the twenty-five N-terminal amino acids of cachectin and tumor necrosis factor (another endotoxin-induced monokine) was demonstrated (102). Moreover, the two proteins exhibited identical physical characteristics, copurified, and served as potent agonists in the tumor necrosis factor assay (102). These data are consistent with the hypothesis that the two proteins are identical. In point of comparison, the TNF concentration required for half-maximal cytotoxic effect in sensitive cell lines is less than 10 pM (103); whereas, the concentration required for half maximal suppression of LPL is about 100 pM.

Figure 2 shows the loss of LPL activity from 3T3-L1 cells when exposed to crude or purified monokine preparations. Recently, Price et al. (104) demonstrated that the loss of LPL activity on exposure of the 3T3-L1 cells to cachectin results from inhibition of enzyme synthesis, as determined by a decreased incorporation of [^{35}S]-methionine into immunoprecipitable LPL. General protein synthesis, as judged by [^{35}S]-methionine incorporation into acid-insoluble protein, was minimally effected by purified cachectin. The half-life for decay of LPL activity was approximately 130 minutes in the presence of either cycloheximide or purified cachectin.

Comparison of the half-lives for the loss of LPL activity in the presence of the pure monokine and cycloheximide suggests that the suppression of lipase activity by cachectin results from suppression of enzyme biosynthesis. This proposed mechanism of monokine action does not imply that both agents act identically. Rather, the loss of LPL activity in the absence of lipase biosynthesis should be similar regardless of the manner in which enzyme synthesis is inhibited. Moreover, it was recently demonstrated that exposure of differentiating adipogenic TA1 cells to crude preparations of

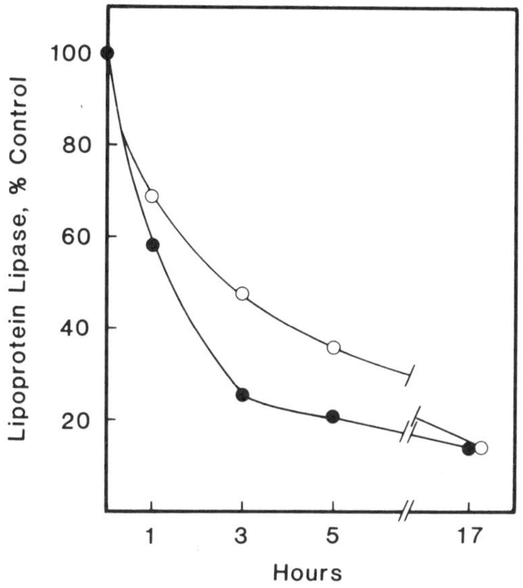

FIGURE 2 Time Course of the Suppression of Lipoprotein Lipase Activity by Crude and Pure Monokine. 3T3-L1 cells were exposed to either crude (○) or purified (●) monokine preparations for various times followed by the determination of lipoprotein lipase enzyme activity. The results displayed represent the suppression of lipoprotein activity in monokine-treated cells compared to control cells which were not exposed to monokine.

cachectin during induction of differentiation, prevented the accumulation of a number of differentially expressed mRNA's (105). One of these was shown to be a mRNA for the key lipogenic enzyme, glycerolphosphate dehydrogenase (105). The effect of this crude monokine preparation was judged to be at the level of transcription. If this also occurs in 3T3-L1 cells, it would suggest that inhibition of LPL synthesis by purified cachectin as shown by Price et al. (104) is also likeley to occur at the level of transcription. The absence of a difference between the $T_{1/2}$ values suggests that pools of mRNA which codes for the lipase are depleted rapidly in the presence of cachectin. Regardless of the step that is blocked, cachectin interacts with adipose cells in a speficic manner and halts the synthesis of the lipase. Thus, these compromised cells would be unable to obtain fatty acids from medium TG which would hamper TG storage.

Cachectin does not appear to be the only monokine capable of suppressing LPL activity. Price et al. (100) were the first to report that a second endotoxin-induced monokine partially suppresses the activity of 3T3-L1 cell LPL in addition to exhibiting a potent interleukin-1 activity. Beutler et al. (106) utilizing recombinant interleukin-1, demonstrated that the lipase could be suppressed by a maximum of 70% relative to control cells. A mechanism of suppression of LPL distinct from that of cachectin/tumor necrosis factor (TNF) was postulated based on the inability of interleukin-1 to compete for the cachectin/TNF receptor. Recently, Price et al. (107) have confirmed and extended these studies by demonstrating that exposure of fully differentiated 3T3-L1 fatty fibroblasts to purified, recombinant murine interleukin-1 resulted in a dose-dependent suppression of LPL activity. The loss of activity reached a maximum of 60–70% of control and appeared to be due to a specific effect on LPL synthesis, in that incorporation of [^{35}S]-methionine into immunoprecipitable LPL was severely reduced. Interleukin-1 had no general effect on protein synthesis as determined by radiolabel incorporated into acid precipitable protein; however, after a 17-hour exposure of the 3T3-L1 cells to this monokine, the synthesis of two proteins (molecular weights, 19,400 and 165,000 daltons) was enhanced several fold. The observed effects on protein synthesis in the adipocytes occur at a interleukin-1 concentration that is similar to the concentration necessary to stimulate [^{3}H] thymidine incorporation into mouse thymocyte DNA.

Endotoxin might induce synthesis and secretion of monokines that possess the ability to regulate the onset of cachexia. In this regard, Pekala et al. (108,109) demonstrated that crude monokine preparation obtained from the conditioned medium of endotoxin-stimulated peritoneal macrophages was capable of a near total (> 80%) suppression of the key enzymes for *de novo* fatty acid biosynthesis, acetyl CoA carboxylase (CBX) and fatty acid synthetase (FAS). Moreover, this same preparation could stimulate lipolysis in these 3T3-L1 cells by activation of hormone sensitive lipase. Purified cachectin and recombinant tumor necrosis factor exhibited only minor (< 20%) inhibitory effects on CBX or FAS and no effect on lipolysis. Recombinant interleukin-1, on the other hand, exhibited no effect on the two enzymes, but markedly stimulated lipolysis (110). Nonetheless, an attractive model for cachexia is presented involving a family of monokines. Cachectin and/or interleukin-1 suppresses the synthesis and activity of LPL, blocking the cell's ability to obtain fatty acids for storage from TG in the extracellular milieu. Additionally, the *de novo* synthesis of fatty acids is inhibited by other monokines and lipolysis stimulated by interleukin-1 leading to a depletion of stored TG with a dramatically reduced ability to resupply. Thus, a number of monokines and perhaps other leukocytic secretory products potentially work in concert to produce cachexia associated with severe trauma, sepsis, and other illnesses in which body wasting occurs. At this time it may be premature to ascribe the name cachectin to a specific monokine responsible for all aspects of cachexia.

Figure 3 depicts a simple diagram of the events initiated by endotoxin in eliciting the suppression of LPL activity in tissues. As both cachectin/TNF and interleukin-1 are synthesized and secreted by the macrophage in response to endotoxin, the adipocyte may be under dual control where both proteins act to suppress synthesis and activity of LPL. Indeed, other monokines may also play a role in this regulation. With this consideration, we term the monokines responsible for suppression of LPL activity, LPL sup-

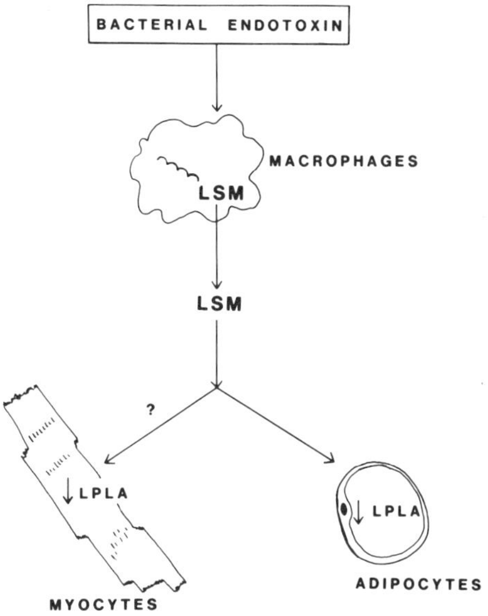

FIGURE 3 The events leading to suppression of lipoprotein lipase activity by endotoxin. LSM is an abbreviation for lipoprotein lipase suppressing mediator(s).

pressing mediators (LSM), simply to identify these proteins with the biological response we are examining.

Little is known concerning the events initiated by endotoxin in macrophages that result in the production and secretion of LSM. Presumably, endotoxin directly or indirectly elicits the synthesis of selected proteins because LSM is not detectable in either supernatant or whole cell sonicates of peritoneal exudate cells which have not been exposed to endotoxin (98).

To date, it has not been possible to induce the appearance of LSM in the circulation for more than several hours. Endotoxin injection into rabbits elicits the appearance of LSM into serum within 15 minutes of injection with peak levels present in about 2 hours (111). Thereafter, LSM levels decline to a baseline within 5 hours. Bagby and coworkers (112) have used suppression of LPL activity in 3T3-L1 cells as a bioassay for LSM in the serum of endotoxin treated rats. LSM was not detected during the 1*st* hour after endotoxin, peaked in 2 to 3 hours, and was nearly absent by the 5*th* hour post-endotoxin. To determine if rats would continue to produce LSM if chronically exposed to endotoxin, rats were infused at a constant rate with endotoxin (50 ug/day) for up to 5 days (113). This procedure only increased the period during which LSM was present in serum from 5 hours to about 8 hours. Six hours of endotoxin infusion produced a similar temporal response. These results indicate that LSM appearance after endotoxin is a transitory phenomenon.

The absence of continual LSM production may be due to endotoxin tolerance. To test this, rats were injected for 5 successive days with endotoxin (112). Prior to and 2 hours after each injection, sera was collected and assayed for LSM. Rats progressively lost the ability to produce LSM and, by the *4th* day, detectable levels of LSM were no longer present 2 hours after endotoxin. For a mediator with LSM activity to cause cachexia, a state would have to be established in which the mediator is continually produced unless the biological lesions they produce are either irreversible or slowly reversible.

To date, LSM has only been demonstrated to be effective against LPL synthesis in adipose tissue or adipocyte-like cells. Kawakami et al. (82) were unable to demonstrate suppression of the heart enzyme in mice with medium from endotoxin conditioned peritoneal exudate cells; yet, heart LPL activity was insensitive to endotoxin when injected into the murine species. In rats and man, muscle LPL activity is also suppressed following endotoxin or during sepsis (56,79,80). As described previously, this decrease is contrary to what one would expect to occur in response to the endocrine adjustments known to occur in endotoxemic and septic animals. The effectiveness of LSM in muscle has been hampered because *in vitro* muscle systems lack the stability necessary to conduct appropriate experiments. However, availability of mediators free of endotoxin will make these studies feasible in the near future.

Undoubtedly, the mediators secreted from macrophages have biological effects beyond their property of suppressing LPL activity. Investigators have ascribed a large range of biological activities to interleukin-1 (114). Based on the finding of Beutler et al. (101,111) that diverse tissues appear to have specific high-affinity receptors for cachectin/TNF, this mediator may also influence multiple aspects of cell metabolism. Thus, it is possible that many metabolic alterations which occur in endotoxemic and septic animals may be due to the appearance of these monokines in the circulation. Their composite role may be to insure adequate mobilization of energy fuels during infection. However, overproduction may be detrimental to animals and play a role in the lethal effects produced by endotoxin administration. Recently, it was shown that immune serum containing antibodies against TNF protected mice from the lethal effects of endotoxin, although the animals were said to become febrile and generally ill in appearance (115). Tempering the biological effects of TNF and other monokines, and possibly lymphokines, may enable animals to cope more successfully during infection.

The suppression of LPL activity and resulting hypertriglyceridemia during endotoxemia and sepsis are not likely to be the principal events responsible for death. However, studying the events leading to this suppression has advanced our understanding of the host response to infection. Since endotoxin leads to the production of mediators that suppress LPL activity in tissues and potentially contribute to the lethal effects of endotoxin, our understanding of the molecular events associated with LPL suppression may provide insights into the cascade of events induced by endotoxin that lead to death.

Plasma Triglyceride Metabolism in Trauma and Sepsis

In the previous section, we saw that trauma and gram-negative sepsis produce divergent responses in LPL activity in some tissues. During the early stage of trauma, muscle LPL activity is increased and the adipose tissue enzyme is decreased, a response similar to other forms of stress. In contrast, some forms of sepsis and endotoxemia suppress LPL activity in both muscle and adipose tissue. The question remains, do these divergent alterations in tissue LPL activity account for changes in plasma TG metabolism? Also, will alterations in tissue LPL activity interfere with TG clearance during hyperalimentation with fat emulsions?

Two mechanisms can potentially cause hypertriglyceridemia associated with infections and some forms of trauma. These are 1) increased rates of TG appearance from the liver, or 2) decreased TG clearance rates by LPL containing tissues. Increased hepatic VLDL production rates and decreased plasma TG clearance rates have both been postulated to occur under some conditions during traumatic and septic challenges. Existing evidence indicates that under appropriate conditions one or both of these phenomena occurs.

Effects of Trauma and Sepsis on Hepatic Triglyceride Output

An increased rate of VLDL production and secretion will increase the appearance rate of plasma TG and tend to elevate plasma TG levels unless a concomitant increase in clearance occurs. Conceptually, fatty acids for TG synthesis in the liver come either from plasma FFA or from *de novo* synthesis using glucose or amino acid carbon. Under most circumstances, TGFA in VLDL are derived from plasma FFA (116). In the fasted state, fatty acids from plasma account for nearly all plasma TGFA. This means that a portion of fatty acids mobilized from adipose tissue are taken up by the liver and incorporated into TG. In the short run, carbohydrate feeding lowers plasma TG concentration by suppressing FFA mobilization from adipose tissue thereby reducing fatty acid delivery to the liver (116,117). With long term glucose infusion, plasma TG concentrations rebound and even increase (116,118). However, even during prolonged glucose administration, plasma FFA appear to remain the major precursor of TGFA.

Unless trauma and sepsis result in shock, plasma FFA concentration and turnover are often elevated (2,3,35,65,66,119,120,121). This, together with increased activities of lipogenic enzymes in the liver (83), has led some to suggest that increased hepatic VLDL output is at least in part responsible for hypertriglyceridemia in trauma and sepsis (66,83,122). In addition, hyperalimentation with glucose as the major energy substrate is often provided to critically ill patients which, if prolonged, can lead to an elevation in plasma TG concentration.

The rate of TG appearance into plasma during traumatic states has not been directly assessed to our knowledge; however, two pieces of information suggest that this rate may be elevated despite normal plasma TG concentrations. First, plasma FFA concentrations are often elevated during trauma (2,3,35,119,120). Second, some investigators report that TG clearance is elevated in trauma patients during nutritional support with artificial fat emulsion (123,124). In this regard, Wilmore et al. (125) reported accelerated fat clearance in thermally injured patients who had normal plasma TG concentration.

Since hypertriglyceridemia is more common during bacterial infections, it is not surprising that more information is available on plasma TG kinetics in septic animals than in animals after trauma. In 1972, Fiser et al. (126) reported that monkeys administered bacteria or endotoxin became hypertriglyceridemic. Although a detailed paper was never published, their data implicated increased hepatic VLDL production and synthesis as being responsible for elevated TG during bacterial infections. At a later time, members of this group published additional results using the same species and similar insults, which indicated that impaired clearance was primarily responsible for elevated plasma TG concentrations during sepsis.

However, it is not clear that increased hepatic TG output can also contribute to hypertriglyceridemia during sepsis. Wolfe et al. (72) simultaneously determined plasma FFA and TG kinetics in normal and hypermetabolic septic dogs. They found FFA and TG concentrations and turnovers to be increased in septic dogs. The increase in TG turnover was shown to be responsible for the elevation of plasma TG levels in these animals since TG clearance was not changed. Furthermore, the increase in TG flux and its resultant oxidation accounted for 17% of total CO_2 production in septic dogs, whereas direct oxidation of plasma TGFA in control dogs was negligible. The increase in FFA concentration and turnover appears to be critical to increased TG turnover. When glucose was infused into their septic animals, FFA mobilization was decreased and VLDL TG turnover was unaffected (72). To our knowledge, no one has studied the effect of prolonged nutritive support with glucose on plasma TG turnover during trauma or sepsis.

Effects of Trauma and Sepsis on Triglyceride Clearance

An increased rate of TG appearance into the plasma compartment during the hypermetabolic state of sepsis should not be taken to mean that this occurs during all stages of sepsis. Hypertriglyceridemia occurs in septic animals and man in the absence of elevated FFA concentrations and turnover (53,56,73,74). During some septic conditions, depressed TG clearance rates due to the suppression of LPL activity are likely to produce this effect. LPL activity is decreased in muscle and adipose tissue of rats administered endotoxin or live E. coli, and in man suffering a bacterial infection (56,59,79,81,83).

Since most LPL in an organism is found in these tissues (127), it is reasonable to expect that such a change would adversely effect TG clearance.

Recently, Bagby et al. (128) studied FFA and TG kinetics in endotoxin-treated rats to determine if hypertriglyceridemia resulted from an increased rate of TG appearance or a decreased TG metabolic clearance rate (MCR). In these experiments, endotoxemic rats exhibited a 3-fold increase in plasma TG concentrations and a decrease in heart and skeletal muscle LPL activity 18–20 hours postendotoxin. Postheparin plasma LPL activity (1 M NaCl inhibitable) in functionally hepatectomized rats was decreased about 50% in endotoxin compared to time-matched control animals. Under these conditions, FFA and TG turnover was determined by constant isotope infusion of [^{14}C]-palmitate bound to albumin and [^{3}H]-palmitate incorporated into rat VLDL-TG *in vivo* using techniques similar to Wolfe et. al. (72). Figure 4 illustrates the fluxes of FFA and TGFA in these animals. Plasma FFA turnover did not differ between endotoxemic and control rats, but endotoxin-treatment significantly decreased TG turnover compared to control values. Decreased TG appearance rate in endotoxin-treated rats implies that either FFA uptake by the liver or VLDL synthesis in the liver is hampered. The absence of an elevated TG turnover, together with increased plasma

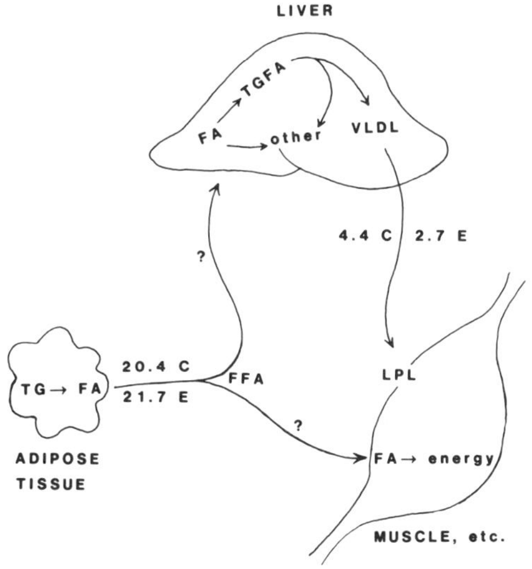

FIGURE 4 Plasma FFA and TGFA kinetics in control (C) and endotoxin-treated (E) rats. Numbers are mean FFA and TGFA turnover rates in μmoles of FA per min.per kg. TGFA turnover was significantly lower in endotoxemic rats compared to control animals ($p < 0.01$). Total FFA uptake by liver is unknown. Thus, extrahepatic tissues derived a minimum of 25% (C) and 14% (E) of their fatty acids from TGFA. As other hepatic pathways use fatty acids, the use of TGFA by extrahepatic tissues became more important.

TG concentrations, indicated that the endotoxin-induced hypertriglyceridemia resulted from suppressed TG clearance. Endotoxemic rats had TG MCR that were less than 20% of control values. Furthermore, it is likely that the reduction of LPL activity in these animals was responsible for impaired clearance. This finding corroborates the earlier work of Kaufmann et al. (70,75) by demonstrating reduced clearance of endogenously produced TG at the prevailing plasma TG concentration present in endotoxemic animals.

This study also demonstrated the relative importance of plasma FFA and TGFA in supplying the fat substrate needs of the rat (128). Plasma FFA account for greater than 80% of total FA flux (FFA + TGFA) in this animal. However, this is somewhat misleading if one considers FA supply to extrahepatic tissues. Comparison of specific activities of [^{14}C] in plasma FFA and TGFA revealed that TGFA came almost exclusively from plasma FFA. This finding is consistent with findings by many other investigators, as reviewed by Hopkins and Williams (116), and means that nearly all fatty acids (FFA and TGFA) originated from adipose tissue. Thus, 12% and 20% of plasma FFA ended up in secreted VLDL-TGFA in endotoxic and control rats, respectively. Unfortunately, measurements made did not allow for determination of total FFA uptake by the liver. Earlier studies indicate that 25%–33% of plasma FFA are removed by the liver in man (129). Furthermore, *in vitro* information indicates that only a small fraction of FFA removed by the liver winds up in VLDL-TG, and a large portion is converted to ketone bodies or oxidized (130,131,132). If this occurs *in vivo*, it means that TGFA may account for a substantial portion of total fatty acid efflux to extrahepatic tissues and accentuates the importance of LPL in directing plasma TGFA to these tissues.

Several laboratories have used artificial fat emulsions to evaluate TG clearance rates during trauma and sepsis. The results are variable, indicating that alterations in TG clearance must depend to some extent on severity and type of injury. Wilmore and associates (125) found a more rapid clearance of Intralipid in burn patients. This observation is consistent with animal studies showing an increase in tissue LPL activity following thermal injury. Rossener (133) studied the clearance of Intralipid in patients after elective surgery, or those who were critically ill. He found the fractional removal rate (K_2) to be increased after surgery but decreased in critically ill patients. Robin et al. (134) found injured and septic patients to display a greater capacity to clear fat during i.v. infusion of Intralipid. This contradicts a parallel study performed by this group which indicated that septic patients had low muscle and adipose tissue LPL activity (56).

Others have observed impaired clearance during sepsis in animals and premature infants. Coran and coworkers (135) reported that puppies made septic by *E. coli* injection were unable to metabolize exogenously administered lipids. Chen (136) determined TG clearance in rats made septic by cecal ligation with puncture. Mean survival time was 33 ± 4 hours and the rats became hypothermic, indicating the severe nature of this insult. Septic rats had elevated plasma TG concentration 6 hours after Intralipid injection compared to control rats. TG clearance and subsequent oxidation was also decreased. Although tissue LPL activity was not measured, it is likely that it was not suppressed in all tissues. Scholl et al. (59) found that rats treated similarly had increases in heart and skeletal muscle LPL activity. Reduced blood flow to LPL-containing tissues may explain impaired TG clearance, but the subcutaneous fluid loading used by Chen (136) should have minimized cardiac output depression (137); however, the presence of hypothermia suggest that this was not completely successful.

Premature septic infants also exhibited a decreased capacity to clear intravenously administered Intralipid. Park et al. (138) found that septic infants possessed higher plasma TG and FFA concentrations than did infants without systemic infections during fat infusion. Since TG levels greater than 1.7 mM probably induce macrophage phagocytosis of fat particles which block the reticuloendothelial (RE) system, reduce bacterial clearance, and impair pulmonary function (139,140,141), they recommended that using less than 2 g fat/kg per day is advisable in infants. The development of hypertriglyceridemia during nutritive support with fat emulsions indicates that such support should be reduced.

Other investigators have also expressed concern over the use of lipid emulsions during total parenteral nutritive support. Heller and associates (62) found that critically ill patients with multiple organ failure and patients after major elective surgery have markedly reduced postheparin plasma LPL activity (50% of normal) yet normal fractional removal rates (K_2) of Intralipid. They suggested that measurement of K_2 may not be useful in evaluating the ability of Intralipid infusion to meet the metabolic needs of critically ill and post-operative patients. Whereas K_2 is not closely correlated with body LPL activity (142), the enzyme is considered to catalize the rate-limiting step in the normal clearance of plasma TG. Thus, a substantial decrease in LPL activity would be expected to interfere with TG clearance from plasma unless it is cleared by an alternative route. The reticuloendothelia system has been shown to clear some lipid emulsions; however, Intralipid appears to be handled like endogenously produced TG-rich lipoproteins in normal subjects (142). It is possible that this may change during sepsis or trauma, so that the RE system may become a more important participant in this clearance. Hulman et al. (143) recently reported that sera from acutely ill patients caused agglutination of Intralipid *in vitro* and that this phenomena was strongly related to the concentration of the acute phase protein, C-reactive protein. They further suggested that if this occurred *in vivo*, these modified particles would either have to be cleared by macrophages or cause microemboli. The latter have been reported to develop in a small percentage of critically ill patients (144,145). Initially, this scenario would result in an increased TG clearance since, in addition to LPL clearance of TG, the RE system would also participate. However, eventually impaired function of the latter system may prevent this pathway of clearance and compromise host defense. Studies should be conducted to determine if agglutination of Intralipid fat particles occurs in the patients during intravenous nutritional support.

We do not want to leave the reader with the impression that use of fat emulsions is not advisable in trauma and septic patients who are unable to receive adequate nutrient support enterally. The potential problems associated with this form of support have merely been emphasized because of the nature of this chapter. Actually, a number of studies point to the efficacy of artificial fat emulsions in the treatment of critically ill patients. Most particularly, their use in combination with glucose produce fewer complications than when glucose is used as the sole energy substrate (142,146,147,148,149,150). It is most likely that defects in clearance will occur in severely septic patients due to suppression of LPL activity and possibly in critically ill patients with high levels of C-reactive protein. Plasma TG metabolism should be monitored when patients are administered fat emulsions during parenteral nutritional support, particularly if they are critically ill or sepsis is expected.

Conclusions

In this chapter, we have attempted to show that LPL activity is increased in heart and skeletal muscle and decreased in adipose tissue in response to stressful states. This pattern of change is consistent with changes that occur in the hormones that normally regulate this enzyme. During stressful states, adipose tissue LPL activity is low due to a reduction of plasma insulin concentrations, the hormone demonstrated to be the primary regulator of LPL production in this tissue. In addition, increased catecholamine levels may play a role in reducing LPL activity in adipose tissue by: 1) suppressing insulin production by pancreatic beta cells, and 2) inactivating LPL activity within the adipocyte. Increased heart and skeletal muscle LPL activity during stress results from increased adrenergic activity, or elevated plasma glucocorticoid concentrations, or a combination of both putative regulators. Their relative importance in regulating muscle LPL activity has not been determined.

During the early stages of shock (not induced by bacterial endotoxins or some forms of sepsis) and trauma, a similar pattern prevails. Whereas, investigations are scarce on this subject, existing information indicates that tissue changes in LPL activity respond to their known humoral regulators during traumatic stress. As the trauma state continues, it is not clear what happens to tissue LPL activity. There is some suggestion that the enzyme in heart and muscle returns to near normal levels despite continual elevation of catecholamines and glucocorticoids. Also, it appears that LPL activity in adipose tissue can still respond to its primary regulator, insulin. Additional, well controlled studies are required to verify these phenomena.

Some forms of infection result in alterations of tissue LPL activity that are not consistent with changes occurring in plasma levels of insulin, glucocorticoids, and catecholamines. That is, despite elevations in glucocorticoids and catecholamines, heart and skeletal muscle LPL activity are not increased and in some cases are decreased. Furthermore, the adipose tissue enzyme does not increase in response to insulin and in some cases is very low. This is the likely cause of hypertriglyceridemia in animals administered bacterial endotoxins or live gram-negative bacteria. This suppression of whole body LPL activity may limit the TG uptake by extrahepatic tissues during hyperalimentation with fat emulsions. The unique response appears to involve modulators of LPL other than the basic known regulators.

In response to endotoxin, macrophages produce and secrete proteins that suppress adipose tissue LPL activity. Whether these proteins adversely effect the muscle enzyme is not known. To date, two monokines have been described that possess this activity: cachectin and interleukin-1. Cachectin appears to be homologous to tumor necrosis factor. This protein was so named because it may be responsible for cachexia associated with infections and other disease states. However, several monokines may play a collective role in this body wasting phenomena. In any case, LPL suppressing mediator(s) (LSM) are present in serum for short periods of time after endotoxin injection or infusion, and animals made tolerant to endotoxin do not contain LSM in their sera. If these mediators are responsible for sustaining cachexia, conditions would have to exist that allow for their continual production. Future studies will be required to identify these conditions.

Research conducted by the authors was supported in part by NIH grants GM 32654 and GM32892.

References

1, Blackburn, G. L. 1977. *Am. J. Clin. Nutr.* 30:1321–1332.
2. Kinney, J. M., and P. Felig. 1979. *In*: Endocrinology. L. J. DeGroot, editor. Grune and Stratton, New York, NY. 1963–1985.
3. Wolfe, R. R., and G. J. Bagby. 1983. *In*: Handbook of Shock and Trauma, Vol. 1: Basic Science. B. M. Altura, A. M. Lefer, W. Schumer, editors, Raven Press, New York, NY 199–216.
4. Spitzer, J. A., and J. J. Spitzer. 1983. *In*: Beneficial effects of endotoxins. A Nowotny, editor. Plenum Publishing Corp., New York, N.Y. 57–74.
5. Cox, T. 1978. *Stress*. University Park Press, Baltimore, MD. 53–73.
6. Beck, L. V., D. S. Zaharko, and S. C. Kalser. 1967. *Life Sci.* 6:1501–1506.
7. Wright, P. H., and W. J. Malaisse. 1968. *Am. J. Physiol* 214:1031–1034.
8. Carlson, L. 1966. *Pharmacol. Rev.* 18:291–301.
9. Cryer, A., S. E. Riley, E. R. Williams, and D. S. Robinson. 1974. *Biochem. J.* 140:561–563.
10. Borensztajn, J., D. R. Samols, A. H. Rubenstein. 1972. *Am. J. Physiol.* 223:1271–1275.
11. Garfinkel, A. S., P. Nilsson-Ehle, and M. C. Schotz. 1976. *Biochim. Biophys. Acta* 424:264–273.

12. De Gasquet, P., and E. Pequignot. 1973. *Horm. Metab. Res.* 5:440–443.
13. Spooner, P. M., S. S. Chernick, M. M. Garrison, and R. O. Scow. 1979. *J. Biol. Chem.* 254:10021–10029.
14. Vydelingum, N., R. L. Drake, J. Etienne, and A. H. Kissebah. 1983. *Am. J. Physiol.* 245:E121–E131.
15. Patten, R. L. 1970. *J. Biol. Chem.* 245:5577–5584.
16. Wing, D. R. and D. S. Robinson. 1968. *Biochem. J.* 109:841–849.
17. Bourdeaux, A. -M., R. Nordmann, and Y. Giudicelli. 1984. *FEBS Lett.* 178:132–136.
18. Ashby, P., D. P. Bennett, I. M. Spencer, and D. S. Robinson. 1978. *Biochem. J.* 176:865–872.
19. Mallov, S., and F. Cerra. 1967. *J. Pharmacol. Exp. Therap.* 156:426–444.
20. Mallov, S., and A. A. Alousi. 1969. *Am. J. Physiol.* 216:794–799.
21. Stam, H., and W. C. Hulsmann. 1984. *Biochim. Biophys. Acta* 794:72–82.
22. Knobler, H., T. Chajek-Shaul, O. Stein, J. Etienne, and Y. Stein. 1984. *Biochim. Biophys. Acta* 795:363–371.
23. De Gasquet, P., E. Pequignot-Planche, N. T. Tonnu, and F. A. Diaby. 1975. *Horm. Metab. Res.* 7:152–157.
24. Cuthbertson, D. P. 1932. *Q. J. Med.* 1:233–246.
25. Kelleher, D. L., B. C. Fong, G. J. Bagby, J. J. Spitzer. 1982. *Am. J. Physiol.* 243:R77–R81.
26. Ryan, N. T. 1976. *Surg. Clin. North Am.* 56:1073–1090.
27. Jaattela, A. 1972. *Ann. Clin. Res.* 4:204–212.
28. Baue, A. E., B. Gunther, W. Hartl, M. Ackenheil, and G. Heberer. 1984. *Arch. Surg.* 119:1125–1132.
29. Wolfe, R. R., M. J. Durkot, and M. H. Wolfe. 1982. *Circ. Shock* 9:383–394.
30. Wilmore, D. W., J. M. Long, A. D. Mason, Jr., R. W. Skrean, and B. A. Pruitt, Jr. 1974. *Ann. Surg.* 180:653–669.
31. Skillman, J. J., J. Hedley-Whyte, and J. A. Pallotta. 1971. *Ann. Surg.* 174:911–922.
32. Hiebert, J. M., Z. Celik, J. S. Soeldner, and R. H. Egdahl. 1973. *Am. J. Surg.* 12:501–507.
33. Sherwin, R. S., H. Shamoon, R. Hendler, L. Sacca, N. Eigler, and M. Walesky. 1980. *Metabolism* 29:1146–1154.
34. Postel, J., Schloerb, P. R. 1977. *Ann. Surg.* 185:475–480.
35. Batstone, G. F., K. G. M. M. Alberti, L. Hinks, P. Smythe, J. E. Laing, C. W. Ward, D. W. Ely, and S. R. Bloom. 1976. *Burns* 2:207–225.
36. Lang, C. H., G. J. Bagby and J. J. Spitzer. 1984. *Metabolism* 33:959–963.
37. Wilmore, D. W., C. A. Lindsey, J. A. Moylan, G. A. Faloona, B. A. Pruitt, and R. H. Unger. 1974. *Lancet* 1:73–75.
38. Aulick, L. H., W. B. Baze, A. A. Johnson, D. W. Wilmore and A. D. Mason. 1981. *J. Surg. Res.* 31:281–287.
39. Ross, H., I. D. A. Johnston, T. A. Welborn, A. D. Wright. 1966. *Lancet* 2:563–566.
40. Ryan, N. T., G. L. Blackburn, and G. H. A. Clowes, Jr. 1974. *Metabolism* 23:1081–1089.
41. Wolfe, R. R., M. J. Durkot, J. R. Allsop, and J. F. Burke. 1979. *Metabolism* 28:1031–1039.
42. Wilmore, D. W. 1976. *Surg. Clin. North Am.* 56:999–1018.
43. Filkins, J. P. 1985. *Fed. Proc.* 44:300–304.
44. Spitzer, J. J., and J. A. Spitzer. 1955. *J. Lab. Clin. Med.* 46:461–470.
45. Wooles, W. R. 1968. *Rad. Res.* 34:596–603.
46. Carton, M., N. Dousset, and L. Douste-Blazy. 1974. *Comptes Rendus Soc. Biol.* 168:905–909.
47. Faliste, R., N. Dousset, M. Carton, and L. Douste-Blazy. 1981. *Radiat. Res.* 87:602–612.
48. Dousset, N., R. Feliste, M. Carton, and L. Douste-Blazy. 1984. *Biochim. Biophys. Acta* 794:444–453.
49. Amr, S., J. P. Thouvenot, N. Dousset, M. Carton, and L. Douste-Blazy. 1977. *Int. J. Radiat. Biol.* 32:181–183.
50. Oehler, G., H. Wolf, F. W. Schmahl, and L. Roka. 1974. *Res. Exp. Med.* 163:31–38.

51. Lehr, L., H. Niedermuller, and G. Hofecker. 1977. *Surgery* 81:521–526.
52. Spitzer, J. A., and J. J. Spitzer. 1972. *J. Trauma* 12:898–902.
53. Bagby, G. J., and J. A. Spitzer. 1980. *J. Surg. Res.* 29:110–115.
54. Bagby, G. J., H. I. Miller, J. A. Spitzer, and J. J. Spitzer. 1981. *Circ. Shock* 8:131–136.
55. Birke, G., L. A. Carlson, and S. -O. Liljedahl. 1965. *Acta Med. Scand.* 178:337–350.
56. Robin, A. P., J. Askanazi, M. R. C. Greenwood, Y. A. Carpentier, F. E. Gump, and J. M. Kinney. 1981. *Surgery* 90:401–407.
57. Borbola, J., A. Gecse, and S. Karady. 1973. *In*: *Adv. Exp. Med. Biol.* A. G. B. Kovach, H. B. Stoner, and J. J. Spitzer, editors. Plenum Press, New York, NY. 33:387–393.
58. Chapman, M. J. 1980. *J. Lipid Res.* 21:789–853.
59. Scholl, R. A., C. H. Lang, and G. J. Bagby. 1984. *J. Surg. Res.* 37:394–401.
60. Carpentier, Y. A., J. Nordenstrom, J. Askanazi, D. H. Elwyn, F. E. Gump, and J. M. Kinney. 1979. *Surg. Forum* 30:72–74.
61. Rogers, M. P., J. Borensztajn, and D. S. Robinson. 1972. *Biochem. Soc. Symp.* 35:83–92.
62. Heller, F., M. Raynaert, and C. Harvengt. 1985. *Am. J. Clin. Nutr.* 41:748–752.
63. Taskinen, M. -R., I. Tulikonra, E. A. Nikkila, and C. Ehnholm. 1981. *Eur. J. Clin. Invest.* 11:317–323.
64. Robin, A. P., M. R. C. Greenwood, J. Askanazi, D. H. Elwyn, and J. M. Kinney. 1981. *Ann. Surg.* 194:681–686.
65. Farshtchi, D., and V. J. Lewis. 1968. *J. Bacteriol.* 95:1615–1621.
66. Gallin, J. I., D. Kaye, and W. M. O'Leary. 1969. *N. Engl. J. Med.* 281:1081–1086.
67. Beisel, W. R., and F. H. Fiser, Jr. 1970. *Am. J. Clin. Nutr.* 23:1069–1079.
68. Griffiths, J., A. C. Groves, and F. Y. T. Leung. 1972. *Surg. Gynecol. Obstet.* 134:795–798.
69. Hirsch, R. L., D. G. McKay, R. I. Travers, and R. K. Skraly. 1964. *J. Lipid Res.* 5:563–568.
70. Kaufmann, R. L., C. R. Matson, and W. R. Beisel. 1976. *J. Infect. Dis.* 133:548–555.
71. Fiser, R. H., J. C. Denniston, and W. R. Beisel. 1974. *Pediatr. Res.* 8:13–17.
72. Wolfe, R. R., J. H. F. Shaw, and M. J. Durkot. 1985. *Am. J. Physiol.* 248:E732–E740.
73. Levin, J., T. E. Poore, N. S. Young, S. Margolis, N. P. Zauber, A. S. Townes, and W. R. Bell. 1972. *Ann. Intern. Med.* 76:1–7.
74. Fiser, R. H., T. D. Schultz, R. B. Rindsig, and W. R. Beisel. 1973. *Biol. Neonate* 22:155–160.
75. Kaufmann, R. L., C. F. Matson, A. H. Rowberg, and W. R. Beisel. 1976. *Metabolism* 25:615–624.
76. Oehler, G., R. Hassinger, F. W. Schmahl, K. Huth, and L. Roka. 1975. *In*: Gram-Negative Bacterial Infections; Pathophysiological, Immunological and Clinical Aspects. B. Urbaschek, R. Urbaschek, and E. Neter, editors. Springer-Verlag, New York, NY 301–305.
77. Bagby, G. J., and J. A. Spitzer. 1977. *Fed. Proc.* 36:504 (abst.).
78. Bagby, G. J., and J. A. Spitzer. 1977. *Physiologist* 20(4):4 (abst.).
79. Bagby, G. J., and J. A. Spitzer. 1980. *Am. J. Physiol.* 238:H325–H330.
80. Bagby, G. J., and J. A. Spitzer. 1981. *Proc. Soc. Exp. Biol. Med.* 168:395–398.
81. Sakaguchi, O., and S. Sakaguchi. 1979. *Microbiol. Immunol.* 23:71–85.
82. Kawakami, M., and A. Cerami. 1981. *J. Exp. Med.* 154:631–639.
83. Lanza-Jacoby, S., S. C. Lansey, M. P. Cleary, and F. E. Rosato. 1982. *Arch. Surg.* 117:144–147.
84. Kelleher, D. L., P. A. Puinno, B. C. Fong, and J. A. Spitzer. 1982. *Metabolism* 31:252–257.
85. Lang, C. H., G. J. Bagby, G. H. Bornside, L. J. Vial, and J. J. Spitzer. 1983. *J. Surg. Res.* 35:201–210.
86. Rouzer, C. A., and A. Cerami. 1980. *Mol. Biochem. Parsitol.* 1:31–38.
87. Mathison, J. C., and R. J. Ulevitzh. 1979. *J. Immunol.* 123:2133–2143.
88. Ulevitzh, R. J., A. R. Johnston, and D. B. Weinstein. 1979. *J. Clin. Invest.* 64:1516–1524.
89. Green, H. and O. Kehinde. 1974. *Cell* 1:113–116.
90. Green, H. and O. Kehinde. 1975. *Cell* 5:19–27.

91. Green, H. and O. Kehinde. 1976. *Cell* 7:105–113.
92. Pekala, P. H., M. D. Lane, P. Watkins, and J. Moss. 1981. *J. Biol. Chem.* 256:4871–4876.
93. Mackall, J. C., A. K. Student, S. E. Polakis, and M. D. Lane. 1976. *J. Biol. Chem.* 251:6462–6464.
94. Student, A. K., R. Y. Hsu and M. D. Lane. 1976. *J. Biol. Chem* 253:4745–4750.
95. Coleman, R. A., B. C. Reed, J. C. Mackall, A. K. Student, M. D. Lane, and R. M. Bell. 1978. *J. Biol. Chem.* 253:7256–7261.
96. Wise, L. S. and H. Green. 1978. *Cell* 13:233–242.
97. Spooner, P. M., S. S. Chernick, M. M. Garrison, and R. O. Scow. 1979. *J. Biol. Chem.* 254:1305–1311.
98. Kawakami, M., P. H. Pekala, M. D. Lane, and A. Cerami. 1982. *Proc. Natl. Acad. Sci. U.S.A.* 79:912–916.
99. Mahoney, J. R., B. A. Beutler, N. Le Trang, W. Vine, Y. Ikeda, M. Kawakami, and A. Cerami. 1985. *J. Immunol.* 134:1673–1675.
100. Price, S. R., A. Bautista, A. Volkman, and P. H. Pekala. 1985. *Fed. proc.* 44:7565 (abst.).
101. Beutler, B., J. Mahoney, N. Le Trang, P. Pekala, and A. Cerami. 1985. *J. Exp. Med.* 161:984–995.
102. Beutler, B., D. Greenwald, J. D. Hulmes, M. Chang, Y. - C. E. Pan, J. Mathison, R. Ulevitch, and A. Cerami. 1985. *Nature* 316:552–554.
103. Kull, Jr., F. C., S. Jacobs, and P. Cautrecasas. 1985. *Proc. Natl. Acad. Sci. U.S.A.* 82:5756–5760.
104. Price, S.R., T. Olivecrona, and P. H. Pekala. 1986. *Biochem. J.* 240:601–604.
105. Torti, F. M., B. Dieckmann, B. Beutler, A. Cerami, and G. Ringold. 1985. *Science* 229:867–869.
106. Beutler, B. A., and A. Cerami. 1985. *J. Immunol.* 135:3969–3971.
107. Price, S. R., S. B. Mizel, and P. H. Pekala. 1986. *Biochem. Biophys. Acta* 889:374–381.
108. Pekala, P. H., M. Kawakami, C. W. Angus, M. D. Lane and A. Cerami. 1983. *Proc. Natl. Acad. Sci. U.S.A.* 80:2743–2747.
109. Pekala, P. H., S. R. Price, C. A. Horn, B. E. Hom, J. Moss, and A. Cerami. 1984. *Trans. Assoc. Am. Phys.* 97:251–259.
110. Price, S. R., S. B. Mizel and P. H. Pekala. 1986. *Fed. Proc.* 45:1719 (abst.)
111. Beutler, B. A., I. W. Milsark, and A. Cerami. 1985. *J. Immunol.* 135:3972–3977.
112. Bagby, G. J., C. B. Corll, J. J. Thompson, and L. A. Wilson. 1986. *Am. J. Physiol.* 251:E470–E476.
113. Bagby, G. J., C. B. Corll, J. J. Thompson, and L. A. Wilson. 1987. (Submitted for publication).
114. Dinarello, C. A., 1984. *Rev. Infect. Dis.* 6:51–95.
115. Beutler, B., I. W. Milsark, and A. C. Cerami. 1985. *Science* 229:869–871.
116. Hopkins, P. N. and R. R. Williams. 1981. *Am. J. Clin. Nutr.* 34:2560–2590.
117. Baker, N., A. S. Garfinkel, and M. C. Schotz. 1968. *J. Lipid Res.* 9:1–7.
118. Wolfe, B. M., and S. P. Ahuja. 1977. *Metabolism* 26:963–978.
119. Carlson, L. A., S. -O. Lijedahl. 1963. *Acta Med. Scand.* 173:25–33.
120. Birke, G., L. A. Carlson, S. O. Liljedahl. 1965. *Acta Med. Scand.* 178:337–350.
121. Shaw, J. H. F., and R. R. Wolfe. 1984. *Surgery* 95:553–561.
122. Fiser, R. H., J. C. Denniston, and W. R. Beisel. 1972. *J. Infect. Dis.* 125:54–60.
123. Carlson, L. A., and S. -O. Liljedahl. 1971. *Acta. Chir. Scand.* 137:123–128.
124. Hallberg, D. 1965. *Acta Physiol. Scand.* 65:153–163.
125. Wilmore, D. W., J. A. Moylan, G. M. Helmkamp, and B. A. Pruitt, Jr. 1973. *Ann. Surg.* 178:503–513.
126. Fiser, R. H., J. C. Dennison, and W. R. Beisel. 1972. *Pediat. Res.* 6:398 (abst.)
127. Bragdon, J. H., and R. S. Gordon Jr. 1958. *J. Clin. Invest.* 37:574–578.
128. Bagby, G. J., C. B. Corll, R. R. Martinez. 1987. *Am. J. Physiol.* (in press).
129. Carlson, L. A., J. Bogerg, and B. Hogstedt. 1965. *In*: Handbook of Physiology, Section 5: Adipose Tissue. A. E. Renold and G. F. Cahill, Jr., editors. American Physiological Society, Washington, D.C. 625–644.

130. Mayes, P. A., and J. M. Felts. 1967. *Nature* 215:716–718.
131. Ontko, J. A. 1972. *J. Biol. Chem.* 247:1788–1800.
132. Ide, T., and J. A. Ontko. 1981. *J. Biol. Chem.* 256:10247–10255.
133. Rossner, S. 1980. *Acta Chir. Scand.* Suppl. 507:220–225.
134. Robin, A. R., J. Nordenstrom, J. Askanazi, D. H., Elwyn, Y. A. Carpentier, and J. M. Kinney. 1980. *J. Parent. Ent. Nutr.* 4:505–510.
135. Coran, A. G., R. A. Drongowski, G. S. Lee, M. D. Klein, and J. R. Wesley. 1984. *J. Parent. Ent. Nutr.* 8:652–656.
136. Chen, W. J. 1984. *J. Parent. Ent. Nutr.* 8:14–17.
137. Smith, L. W., S. L. Winbery, L. A. Baker, and K. H. McDonough. 1986. *Am. J. Physiol.* 251:H405–H412.
138. Park, W., H. Paust, and H. Schroder. 1984. *J. Parent. Ent. Nutr.* 8:290–292.
139. Nordenstrom, J., C. Jastrand, and A. Wiernik. 1979. *Am. J. Clin. Nutr.* 32:2416–2422.
140. Bradfield, J. 1980. *Lancet* 2:1180.
141. Palmblad, J., O. Brostrom, A. M. Uden. 1980. *Lancet* 2:1138.
142. Wretlind, A. 1976. *In*: Fat Emulsions in Parenteral. H. C. Meng, and D. W. Wilmore, editors. American Medical Association, Chicago, IL. 109–122.
143. Hulman, G., H. J. Pearson, I. Fraser, and P. R. F. Bell. 1982. *Lancet* 2:1426–1427.
144. Forbes, G. B. 1978. *J. Clin. Path.* 31:765–771.
145. Hessov, I., F. Melsen, and A. Haug. 1979. *Arch. Surg.* 114:66–68.
146. Jeejeebhoy, K. N., G. H. Anderson, A. F. Nakhooda, G. R. Greenberg, I. Sanderson, and E. B. Marliss. 1976. *J. Clin. Invest.* 57:125–136.
147. Bark, S., I. Holm, I. Hakansson, and A. Wretland. 1976. *Acta Chir. Scand.* 142:423–427.
148. Kirkpatrick, J. R., M. Dahn, M. J. Hynes, and D. Williams. 1981. *Surgery* 89:370–374.
149. Kirkpatrick, J. R., M. Dahn and L. Lewis. 1981. *Am. J. Surg.* 141:116–120.
150. Jeejeebhoy, K. N., E. B. Marliss, G. H. Anderson, G. R. Greenberg, A. Kubsis, and C. Breckenridge. 1976. *In*: Fat Emulsions in Parenteral Nutrition. H. C. Meng and D. W. Wilmore, editors. American Medical Association, Chicago, IL. 45–54.

Chapter 11

COMPARATIVE BIOCHEMISTRY AND PHYSIOLOGY OF LIPOPROTEIN LIPASE

Anthony Cryer

As noted elsewhere (1), the necessity for a vascular transport system emerges along with the increased size that is attainable when digestive, respiratory, and excretory functions become discernible as separate entities (2). Particularly, where comparative data is available, it would appear that where closed vascular systems bounded by endothelium exist, the transport of lipid within the plasma compartment occurs with the lipid in the form of lipoproteins (3). The structure, function, metabolism, and interrelationships of these lipid transport particles have been the subject of extensive review, both in this volume and elsewhere (4–14). Lipoprotein lipase (LPL), as one of the pivotal enzymes involved in the metabolism of these lipoproteins, has received attention from diverse sources and as the subject of such scrutiny, it is timely to examine the similarities and differences that emerge from a comparative review of the enzyme. Obviously, pitfalls await the unwary who embark on such a proposed synthesis of information taken from what are sometimes vastly different sources. However, by trying to compare like with like, and by being only mildly speculative, the present

Chapter will attempt to analyze the situation in such a way as to stimulate others to throw more light on this relatively neglected area.

Occurrence of Lipoprotein Lipase

The demonstration of a tissue activity with the functional characteristics of LPL has been undertaken in a surprisingly wide range of species. The enzyme has been shown to be present in the tissues of, among others, man (15–27), non-human primates (28) and monkeys (29). Also, in addition to our own comparative survey of LPL activity in the tissues of 10 species (30), the enzyme has been reported to occur variously in the tissues of rat (30–36), mouse (30,37–40), ferret (30,41), hamster (30,42), guinea pig (30,43–47), ground squirrel (48), pig (30,49–52), cow (30,53–55), sheep (30,56), goat (57,58), rabbit (30), chicken (59–64), turkey (65), duck (66), pigeon (30,67), and rainbow trout (68). This range of species has been extended from time to time by claims that an enzyme similar to mammalian and avian LPL is present in, for example, insects (69), but the variability of assay conditions and criteria for characterization (see later) often make such studies difficult to assess. The enzyme is widely distributed in the animal kingdom and can be found in a wide range of tissue and cell types. In addition to its presence, as a significant functional activity, in the tissues described individually in other Chapters in this volume the enzyme has been shown to be present in a variety of other tissues, tissue cell types, and in milk (see Chapter 2 and ref. 27,47,70–74). The other tissues in which the presence of LPL is best substantiated include; lung (30,33,75–78), in which the pulmonary macrophage contributes a significant proportion of the total activity (79) (see later), aorta (54,64,80–82) and other vascular tissue, diaphragm (30,83), placenta (45,84,85), uterine tissue (86), and corpus luteum (87,88). Although most of the detailed analysis of adipose tissue LPL has concentrated on white adipose tissue, it is also clear that the enzyme plays an important physiological function in brown adipose tissue (36,75,89–94). A number of reports have also appeared which indicate that functional LPL activity is present in fetal liver (95,96) and in the brain (97–99) of experimental animals. An enzyme with the characteristics of LPL has also been detected in avian liver (100), where it exists together with the other recognized hepatic triglyceride lipase.

The enzyme has further been detected and studied in a wide range of isolated cells including, adipocytes from the white adipose tissue of a number of species (101–109), cardiac myocytes (110–116), granulosa cells (117,118), mammary acinar cells (119–121), and tumour cells (122,123). Recently, great interest has also centered on the macrophage as an important cell type expressing functional LPL activity (see later) (79,124–132).

In addition to the activity found in isolated cells, a number of cultured cell strains and established cell lines have also been shown to exhibit LPL activity. The most carefully studied examples include: The 3T3-L1, clones of mouse embryonic fibroblasts which undergo an adipose conversion *in vitro* (133,134,135–139); preadipocyte cell lines isolated from adipose tissue [ob17 (140–143), ST 13 (144,145)], preadipocyte cell strains of similar origin (146–158), cultured heart cells (159–161), and vascular smooth muscle cells (162).

In each of the cases described, it has been suggested almost invariably that the presence of LPL activity confers the capacity for triglyceride uptake (see later) by the tissue and cells studied. The corollary to this, of course, is that organs which do not have LPL cannot utilize lipoprotein triglyceride fatty acids and have to depend on glucose and albumin-bound non-esterified fatty acids for their metabolic fuel. It has been shown, for example, that the small intestine, being without the enzyme, is unable to use triglyceride fatty acids (163).

The Comparative Molecular Properties of Lipoprotein Lipase Purified from Various Sources

With so many sources of LPL available, it is not surprising that attempts have been made to purify the enzyme from a number of them. Many of the earlier studies employed postheparin plasma as a rich source of enzyme activity. Although this source provided what were thought to be enzyme preparations of high purity (164,165), further studies revealed that the major protein present was in fact antithrombin III, with LPL being only a minor component (166–168). Although more recently LPL preparations from post-heparin plasma have become available which have no immunodetectable antithrombin III present, they too are still less than homogeneous in their protein content (169). Tissue sources of the enzyme have, however, produced what appear to be the most useful preparations of LPL and which may therefore become the subjects of comparative analysis. Notwithstanding the difficulties surrounding the comparison of measured enzyme activities that will be considered later, the two most currently accessible comparators for LPL preparations are molecular weight and specific activity (see Table 1). With regard to molecular weight, the most popular means of determination has been the use of polyacrylamide gel electrophoresis in the presence of sodium dodecylsulphate; thus mostly the values which may be compared are monomer molecular weights. However, evidence from electrophoretic studies done under more physiologically relevant conditions (170) and from the study of enzyme *in situ* using radiation inactivation (171) suggest that the functional unit exists as a dimer of identical subunits *in vivo*.

From the examples listed in Table 1, it is clear that where consistent methodology has been applied, the enzyme from all sources has a molecular weight between 48- and 67,000. The significance of any true differences between the molecular weights of the enzyme protein from different sources is not easy to assess. Nevertheless, as reviewed by Nilsson-Ehle (186), these estimates, together with rather incomplete amino acid composition data and immunological studies (60,187–189) do suggest considerable similarity,

TABLE I The comparative molecular properties of lipoprotein lipase isolated from a variety of sources

Species	Tissue	Molecular weight	Specific activity (μMol/h/mg)	Reference
Rat	Heart	60,000	300	172
		34,000	600	173
		37,500	2400	174
		54,600	300	176
	White	60,000	330	175
	Adipose	56,000	5–15,000	177
		ND	900	178
		ND	220	179
	Brown Adipose	67,000	1800	91
Porcine	Heart	73,000	600	51
	White	60–62,000	3600	50
	Adipose	60,000	3000	181, 182
Chicken	White	60,000	10,800	62
	Adipose	61,000	21,000	64
Human	Milk	63,000	2250	72
		ND	5000	27
Bovine	Milk	60,000	18–42,000	183
		48–51,000	37,000	170
		55,000	25–28,000	184
		41,700 / 47,500*	ND	185
	Aorta	60,000	3600	54
Guinea-pig	Milk	62,000	34,200	47

ND: either not detected or not possible to calculate readily from data given. *Determined from partial specific volume measurements and from gel exclusion chromatography in guanadinium chloride.

if not identity, between the enzymes present in different tissues of the same species. However, less similarity is found when enzymes derived from a variety of species are compared. The specific activities given in Table 1 also indicate that, although all LPLs share the same relatively low specificity for substrate with a strict positional specificity (190–193) and an absolute requirement for apo CII activator (194–196), the proteins from different sources, at least superficially demonstrate quite disparate catalytic efficiencies *in vitro*. Whether such differences reflect technical variation or contribute to real differences in the functional activity of LPL as a system facilitating the transport of triglyceride fatty acids into tissues *in vivo* remains unknown (see 197). The possibility that the two apparent forms of the enzyme, distinguishable by gel permeation chromatography, represent functionally or locationally distinct entities in tissues (198–200) has now been abandoned following the demonstration that the previously reported differences in molecular weight were due to artifactual association wiith residual lipid (201).

From a comparative standpoint, it is clear that all the LPL enzymes so far studied are glycoproteins with a carbohydrate content variously estimated between 3 and 10% by weight (for references, see Table 1). Whether differences in the structure of the carbohydrate present contributes to the apparent species-related differences in molecular weight and activity is not known. Furthermore, the involvement of glycosylation in the conversion of an inactive precursor enzyme to the fully active secretory product in all situations is not yet totally clear (142).

Lipoprotein Lipase Activity Determinations and the Problems of Comparability

Clearly, mammalian tissues and cells contain a number of lipase activities (202–207). Some of these enzymes are confined to single tissue sources, whereas others like LPL are more widely distributed. In considering the comparability of studies on LPL, it is important to consider the conditions under which optimal measurements of activity can be made and to define the essential properties that LPL must exhibit. Table 2 shows a comparison of the properties of LPL with the properties of other known mammalian lipases. Clearly, most of the lipases listed demonstrate relatively catholic tastes with regard to substrate. Although the rate of esterolysis may be quite different with each of the substrate species, the enzymes show a common preference for *sn* 1(3) fatty acid cleavage. Virtually all the enzymes have a serine residue involved in the active site together with a reactive histidine and demonstrate a serine-esterase-like activity with acyl-enzyme intermediates being formed during catalysis. As is pointed out elsewhere in this volume, the only truly characteristic feature of LPL is its requirement for apolipoprotein CII for full activity expression. Although the inhibition of activity in the presence of high NaCl concentrations has previously been considered diagnostic with regard to the identity of LPL, this inhibition is variable (277) and is not a true active site inhibition but is exerted rather

TABLE II Comparison of the enzymological and molecular properties of lipoprotein lipase with those of other mammalian tissue lipases

	Lipoprotein Lipase	Lingual Lipase	Pancreatic Lipase	Pancreatic Carboxyl Ester Lipase	Hepatic Endothelial Lipase	Lysosomal Acid Lipase	Hormone-Sensitive Lipase
Occurrence/Distribution	Extra-hepatic tissues	tongue	pancreas	pancreas	liver	wide cell-type distribution	Adipose tissue (adrenal cortex, corpus luteum)
Substrates	TAG (208) DAG (209) MAG (210,211) PC (212–215) PE (216,217) p-nitrophenylesters (218–219) Tween (210) Palmitoyl CoA (220)	TAG (202) DAG (202)	TAG (203,221) s-fatty acylthiols (222) nitrophynelesters (223)	CE (204) p-nitrophenyl-acetate (224,225) PL (226) TAG (226) DAG (226) MAG (226,227) substituted arylacetates (225,228)	TAG (229) DAG (230) MAG (231) PE (232–4) Acyl CoA esters (235) Esters of primary alcohols with fatty acids (236)	TAG (206) DAG (237) CE (238) fluoro and chromogenic acyl esters (239)	TAG DAG, MAG CE (207,240)
pH optimum	8–9 (12,50,241,242)	4.4–5.4 (243,244)	7–8 (203)	5.5–7.4 (204)	8–8.5 (205)	4–5 (206)	6–8 (207,245)
Positional specificty	TAGsn 1(3) > sn2 (209,191,246) sn1 > sn3 (192,246,247) MAG sn1(3) (209,191,246)	TAGsn3 (202) (248)	TAGsn1 only (249)	TAG sn-1(3) and 2 (250,226)	TAGsn1 > sn3 (251) sn1 of PL (234)	Not distinguished for TAG (206)	TAGsn1(3) > sn2 (207)
Activity modifying proteins	Apolipoprotein CII (194–196) Hen's egg activator proteins (252,253)	None known (202)	Colipase (254)	None known (204)	Contradictory reports viz. C apo-proteins (255,256) AI and AII (256,257)	None known (206)	Activation by cAMP dependent protein kinase phosphorylation (207)
Effect of NaCl (1M)	inhibition (258,259,260)	–	–	–	Slight inhibition (229,261,230)	–	–

Product inhibition *in vitro*	Highly sensitive to FFA (262) and MAG (263)	Sensitive to FFA (202)	—	—	—	—	Sensitive to FFA (207)
Inhibitory modifiers	DFP (173) PMSF (173) BNPC (190) DNPP (12) Boronic acid (264) Benzene boronoic acid (265)	—	DNPP (266) DEPC (267) boronic acid (270)	DFP (268) PMSF (268)	Boroxic acid (205) Benzene boronic acid (205)	DFP (no effect) (269) MM (206) iodoacetate (206) PCMB (206)	DFP (240) $HgCl_2$ (240) NaF (240) MM, PCMB dithiopyridine (207)
Active site residues	His (12) Ser (12)	—	His (270) Ser (for substrate absorption) (203)	Ser (268)	Ser (205) His (205)	Cys (206)	Ser (207) Cys (207)
Suggested reaction mechanism	serine-esterase nucleophilic catalysis; acyl enzyme intermediate (12)	—	esterolytic-cleavage: acyl enzyme intermediate (203)	serine-esterase acyl enzyme intermediate (204,268)	—	—	serine-esterase; acyl enzyme intermediate (207)
Stabilizers of activity	detergents (271) glycerol (177)	Stable	Stable	Stable	detergents (205)	—	detergents, glycerol, EDTA,-SH group protectors (272)
Specific activity (μmol/mg/h [highest])	42,000 (183)		5000 (273)	4800 (204)	45000 (274)	60–160 (276)	12000 (272)
Tissue activity (μmol/g/h)	2–6300 dependent on source (30)	c40/ml of gastric aspirate (202)	18,000–78,000 dependent on species. (203,204)	c100 (204)	(see 275)	0.02 (206)	40 (272)

Abbreviations: TAG, triacylglycerol; DAG, diacylglycerol; MAG, monoacylglycerol; PC, phosphatidylcholine; PE, phosphatidyethanolamine; CE, cholesterylester; PL, phospholipid; DFP, di-isopropylfluorophosphate; PMSF, phenylmethanesulforylfluoride; BNPC, n-butyl (p-nitrophenyl) carbamide; DNPP, diethy-p-nitrophenylphosphate; DFPC, diethylpyrocarbonate; MM, methylmaleimide; PCMP, p-chloromercuribenzoate; His, histidine; Ser, serine; Cys, cysteine.

at the level of changes in the physical state of the enzyme molecule (259,260). Although many studies have sought to distinguish LPL from, for example, hepatic endothelial triglyceride lipase on the basis of sensitivity to salt inhibition, because the effect of the salt varies with the other compositional details of the assay systems, this criterion cannot be considered a satisfactory basis for making identifications (see 278). From the foregoing, it is clear that when comparisons involving tissue LPL activities are to be made, the nature and comparability of the activity assays employed in different studies is of the upmost importance. Various methods of assay for lipoprotein lipase activity have been developed and used (see also Chapter 3). Generally, they fall into four main groups: 1) Assays which use the physiological lipoprotein triglyceride substrate, present in the form of either chylomicrons or very low density lipoproteins, and which rely upon the measurement of fatty acid or glycerol release by titration or chemical means (279). 2) Assays as in group 1, but in which commercial artificial triglyceride emulsions (e.g. Intralipid) are used (280). 3) Assays like those in group 1, but where the fatty acids are determined enzymatically (281) using either spectrophotometric (282) or fluorometric methods (283). 4) Where radioactive triglyceride, labelled in either the fatty acid or glycerol moiety, has been incorporated into an emulsion and used as substrate, the release of radioactive fatty acid or glycerol then being measured (280, 284–286).

Almost invariably, the originators of each type of assay system go to considerable lengths to validate the procedure in relation to certain criteria characteristic of LPL activity. However, very few comparative studies on the simultaneous assay of the enzyme using a variety of procedures exist. At best, the comparative needs of assays for LPL and hepatic endothelial lipase are usually addressed (287–290).

Although some studies have considered aspects of such a comparison of assay methods (291) and revealed the importance, for example, of the purity of the triglyceride used and the repeated daily preparation of fresh emulsions, the study undertaken by Riley and Robinson (280) some twelve years ago remains the only major comparative study of LPL assay methods. These authors compared each of the procedures with the outcome obtained when chylomicrons were employed as the substrate particle. Primarily it was found that, with a variety of enzyme sources, the absolute activities and the characteristics of the activity were virtually identical when either chylomicrons or Intralipid (a commercial triglyceride emulsion stabilized with phospholipids) were used. By contrast, the use of emulsions prepared with radiolabelled triglyceride and stabilized with phospholipid produced activity measurements which, although similar in pattern when different enzyme sources were studied, were significantly lower, in absolute terms, than those seen with either chylomicrons or Intralipid. Furthermore, the effects of salt inhibition were less clear cut with such radioactive substrate mixtures. These observations were confirmed when other stabilizing agents were used during the preparation of the substrate emulsions. Clearly, in that we have drawn similar conclusions from our own comparative study of a selection of assays (Jones, Casey and Cryer, unpublished observations) these observations, although not detracting from the internal consistency of particular studies, do not make the task of comparing data between laboratories any easier. Although it is highly unlikely that a universally accepted standard assay format for the measurement of LPL activity could be agreed upon, it would seem sensible that the validation of each assay method used should include, in addition to the accepted criteria, a comparison between the absolute values obtained, under a variety of conditions, with the substrate in question and the physiological substrate derived from the species under study.

Apart from the variability inherent between various assay formats, a further difficulty is encountered when different studies are compared. Namely, the nature of the preparation in which the activity is measured. As far as postheparin lipolytic activity in serum is concerned, this is a composite activity of enzymes derived from both hepatic and extrahepatic sources (30,264), and the problem is not one of the form in which the activity is presented, but in selectively determining the proportion of the activity which is identifiable by its susceptibility to the action of apo-CII (194), or by its specific immunoreactivity (292). With tissue samples, however, a number of procedures have been used to produce preparations which can be processed quantitatively and which are free of interfering lipase activities. Most common among the procedures have been the use of heparin-containing media to extract the enzyme from fresh tissue into solution, the use of whole homogenates, and the use of homogenates of acetone-diethyl ether dried tissue samples. In our own study (293), these latter two preparations were compared directly, and acetone-diethyl ether dried powders clearly yielded much higher activities on assay than did fresh tissue. This is not surprising for a number of reasons not least of which is that virtually all the intracellular LPL activity is entrapped in membrane vesicles following tissue disruption (112,142,176). Furthermore, whereas the identity of the activity was readily demonstrated with acetone-diethyl ether dried preparations in all cases, this was not so with fresh tissue homogenates. Problems also exist with the use of heparin eluates of tissue in that not only does soluble LPL exhibit a considerable instability under such conditions, but also the proportion of activity eluting from different tissue samples under the conditions used is rarely if ever assessed.

Despite these methodological problems, it is still possible and useful to adduce comparative information relating to the functional significance of tissue LPL activity and its response to stressors in different species and cell types. A detailed consideration of such information makes up the remainder of this review.

Functional Significance of Lipoprotein Lipase Activity in Tissues and Cells

Clearly, the presence of functionally active LPL in the tissues of animals must be considered essential to the harvesting of plasma triglyceride fatty acids and their uptake into peripheral tissues. Although hitherto much of the evidence in favor of this relationship has been circumstantial (197,279), direct evidence has been forthcoming more recently from both clinical and laboratory studies. Clinical studies have revealed that familial Type I primary hyperlipoproteinemia (294), which is characterized by hyperchylomicronemia, is associated with a reduced or absent postheparin lipolytic activity response and usually an absence of enzyme activity in adipose tissue biopsy samples. A similar hypertriglyceridemia may also be seen in patients where tissue enzyme activity is normal, but where there is a lack of apolipoprotein CII for enzyme activation (295–297). LPL deficiency *per se* has also been demonstrated in experimental animals, where it produces equally dramatic consequences (39). In mice for example, a so-called combined lipase deficiency (cld) occurs which is carried as a recessive mutation within the T/t complex of chromosome 17(39). Mice homozygous for this defect display severe functional deficiencies of LPL and the related hepatic endothelial triglyceride lipase. They develop massive hyperchylomicronemia and die within 3 days if they are allowed to suckle. Recent elegant studies have revealed that the tissues of cld/cld mice do in fact synthesize a LPL-like molecule, but that it has a severely subnormal catalytic activity (298). In addition to the evidence that can be adduced from the study of such deficiency conditions, direct evidence for the role of LPL in the removal of plasma triglycerides has come from experiments *in vivo* in which animals have been treated with anti-LPL serum. Thus, for example, when LPL activity was blocked immunochemically in roosters, there was a consequential dramatic increase in plasma very low density lipoproteins (60) with a decrease in plasma low density lipoproteins (299). Such evidence, together with other related studies of lipoprotein metabolism (300), implicates LPL specifically in the transformation of very low to low density lipoproteins with the concomitant removal of plasma triglycerides, and reemphasizes the endothelial localization of this structural activity (301).

With regard to the foregoing, the highly pertinent comments of Vernon and Clegg (197) are of particular significance. They point out that "while demonstrating the involvement of LPL in whole animal lipid metabolism, such experiments *in vivo* do not indicate the quantitative contribution made by the enzyme to plasma triglyceride turnover in different tissues and different locations." These authors reanalyzed available data (34,302–309) and attempted to reconcile measured rates of tissue triglyceride uptake *in vivo* with the measured activities of LPL. Their conclusions, which are generally supported by other available evidence, include the following (197): 1) The total tissue and particularly the extracellular component of total tissue LPL activity in all cases exceeds the rate of fatty acid uptake into tissues, whether this latter is measured *in vivo* or *in vitro.* 2) From the evidence arising from work in Scow's laboratory (e.g. 310,311), it is clear that only a proportion of the fatty acids released by the action of tissue LPL activity is taken up directly by the tissue in question. Indeed, in perfused organ studies, up to

45% of the triglyceride hydrolysis products appeared in the perfusate (309,310). 3) It is clear that *in vitro* and probably *in vivo* also, very low density lipoprotein triglyceride and chylomicron triglyceride are equally good as substrates for LPL and, in the fed animal at least, the enzyme activity present in, for example, adipose tissue is not saturated with its substrate and therefore not working at its maximal velocity. Thus lipoprotein triglyceride uptake rates in tissues will not only be modified by the amount of LPL activity present, as reviewed repeatedly (e.g. 312), but also by alterations in the concentration of substrate delivered to the tissue enzyme by the circulation. However, in most studies (including those on humans), the fractional removal rate from plasma of triglyceride-rich lipoproteins is correlated positively with the amount of available LPL activity (313) with saturation of the common mechanism only occurring under pathological conditions of hypertriglyceridemia (314).

Despite the obvious importance of lipoprotein triglyceride fatty acids in overall energy metabolism, studies on their contribution to the energy economy of the whole body or individual tissues *in vivo* are limited. These limitations are generally attributable to methodological difficulties and to the problem of distinguishing between the fates of albumin-bound nonesterified fatty acids and fatty acids derived from circulating triglyceride by the action of LPL. Clearly, the contribution of triglyceride-derived fatty acids is a potentially significant part of total fat oxidation in that in many studies (e.g. 315), only about one-third of the total rate of fat oxidation (as determined by indirect calorimetry) can be accounted for when labelled fatty acids are used to measure the rate of plasma non-esterified fatty acid utilization (oxidation). The distinction between the oxidation of triglyceride-derived fatty acids and plasma (albumin bound) non-esterified fatty acids is an important consideration when interpreting the potential significance of the relative changes in LPL activity that occur in different tissues under varying physiological conditions (see later also). These problems have been addressed recently in a study by Wolfe and Durkot (316). They considered the possibility that if the main route of very low density lipoprotein-fatty acid oxidation was through entry into the plasma non-esterified fatty acid pool, then changes in LPL activity in individual tissues would be of much less importance in determining the nature of substrate oxidation in that tissue than if the very low density lipoprotein fatty acids were taken up directly and oxidized in the tissues in which the enzyme acted. From their study, carried out in the rat, it was concluded that the direct oxidation of fatty acids in very low density lipoproteins played an important role in the energy metabolism of the rat, accounting for a percentage of the total CO_2 production (approximately 16%) that was equal to the amount that arose from the oxidation of plasma non-esterified fatty acids. Most significantly, in the present context, it was also clear that the oxidation of very low density lipoprotein-derived fatty acids did not involve their prior entry into the plasma non-esterified fatty acid pool. This not only substantiates the importance of plasma triglyceride dynamics, but adds weight to the previous suggestions that the complementary and reciprocal LPL activity changes that occur in different tissues gives the enzyme an important directive role with regard to the tissue fates of circulating triglycerides (312,317).

The major fate of triglyceride fatty acids taken up by a number of tissues (e.g. cardiac muscle, skeletal muscle and diaphragm), as intimated above, is their direct oxidation, the rate of which may in turn be correlated with uptake rates and LPL activities determined *in vitro* (e.g. 32,318). Of the other tissues that contain a functional LPL, a function for the triglyceride fatty acids that are made available through its action, has been documented in a number of cases. For example, in the case of adipose tissue the major fate of the triglyceride fatty acids that are taken up, is intracellular storage as triglyceride in adipocytes (154,317). In the lactating mammary gland, their major fate appears to be incorporation into secreted milk lipids (319) with which the enzyme seems to be found fortuitously in whole milk (70–74, 278) where it exerts little or no action. In the lung, in addition to their oxidation, triglyceride fatty acids taken up through the action of LPL also provide part of the fatty acid requirement for surfactant production (33,320,321). With regard to the macrophage, a considerable proportion of both lung and arterial LPL activity probably resides in this cell type, where it has been suggested to function in a number of ways. It may be involved in the energy metabolism of the cell (128); it may function as a part of the cells scavenging role (128); or the enzyme may be one of the facets of the macrophages' roles as a secretory cell (130,322). The second two functions would be consistent with the suggested role of the macrophage in atherogenesis (323), where it might contribute to the formation of atherogenic triglyceride-rich lipoprotein remnants at or near the endothelium (324).

Comparative Aspects of Lipoprotein Lipase Activity Changes

In the following section, aspects of the changes in LPL activity that occur in response to specific stimuli are considered. However, because most experimental studies concentrate on the use of a small range of experimental animal species, before considering the details of such responses it is appropriate to consider whether all species are likely to modulate their LPL systems in a similar fashion. Although many studies on individual species of varying types exist (21,22,26,31,41,43–46,52,55,58,59,63,66,67), for the reasons mentioned above direct comparisons between such studies are generally dangerous. Very few studies exist in which comparisons on the basis of species differences have been addressed directly, and only limited responses have been studied (30). However, from the data that is available, in mammals at least, the concerted changes in tissue LPL activities that occur in response to, for example 24 hour starvation, are very similar, although it must be stressed that a far from complete picture exists. The general pattern is similar when avian species are considered, except that the overall differences that are observed between the specific physiological states are smaller in magnitude than those seen for mammals (see also 63,66).

Lipoprotein Lipase Activity Changes in Response to Physiological Stimuli

Gender

Specific studies on the effects of gender on the LPL system are relatively few in number. It is quite clear, however, that the rate of very low density lipoprotein triglyceride clearance is greater in the female rat than in the male (302); the $t^{1/2}$ for removal being 30 and 44 minutes respectively. In humans, this general situation also pertains and may be related to the higher activities of LPL seen in the (consequentially?) larger adipocytes found in the adipose tissue of women (303). Clearly, it is oversimplistic to equate the differences in plasma triglyceride turnover mentioned above with measurements of total tissue LPL activity, not least of all because of uncertainties surrounding the distribution of functional activity within tissues *in vivo*, and the contribution made by various tissues to plasma substrate removal (see 197 for review). Furthermore, only limited data exists in which the tissues of males and females have been compared directly. In our own study (30 and unpublished observations) for adipose tissue sites in mouse and hamster, the enzyme activities of females were consistently elevated over those of matched males. This was certainly not the case in rats, where the situation was reversed. In the muscular tissues of animals of each of the three species, gender did not have an effect on the LPL activity present, although activities in lung tissue were consistently higher in females. In the avian species studied in this work, no gender-related differences were discerned in any of the tissues examined. Clearly, the differences that have been noted are relatively insignificant, particularly when compared to those induced by other physiological variables. The gender of animals studied will, therefore, not be considered further in this chapter.

Age

A number of observations have indicated that the rate of plasma lipoprotein triglyceride removal from chylomicrons and very low density lipoproteins in both aged humans (325–327) and rats (328,329) is depressed. Consideration has, from time to time, been given to whether this relates to any overall changes in tissue LPL activities. Although total postheparin lipolytic activity has been demonstrated to decline significantly with age in humans (330), it is not known whether such a difference is due to a decrease in released tissue LPL, or hepatic triglyceride lipase activities, or both. Although a number of studies on rats have looked at tissue LPL activity over adult life, few can be said to have studied any animal beyond what might be termed "middle-to late-middle age". In general, no changes in either adipose or muscular enzyme activity (331,332), or that found in the aorta

(333) are manifest with increasing age (up to the limit mentioned) with diet (see later) being a more important determinant of activity (332). This also seems to be the case for hepatic triglyceride lipase activity (332). However, a fully controlled study extending into true old age, with particular attention to the different adiposal and other tissue sites, remains to be reported.

Development

The ontogeny of the LPL system in a variety of experimental situations has been the subject of considerable interest, particularly as it relates to the development of various tissues and to the effects of neonatal nutrition on the efficiency of metabolic control later in life. Although this area has been the subject of previous review (33,154), it deserves further consideration in the context of this comparative overview.

The main sources of calorie provision change markedly both at birth and at weaning. At birth, the transition in most species is from primarily carbohydrate and fatty acids to predominantly triglyceride. At weaning, this is replaced by an adult diet of variable composition.

With regard to the accretion of lipids from the plasma, it is now generally accepted that in a wide range of suckling animals, the main source of energy is fat derived from maternal milk. In the rat, for example, 70% of all its metabolic energy is derived from milk lipids (334). Of these milk lipids, 97% are triglycerides, 65% of which contain long rather than medium chain fatty acids (335). Whereas the medium chain fatty acids find their preferential utilization by the liver (e.g. 336), the long-chain fatty acids contained in triglycerides will be directed towards the extrahepatic tissues. Thus, by controlling the supply of long-chain fatty acids at the tissue level, LPL must be assumed to have an important function in the growth and maturation of individual organs. With regard to the circulating substrate for LPL in neonates, the rat is the most closely studied species, although some studies of human neonates have appeared (337). In rats, serum triglyceride concentrations increase within hours of birth, remain high in the neonate, increase progressively through suckling, and then fall to reach adult levels after weaning (338). The nature of the lipoprotein carriers of serum triglycerides has been determined in this species (339), and it has been shown that even at the earliest post-natal stages, the triglyceride in the plasma is able to act as a substrate for LPL since adequate levels of apolipoprotein CII are present (340).

Studies on the development of LPL activities in tissues indicate that they are regulated by local factors, and the enzyme behaves characteristically in each tissue. Before consideration of any of these tissue specific changes, it is relevant to ask what is the relative importance of the groups of tissues containing LPL in the removal of serum triglycerides during development? This question was addressed in the rat by De Gasquet and his colleagues (341). They concluded from their study that in the adult, the main contributor to total body LPL activity (and plasma triglyceride removal) was white adipose tissue in fed rats and muscle in fasted rats. In suckling pups, however, regardless of the nutritional state, muscle enzyme contributed 63–85% of the total and white adipose tissue less than 25%. Furthermore, they adduced from this that the clearing of circulating triglyceride-rich lipoproteins during suckling largely depended on muscle LPL. Of the other tissues contributing to total LPL activity, these authors indicated that between birth and weaning brown adipose tissue contributes between 10 and 15% of the whole, but that after weaning this fell to relatively low levels (1–2%). The lungs and kidney represented approximately 3–7%.

Using the rat as a model and taking the muscular tissues first, the activity of cardiac muscle LPL is very low in the fetus (341,342,89), but rises to adult levels during suckling. This pattern reflects the overall cellular development of the heart that takes place (343) and the progressive increase in long chain fatty acid oxidation by the heart over this period. It has been suggested that "association of the increase in the capacity for palmitate oxidation with the postnatal emergence of LPL in heart muscle is plausible", and that increased oxidative capacity is also related to cardiac mitochondrial maturation (344). The low activity of LPL present in fetal skeletal muscle emerges to a relatively high neonatal level within hours of birth (89,341). This peak of activity is followed by a further peak in the early—to mid-suckling period. These increases provide the necessary fuel for the increase in the capacity for fatty acid oxidation that occurs in skeletal muscle during the neonatal period (344). The high capacity for triglyceride hydrolysis by the muscle mass of suckling rats may contribute significantly to the high free fatty acid concentrations present in the plasma at this stage of development (341). As illustrated by Scow and colleagues, up to 40% of triglyceride fatty acid liberated by LPL action at the endothelium may enter the plasma rather than the tissues and thus become available for utilization elsewhere (311).

The changes that occur in the total activity of LPL in white adipose tissue from various sites during development has received considerable attention (146 for review). However, because in many situations the reports have been inconsistent, it has been difficult to make comparisons. Certain consistent threads may nevertheless, be identified. In many species, the fatty acids derived from plasma lipoprotein triglyceride are the predominant source of fatty-acyl components present in the stored lipid of adipocytes (345), with fatty acid synthesis *de novo* generally making a relatively minor contribution (346). Despite this generalization, white adipose tissue can have an important role in the synthesis of long-chain fatty acids in some species. Pigs (347), sheep (348), and cattle (349) for example, synthesize most of their fatty acids in adipose tissue. This situation may be contrasted with that of the mouse (350) and rat (351) where both liver and white adipose tissue are involved; and with the chick (352), pigeon (353) and human (354), where fatty acid synthesis is almost exclusively a hepatic function. Although as intimated previously, the total activity of tissue LPL may not relate directly to triglyceride fatty acid uptake capacity into adipose tissue cells under all conditions, heparin-induced release rates for the enzyme *in vivo* have been suggested as an alternative (355), and under most conditions, where useful comparisons can be made, the correlation between the two variables holds (317).

In the rat, the pattern of change in adipose tissue LPL activity is remarkably similar when anatomically-distinct depots are compared. In general, the small amounts of immature triglyceride-poor white adipose tissue present at birth contains significant levels of LPL activity (356,357). During the first 6 hours of life, however, a time when no accumulation of triglyceride occurs in the tissue, the enzyme activity declines significantly in a response that is probably related to a fall in plasma insulin levels within the first 6 hours of birth (358,359). During the 6–24 hour period of postnatal life, both the LPL and triglyceride content of the tissue increases substantially. This increase is sustained progressively over the first 10 days of life such that levels of activity 2–4 times greater than adult levels are achieved by mid-suckling. Following the 10th day of life, the enzyme activity in all depots falls progressively over the remainder of the suckling period, reaching minimum levels on day twenty. Thereafter, the activities rise again and remain relatively high for the period up to about 8–10 weeks of age after which they decline to the relatively constant adult level by the 20th week of life. It is clear that in the first 10 days of life, the relatively small increases that occur in adipose tissue mass occur substantially as a result of active cellular hyperplasia, together with a modest increase in the size of recognizable fat cells (338,360). Thus, although the changes in LPL activity per recognizable adipocyte correlate with the rate of lipid accretion by the tissue over this period, it is clear that a proportion of the total tissue activity is dependent upon the emergence of the enzyme in predetermined, but hitherto undifferentiated adipocytes present in the tissue (147,361,362) (see later also). The decline in adipose LPL activities during the second half of suckling are less easily related to the aspects of cellularity and lipid accretion mentioned above. In the first case, the total lipid content of most depots continue to increase over this period (338). Pad growth also continues (338,341) as does adipocyte size, although adipocyte numbers do not alter substantially (338). A number of possible explanations for this may be advanced. The high lipogenic capacity of late suckling adipose tissue, together with a low rate of intracellular triglyceride turnover in adipocytes, coupled with the high levels of serum free fatty acids generated by the high capacity of the muscle LPL system at this time, may all combine to maintain the rate of storage of caloric excess in adipose tissue. During this time, the low adipose and high muscular LPL activity serve to direct the high level of dietary-derived triglyceride to tissues where high rates of oxidative metabolism must be fueled by lipid. Following weaning in the rat, average adipocyte size increases substantially in a fashion which is related to the activity of LPL expressed on a per cell basis (362). Thus "lipid-filling" of differentiated adipocytes again seems related to the activity of this enzyme.

The effect of litter size on the developmental changes in adipose tissue LPL activity has been studied in the rat (338,360). From such studies, it was clear that the enzyme activity in all white adipose depots, when studied from weaning to one year of age, were unaltered by variations in litter size. However, LPL activities per 10^6 cells were higher in males reared in small litters compared with those reared in large litters. Interestingly, this difference was not exhibited in females. The persistent hyperinsulinemia of animals reared in small litters may contribute to these differences as intimated from these studies (see later).

When other species are considered, the sparce data available appears to indicate a somewhat more complex picture. For example, during growth and dietary manipulation in ruminants, LPL activity in different adipose depots seems to behave differently. In the early postnatal development of ruminants, the growth of adipose tissue is due to both cellular hypertrophy and hyperplasia (363). Although adipocyte hypertrophy is the major mechanism in the fattening of ruminants grown to market weight, evidence is accumulating that preadipose cells can proliferate postnatally, even in mature animals (152,364). The relation of adipocyte hypertrophy and LPL activity in ruminants has received a certain amount of attention. For example, it was found (365) that in developing sheep the deposition of exogenous fat in the different adipose depots correlated closely and positively with the changes in LPL activity that occurred. Furthermore, the close relationships between feed-type, genetic background, and depot site on lipid accretion and LPL activity in the bovine have also been reviewed (363). In pigs, the available data suggests that LPL activity in adipose tissues is relatively high at birth and increases dramatically during the early neonatal (suckling) period (366) when lipogenesis *de novo* is low in the tissue but lipid accumulation is rapid. The relationship between LPL activity and lipid accumulation is close in this species as well and is maintained throughout the important period of fattening.

Of the tissues remaining in which the ontogeny of LPL has been studied, particularly in the rat, brown adipose tissue is of significant developmental importance. Its importance as a thermogenic organ, particularly in the early part of life has been demonstrated clearly and reviewed fully elsewhere (367,368). The normal fuel for thermogenesis is free fatty acid derived from stored triglyceride. It has been suggested that plasma free fatty acids do not serve as a substrate for thermogenesis (369), and that the rate of fatty acid synthesis in brown adipose tissue is low in suckling (370) and only becomes significant following weaning (371). From these observations, it seems reasonable to suggest that plasma lipids derived from mother's milk must be the source of thermogenic fuel during suckling. Consistent with these observations is the high level of LPL activity present in the brown adipose tissue of suckling rats (89). The activity in brown adipose tissue exhibits two peaks of activity at 2 and 12 days of age with a fall to relatively low levels by weaning. The high total and heparin-releasable (90) LPL activity present in the tissue during suckling may therefore provide a mechanism whereby, because of the tissue enzymes' significant (10–15%) contribution to whole body LPL activity, a preferential utilization of circulating triglyceride fatty acid either as oxidizable fuel for thermogenesis, or as a source for the intracellular triglyceride stored by the tissue could be envisaged. Such changes in thermogenic fuel provision may in turn be related tentatively with coincident behavioral changes [eg. exploratory activity which occur at mid-suckling (372)].

Another organ in which LPL appears to have a specific developmental role, is the lung. In the case of the rat lung, LPL activity has been detected up to 5 days before birth. The activity increases markedly during the last few hours *in utero* and during the first day of extrauterine life (89,341,373–375). The enzyme activity is thus elevated during the period of lung development when rapid rates of pulmonary surfactant synthesis occur (376). It has been suggested that this increased perinatal pulmonary LPL activity may provide a source of diglyceride for the dipalmitylphosphatidylcholine production necessary for pulmonary surfactant formation (89,377). If this is the case, it is clear that even before birth the very low density lipoprotein triglyceride present in the fetal rat circulation (378), in addition to free fatty acids, could be utilized for prenatal surfactant synthesis. It is also tempting to speculate that a relationship exists between the precocious increase in LPL activity produced by the administration of dexamethasone *in utero* (379) and the morphological and functional changes induced in the lung by the same stimulus. Such changes include the enhanced differentiation of type II pneumocytes, enhanced pulmonary function, and an increase in the levels of total and disaturated phosphatidylcholine in the fetal lungs and alveolar spaces of a number of species (380).

Two other organs deserve attention here in that they are normally regarded as having little or no LPL activity in the adult, but do express the activity at specific developmental stages. It has been suggested that LPL may play a special role during the development of the brain (97–99). Such a suggestion, based on studies in the rat, derives from the observation that LPL activity is low or absent in the brain except during the first ten days of extrauterine life, during which time there is a dramatic increase in brain weight and cholesterol content (381). This, together with other enzymic changes (382), has led to the view that the provision of fatty acids for brain phospholipid production may, at this stage of development, be dependent on an active LPL system in this organ.

The presence of LPL in fetal and newborn liver has also been demonstrated (95,96) and here too the activity is not expressed in adults. However, a convincing suggestion as to the specific functional role for this activity in animals at this stage of development has not, as yet, been advanced.

Most of the work on the development of the LPL system in humans has been confined to observations on the efficiency of plasma lipid clearance since, although some observations on postheparin lipolytic activities have been made (383), individual tissue activities are not available. In the case of premature infants of gestational ages less than 32 weeks, the efficiency of lipid clearance is less than for their more mature counterparts (384–386). For the human, the suggestion has been made (387), on the basis of the similarity as regards impaired triglyceride clearance between premature, small-for-gestational-age, and marasmic individuals (385,388–389), that a critical mass of adipose tissue is probably necessary for the normal development of the metabolism of circulating triglycerides.

Diurnal and other cyclical biorhythms

During the diurnal cycle in many species, feeding is intermittent. This is reflected in predictable and cyclical changes in hormonal status (see later). In rats, for example, where feeding is a nocturnal activity, changes in plasma insulin concentrations tend to be reflected in changes in adipose tissue LPL activity (390–392). The particular pattern of a mid-afternoon minimum in activity with a maximum approximately 4 hours following the commencement of feeding is particularly noticeable in animals in which daytime nibbling is avoided by adaptation to a strict meal-eating regimen (31,393). Clearly, in the short-term control of triglyceride synthesis and storage in adipose tissue, these changes in LPL are of paramount importance, with the enzymes of intracellular triglyceride synthesis themselves only being subject to intergrative control over the longer-term (394). Such rapid changes in human tissue LPL activities also occur when the diurnal cycle is related to the frequency and composition of meals (22,395).

Although a seasonal variation in the tissue activities of LPL has been suspected for animals (and clearly this may relate to the seasonal deposition of adipose in hibernating or migratory species), it has also been shown that there is a seasonal variation in the activity of human subcutaneous adipose tissue (396).

The cyclical changes in LPL activity that occur in females during the oestrus cycle, pregnancy, and during lactation are considered below.

Hormonal, nutritional and miscellaneous challenges

As indicated many times, the levels of tissue LPL activity change in response to a wide number of stimuli (312). Before considering the various systems in which the effectors mediating such responses have been studied *in vitro*, the changes observed when the intact animals or human has been challenged will be considered here.

Insulin. A considerable body of evidence, both circumstantial and direct, is now available to substantiate the view that insulin is a major physiological regulator of tissue LPL activities. In rats, there is a strong positive correlation between adipose tissue LPL activity and plasma immunoreactive insulin concentration measured under a wide variety of conditions (34), including during the diurnal cycle (391). The activity of the enzyme in adipose tissue is also low in alloxan diabetic animals (397). This deficiency in the adipose tissue activity of diabetic animals can be restored to normal by the administration of insulin (398). Although some studies have indicated that insulin has no effect on the LPL activity of muscle tissue (399), the enzyme has been shown to be depressed in the hearts of rats made diabetic either with alloxan (400) or streptozotocin (401). In both situations, insulin treatment led to a restoration of normal myocardial activities with the effect being dependent on protein synthesis (401). Clearly, in diabetes, such a general lowering in the capacity of peripheral LPL may be considered a likely major factor limiting peripheral very low density lipoprotein uptake (402). However, recent studies have additionally indicated that the very low density lipoprotein isolated from the plasma of diabetic animals (which are relatively apolipoprotein E-deficient) are removed more slowly from the circulation, even when they are administered to normal animals (403). The independent stimulatory effect of insulin on adipose tissue LPL activity has also been demonstrated clearly in humans using a euglycemic clamp technique (404).

Corticosteroids. Under certain conditions the administration of glucocorticoids to rats has been shown to induce an increase in adipose tissue LPL activity (405). However, other studies have not demonstrated such a relationship (406), the nature of which may be dose dependent (407,408). Glucocorticoid administration has also been shown to produce an increase in LPL in lung and muscular tissues (77,399,405,406,409). Although the therapeutic use of corticosteroids in humans has been known for some time to produce hyperlipoproteinemia (410), the mechanism responsible has not been fully elucidated.

Other steroidal hormones. In general, the administration of estrogenic steroids produces a marked reduction in adipose tissue LPL activity in the rat with no effect on skeletal muscle activity (411–415). It has been suggested that a similar decline in tissue enzyme activity may be involved in the decreased rate of triglyceride clearance in humans with high induced concentrations of estrogens (416,417). Additionally, the high LPL activity of adipose tissue in pregnant rats has also been attributed to the low level of plasma estrogens in this species under these conditions (387). Low estrogenic steroid levels in ovariectomised ground squirrels are, however, associated with low adipose tissue LPL activities (48).

Further studies have indicated that dehydroepiandrosterone (DHEA) also has an effect on the LPL system. DHEA causes a weight loss without any effect on food intake, and produces a reduction in adipose tissue LPL in both lean and obese Zucker rats (418). This decline in activity seems to be independently determined in that other hormonal changes were minimal in response to the administration of DHEA. On the other hand, progesterone administration has been shown to increase adipose tissue LPL activity, in a response which is not dependent on changes in food intake (419).

Thyroid hormones. Although certain studies have indicated that animals rendered hyperthyroid by feeding diets containing iodinated casein have elevated cardiac LPL activities (420), others have indicated a similar response in hypothryoid (421) animals. In the latter study, the effects of hypothyroidism appear to be at least partly distinct from the induced effects on food intake that occur under those conditions. Where it has been studied, the increase was suggested to be due to a reduced rate of enzyme degradation both intra- and extra-cellularly (421). Similarly, adipose tissue LPL activities have been shown to be elevated in hypothyroid (421) and thyroidectomized (422) rats, as have postheparin LPL levels (422). In contrast, hypothyroidism in humans has been shown to be associated with reduced levels of both adipose (423) and skeletal muscle (424) activity, this being in turn associated with a significant hypertriglyceridemia.

Chronic thyroxine treatment of rats has been shown to have no effect on the LPL activity of brown adipose tissue (90).

Catecholamines. Although many studies *in vitro* have implicated catecholamines in the prevention of insulin-induced increases in white adipose tissue LPL activity, few studies have addressed this relationship using observations *in vivo*. Indeed, microsurgical denervation of white adipose tissue in the rat is without effect on LPL activity (425), even though the norepinephrine content of the denervated pad is between 0 and 10% of that seen in the enervated contralateral pad. Species differences may however exist (426) in that although rat white adipocytes have beta-1 receptors on their surfaces, they do not have the alpha-2 receptors, the activation of which inhibits lipolysis, which are well characterized on the adipocytes of other species (eg. man, hamster) (427). Much of the evidence in support of a role for catecholamines in the control of white adipose tissue LPL activity comes from studies *in vitro* and will be considered later as will other agonists operating via cAMP.

As far as the activity in brown adipose tissue is concerned, there seems to be clear evidence of an involvement for norepinephrine. Thus, in addition to the effect norepinephrine has on lipolysis and thermogenesis in brown adipose tissue via a cAMP mediated mechanism (368), administration of the neurohormone to both control (92,392) and cold exposed (36) animals produced an increase in the LPL activity of the tissue. Although other workers have seen a high LPL activity in brown adipose tissue depleted of norepinephrine by reserpine treatment (428), it has been considered feasible (36) that a transient increase in agonist concentration may result from the inhibition by the drug of norepinephrine reuptake, and thereby produce the observed rise in enzyme activity.

In muscular tissues, a stimulatory effect of catecholamines has also been invoked (32) with a particularly noticeable effect on the distribution of the activity between the cardiocyte and endothelial sites (429–432).

Glucagon. Because of the generally reciprocal action of glucagon and insulin on white adipose tissue metabolism, glucagon is generally accepted to have a depressive effect on LPL activity in this tissue (see 312). There are however conflicting reports on the effect of this hormone on, for example, cardiac muscle activity (433,405,434); although as with the catecholamines, this hormone additionally appears to affect the proportion of total tissue activity that is involved in triglyceride fatty acid hydrolysis (435,436).

Growth hormone. Although a small number of studies suggest that growth hormone may affect tissue LPL activities *in vitro* (see later), few controlled studies *in vivo* have been reported. However, it is clear that when growth hormone deficient humans are treated with growth hormone, both postheparin LPL and hepatic triglyceride lipase activities decline (437).

Prolactin. Clearly not only does LPL activity rise in mammary gland following parturition under the influence of prolactin (44,438), but the activity in adipose tissue declines under the same conditions. Thus, the direction of triglyceride fatty acids to adipose in pregnancy is shifted on parturition to the mammary. Some of the consequences in adipose tissue have been described elsewhere (439).

Toxins. Although studied previously in relation to the hypertriglyceridemia associated with endotoxemic shock (440), the LPL activity of tissues has been studied most extensively following treatment with cholera toxin because of the action it has as an irreversible agonist of cyclic AMP. In the two main studies using this agent, generally compatible observations were made. In the study by Knobler et al., (441) the persistent effect of the agent on the activity of adenylate cyclase resulted, at 16 hours after administration, in a large increase in cardiac LPL activity together with significant increases in lung and diaphragm activities which were also reflected in measurable levels of activity being detected in the serum of the treated animals. Simultaneously, the activity present in white adipose tissue fell to one third of the control level. The effect of cholera toxin on the heart LPL activity was maximal at 8 hours following its administration and persisted for 24 hours, with the increase in intracellular cAMP concentration being maximal at 1 hour with a return to basal levels over a 16 hour period. It was also quite clearly shown in this study that the nutritional status of the animals studied did not have any effect on these cholera toxin-induced changes previously noted. In the other, more recent, study (406), cholera toxin was shown to increase muscular LPL activity while causing a decline in the adipose tissue activity and the activity of the hepatic endothelial triglyceride lipase. These changes were accompanied by increases in the plasma concentrations of insulin and corticosterone, but were unaltered when cholera toxin was administered to adrenalectomized animals.

Other effects not directly related to known hormonal or nutritional changes. Before considering in detail the effects of nutritional factors on tissue LPL activities, a number of other known effectors of this parameter might be mentioned. First, certain drug treatments are known to affect the activity, for example, clofibrate is known to decrease white adipose tissue LPL activity and increase that in cardiac tissue. The net effect being no change in postheparin LPL activity which leads to the conclusion that the hypotriglyceridemic effect of the drug is not due to an enhanced rate of extrahepatic lipoprotein triglyceride removal (442). Second, one of the consequences of whole-body irradiation appears to be to induce a deficiency in extrahepatic LPL and a consequential dyslipoproteienaemia (443). Third, infections of hamsters with the tapeworm, *Spirometra mansonoides*, produce an increase in adipose tissue LPL activity (444) which is associated with the chronic insulin-like effects of infection on metabolism. The hypertriglyceridemia associated with infections of *Trypanosoma brucei* and *plasmodium berghei* may alternatively be associated with the suppression of adipose LPL by a factor released specifically from peritoneal exudate cells under the influence of the hepatoprotozoans (445). It is not known whether such a factor is similar to cachectin, a hormone known to suppress LPL activity in adipose and which is secreted by endotoxin-induced RAW 264.7 cells in culture (138,446).

Nutritional and dietary effectors. Although the changes in LPL activities that occur during the feeding-starvation-refeeding cycle are governed by the hormonal changes that accompany such cycles, the nature and composition of the diet also has significant effects on the activity of the enzyme in tissues. The tissues studied most extensively in both animals and humans in this regard are white adipose tissue and skeletal muscle. In the fed state, a large proportion of the triglyceride fatty acids removed from the plasma are taken up by adipose tissue. The activity of LPL under these conditions, in white adipose tissue is high after feeding and conversely is low during fasting. Skeletal muscle is also quantitatively important in plasma triglyceride fatty acid removal under a variety of conditions (447,448). Here, the fatty acids acquired are especially important as a fuel source in muscle masses containing a large proportion of slow twitch, red fibres. In fact, LPL activity is much higher in red than in white skeletal muscle (399,449) and is also more responsive in terms of activity increase during fasting.

The acute and more chronic effects of dietary composition on these situations have been studied in both man (450) and experimental animals. In man, the refeeding of carbohydrate to the fasting individual results in a rapid (within 2 hours) increase in adipose tissue LPL activity which is not seen when an equicaloric amount of fat is given (395). In experimental animals, this rapid effect of carbohydrate is also manifested as a precipitous decline in cardiac LPL activities (451). The feeding of fat to the rat produces an increase in the heparin-releasable fraction of cardiac LPL activity which is exaggerated if glucose is given prior to the fat load (409). This fat-induced increase is absent in adrenalectomized rats but is mimicked by corticosteroid replacement, which suggests the possible pathway of hormonal mediation for the fat feeding effect.

Following a fast, the effects of refeeding on tissue LPL activity may be prolonged. At least one study has indicated that in rats, following a 3 day fast, refeeding *ad libitum* produced normal adipose tissue LPL activities within 3 days. However, these activities overshoot normal fed values to become elevated by 100% at 10 days following the initial refeeding (452). It was not until 20 days had elapsed that normal (fed) adipose tissue LPL activities were regained. Two further points of interest emerged from this study. First, in animals that were fed *ad libitum*, the adipose LPL activity returned to normal over the same time course as fat cell size was regained and in which refeeding-induced adaptive hyperlipogenesis in adipose and liver has been observed (453). Second, restriction in the amount of food allowed on refeeding prevented the LPL activity overshoot.

With persistent changes in dietary composition, not only does the rate of triglyceride-rich lipoprotein removal from the plasma alter (eg. 454,455), but the tissue levels of LPL activity also change significantly. For example, when rats have been fed diets high in either carbohydrate or fat, the effects on adipose and muscle LPL are consistent with their having significant effects on the kinetics of plasma triglyceride removal (456). Thus in carbohydrate fed animals, relative to normal controls studied in the same nutritional state, adipose tissue enzyme activity was elevated, whereas, that in skeletal and cardiac muscle was low. In fat-fed rats, the LPL activity of adipose tissue was elevated somewhat but was particularly high in the muscular tissues studied. This differential response in the tissues has also been observed in humans (457) where carbohydrate rich diets depress skeletal muscle LPL activity while a fat and protein enriched diet increase it. It is of interest in this context that in a number of situations in which human skeletal muscle glycogen reserves are depleted, the LPL activity of the tissue is enhanced (457–459).

Attempts have been made to establish the factors involved in the response of tissue LPL activities to fat feeding. Specifically, it has been suggested that gastric inhibitory polypeptide (GIP), the plasma concentration of which increases 4 to 5-fold on fat feeding, may play a role which could involve a direct regulatory effect on enzyme activity (464). It has been suggested (12,465) that other gastrointestinal hormones, released into the circulation following fat feeding (eg. gastrin, secretin, vasoactive intestinal peptide, and pancreozymin), may also be involved in the induced changes in tissue LPL activities.

Other specific changes in diet composition have also been reported. Of these, saturated or unsaturated fatty acids (43,455,460), cholesterol (461), and erucic acid (462,463) have received particular attention-although the significance of the effects of these, and other, dietary components on animals or humans fed on normal balanced diets, is unclear.

The Distribution of Tissue Lipoprotein Lipase Within and Between Cells

Intracellular distribution of LPL

As considered elsewhere, although tissue LPL exerts its physiological function at the capillary endothelium (1) it can also be recovered from adipose tissue and cardiac muscle with isolated adipocytes (101,104) and cardiac muscle cells (110,111,114) respectively. Much evidence also exists (1,312) to indicate that the enzyme present at the endothelium does not originate there (466), but is synthesized and exported by the tissue parenchymal cells. It is of significance, therefore, to investigate the intracellular distribution of the enzyme in order to determine whether this is consistent with it being a secretory/exportable component of such cells. The most useful studies in this regard are those in which isolated parenchymal cells, rather than whole tissue, has been fractionated.

In the case of mature tissue-derived adipocytes, although the relative proportions distributed between the fractions vary from study to study, it is clear that the plasma membrane and microsomal membrane fractions contain the highest enrichments of the enzyme (176,467). The activity present at the plasma membrane, where it is also detectable immunometrically, is fully patent (176) and able to catalyze lipoprotein triglyceride breakdown (106,107) in a manner which is sensitive to modulation by C apoproteins (108). In earlier studies however, a high proportion of the cellular activity was found in the cytosol (467). This location now appears to be artifactual (176) and due to the harsh cell isolation (468) and homogenization procedures used. Indeed, using a particularly well controlled homogenization technique and Ob17 adipocytes grown in culture, no soluble activity has been detected, with the enzyme being exclusively confined within a variety of cell-derived membrane structures (469). Furthermore in the latter study, no patent LPL activity was detected in carefully homogenized cells, which, when subjected to isopycnic centrifugation, revealed that a large proportion of the enzyme was located in the Golgi apparatus. Previous immunofluorescence localization studies (141) with Ob17 cells did, however, indicate that a topographically distinct pool of cell surface enzyme was also a feature of the distribution of LPL in this adipose cell type as well. The intracellular distribution of LPL within membranous structures is of particular significance in adipocytes in that this situation ensures that, unlike hormone-sensitive lipase (470), the enzyme does not come into contact with the intracellular triglyceride present. Clearly, for adipocytes, a secretory fate for LPL is indicated by these intracellular localization studies.

Despite early interest (420,471), only very few studies have appeared on the localization of LPL within, for example, cardiac muscle. However, in a study comparing the distribution of enzyme in fractions obtained from either whole cardiac tissue or cardiac muscle cells derived from it, we (112) showed that, in this cell too, the subcellular localization was consistent with LPL being a secretory product of the cells. Furthermore, evidence was presented (112), indicating that a proportion of cellular activity was present at the plasma membrane in this cell-type also.

In both adipocytes and cardiac muscle cells, comparison of the differences in the enzyme's distribution between subcellular fractions obtained from either fed or starved animals substantiated the proposed secretory fate of the enzyme, and indicated that changes in the rate of flux through the intracellular pools occurred during the starvation/refeeding cycle (176,467).

A further complementary study has appeared, in which the subcellular distribution of LPL among the fractions obtained from lactating rat mammary gland is reported (119). In this case too, although significant levels of soluble cytosolic enzyme were found, substantial proportions of the total activity were found associated with membranous structures having buoyancies and marker enzyme characteristics consistent with their being of plasma membrane and endoplasmic reticulum origin. In a manner consistent with the other tissue cell types studied, the plasma membrane enzyme activity was at least partly derived from cell surface structures characteristic of the secretory mammary epithelial cell type.

Distribution of lipoprotein lipase between cells

From the foregoing, it is clear that because LPL is a secretory product of tissue parenchymal cells and exerts its function at the capillary endothelium, a number of pools of enzyme must exist in tissues. Such pools have been studied in a number of ways and at least three must be distinguished: 1) within cells, 2) extracellular and en route to the endothelium, and 3) bound extracellularly to the endothelial cell surface. This classification does not exclude the possibility of other pools, however.

In simplistic terms, the presence of intracellular enzyme in cells from tissues distinguishes this pool from those that are extracellular (see above). However, more detailed information on distribution is available and particularly the perfused heart *in vitro* has been a useful model in this regard.

Most of the earlier studies using perfused hearts concentrated on distinguishing the proportion of activity that was readily released when heparin was present in the perfusate (presumed to be at or near the endothelial cell surface), and that which was residual in the tissue following heparin treatment, presumed intracellular [eg. 32]. More recent information using this approach has confirmed the precursor-product relationship between the two enzyme pools (472), although some evidence has indicated that the precursor may be a relatively low affinity and less active form of the high affinity, functional endothelial bound form (473). The most sophisticated use of the technique using heparin helped reveal slightly more of the situation. Using a procedure that allowed separate collection of coronary and interstitial effluents from perfused hearts, Jansen and his colleagues (474) were able to show the presence of LPL in postheparin interstitial effluent and in the corresponding coronary effluent. Although the lipolytic activity present in the coronary effluents from the hearts of fasted rats were higher than those for fed rats, the opposite was true in the case of the activity present in the interstitial effluents. Whether the enzyme appears in the interstitial compartment of the heart under normal conditions *in vivo*, when significant concentrations of free heparin are absent (475–478), is unknown. What is more clear is that enzyme present, albeit transiently, at the endothelium is lost from this site at a rapid rate. For example, it has been shown that when hearts have been perfused under constant and controlled conditions for 1 hour at 37°C, their capacity for functional triglyceride removal from either triglyceride emulsions or lymph chylomicrons present in the perfusion medium was lost at a rate of 2% of the original activity/minute (479). Indeed, the presence of serum in the perfusate enhanced this presumed rate of active LPL disappearance. That this loss is associated with a release of LPL into the perfusate in the absence of heparin was illustrated recently by Bagby (480), who showed that over a 60 minute perfusion, rat hearts lost 2.1U/g of active LPL in this way per minute. This continuous release of endothelial LPL into the vascular compartment was compared with the fractional release rate for other intracellular enzymes. It was found that LPL had a fractional release rate of 1.3%/minute, whereas the equivalent parameter for alkaline phosphatase and creatine kinase under the same conditions were 0.002% and 0.03%, respectively. From these data, it was calculated that the endothelial (extracellular) pool of LPL activity had a $t_{1/2}$ of 10 minutes compared with the $t_{1/2}$ of 42 minutes calculated for the intracellular enzyme. From these types of data, we must assume that under most circumstances, the flux of enzyme molecules through the extracellular compartment prior to endothelial surface sequestration must be rapid and of large capacity.

The removal of active enzyme from the vascular compartment by the liver is also very rapid, injected LPL having an initial vascular $t_{1/2}$ of only 1 minute (481,482).

The heparin-independent release of LPL from organs perfused *in vitro* would appear to have a parallel *in vivo* in that low but measurable levels of activity have been found in the plasma of both animals and humans (see 483). In two recent studies (483,484), it has been estimated that the LPL activity in the circulation represents between 0.5 and 1% of the functional pool of enzyme present at the endothelium. The level in the plasma varies with stage of development (483) and nutritional state (484), is elevated by hypertriglyceridemia (483), and the removal of activity from plasma is dependent on hepatic function (483,484).

The Nature of the Endothelial Binding of Lipoprotein Lipase

Clearly, the binding interactions that occur at the endothelium are many and varied (485), and LPL is only one of many physiologically important molecules that have been studied extensively with regard to their interactions with the endothelial cell surface. Other such molecules include thrombin (486,487), plasmin (488), lipoproteins (489–491), glycosaminoglycans (492), and hormones (493). Some of these molecules appear to have specific receptors, while others bind through components of the surface which are multifunctional. LPL appears to fall into the second category. Its binding to the endothelial surface occurs through interaction with the heparan sulphate present which is also involved in a number of the characteristic interactions at this site (494). Evidence for the involvement of endothelial cell surface heparan sulphate in the sequestration of LPL has accumulated over the last decade from observations made both *in vitro* and *in vivo*. Much of this evidence is reviewed elsewhere in this volume and in the related literature (see for example 1,312,495). However, it is worth repeating that direct evidence for the involvement of heparan sulphate in LPL binding has now been acquired by the use of cultured endothelial cells (496,497) or intact endothelium (498) and specific glycosaminoglycan-degrading enzymes.

Qualitatively, it is clear that LPL binds to the endothelium via interaction with cell surface heparan sulphate. The quantitative aspects of this situation are also worthy of consideration. Using monomer molecular weights for LPL, a variety of estimates have been given for the number of enzyme molecules present at the surface of individual endothelial cells. The values calculated from indirect data (490) are in good agreement with those obtained by direct measurement (496,498) with figures in the region of 3×10^6 molecules/cell being quoted. When the numbers of lipase molecules that bind per cell have been compared with the number of chains of heparan sulphate plus heparin-like glycosaminoglycan present, an apparent ratio of 1 enzyme molecule to 4 available glycosaminoglycan chains emerges (498). Recent evidence has suggested, however, that LPL molecules may exist as dimers *in vivo* (170,171,499). It seems more likely then that, from a knowledge of the effective chain length necessary for enzyme dimer to heparin or heparan sulphate binding (Mr 10–17,000) (500), and the known size of endothelial heparan sulphate glycosaminoglycan chains (Mr 26,500 ± 2,500, as core protein associated doublets; H.B. Streeter and F.S. Wusteman; personal communication), that on average 1 in 8 of the carbohydrate chains are in association with LPL dimers. Furthermore, it is probable that the glycosaminoglycan binding site present on each of the monomeric components of the native complex are in association with the same carbohydrate chain (500). It may also be significant that the heparan sulphate chains are clustered on the endothelial surface, since they are anchored through covalent linkage to a core protein. Current evidence would suggest that each proteoglycan molecule may contain up to four glycosaminoglycan chains (501,502). Thus, on average about half of the heparan sulphate proteoglycan molecules at the endothelium would have a LPL dimer associated with them.

Further calculation from such figures suggests that not only does the heparan sulphate-mediated binding of enzyme to the whole endothelium (503) have the capacity to accommodate more than sufficient enzyme to account for observed plasma lipoprotein triglyceride removal rates *in vivo*, but that it is also compatible with the necessary geometry of interaction with substrate molecules that are packaged in supramolecular complexes many times larger than the enzyme itself.

It is generally accepted that the binding of LPL to glycosaminoglycans *in vitro* (504) or endothelial cells *in vitro* (496,498) and *in vivo* (505) does not affect the overall kinetic properties of the enzyme otherwise observed when the enzyme is in solution (495). Particularly, the enzyme is activated by apo CII when bound, although some of the previously reported inhibitory actions of other apo C peptides are not discernable under these conditions (506). Indeed, even immobilization of LPL by covalent linkage to CH-Sepharose using carbodiimide does not compromise its activity or the stimulation of activity produced by apo CII (507). In this situation also, apo CIII does not bind to the enzyme or compete with apo CII for binding.

In addition to any other role in the operation of the LPL system that is served by the endothelial cell, it has been suggested that the cells can enhance the stability of the enzyme *per se*. This action, which is probably mediated through a membrane lipid has not been fully investigated, but it has been suggested that such a stabilization of the enzyme by the cell may help preserve its function *in vivo* (508). That the state of the endothelial membrane may be critical to the function of LPL is also illustrated by the finding that with rat heart endothelium-bound enzyme, the presence of 15-hydroperoxyarachidonic acid reduces the maximum velocity of chylomicron-LPL interaction (509). Such an effect of the peroxide cannot be demonstrated with enzyme in solution, and it is therefore possible that it is the effect of the peroxide on the membrane that leads to a disturbance of the functional activity of the enzyme at the endothelium.

In light of the specific binding that exists between the endothelial cell and LPL, it is of significance to consider what role this cell-type may have to play in the metabolism of the enzyme. This is pertinent not only because the enzyme arises from non-endothelial sources but also because it is clear (as previously described) that a proportion of the bound enzyme is continuously being lost from the cells by release into the circulation (479,480).

Using bovine milk enzyme as the model (see Chapter 2), it has been shown that LPL has a half life of several hours when it is in association with a variety of common cell types including endothelial cells (510). However, there is a dramatic difference in the ratio of binding to degradation when cells that synthesize the enzyme are compared with those (including endothelial cells) that do not (511). Thus, it has been observed that in heart cell and preadipocyte cell cultures, both of which synthesise LPL, the ratio of enzyme catabolized intracellularly to that bound extracellularly was high at all the time points examined. On the other hand, much less of the bound enzyme was taken up and degraded by either fibroblasts or endothelial cells. These data are consistent with the view that, although capable of binding LPL efficiently, endothelial cells catabolize the enzyme slowly, further suggesting that loss into the vascular space may be the most important route of extracellular enzyme disposal. Whether the differences in interiorization and degradation of lipoprotein lipase between adipocytes and endothelial cells is specific for the enzyme is unknown. However, that it might be so is indicated by the observation that adipocytes (512) and endothelial cells (513) both have the capacity for active endocytosis.

Regulation of the Lipoprotein Lipase System

The LPL system is subject to regulation at many levels (312). In order to simplify the overall consideration, only those aspects involving the synthesis, activation, inactivation/degradation, and intra-/intercellular translocation as they relate mainly to the system in adipose and muscle will be addressed here.

The regulation of the synthetic rates of enzymes is one of the important mechanisms for the control of cellular metabolism, and there have been several attempts to explain the relationship between LPL activity and the rate of total protein synthesis. Some studies, for example, have clearly demonstrated a relationship between total protein synthesis and LPL activity in both adipose tissue and heart tissue (514–517). Early studies *in vivo* showed that the injection of protein synthesis inhibitors resulted in a rapid decline in the activity of the enzyme in both adipose tissue [$t\frac{1}{2}$ = 1–2 hours (514)] and heart [$t\frac{1}{2}$ = 1–2 hours (516)] and suggested that the enzyme activity is normally maintained by a balance between rapid rates of synthesis and degradation. Evidence consistent with such a view has also come from studies in which anti-LPL immunoglobulin was used to determine whether the difference in adipose tissue enzyme activity between fed and starved rats is related to the rate of enzyme synthesis and the total amount of enzymes protein present. These studies (518) suggest that the decline in adipose tissue activity of rats fasted for 24 hours when compared with fed rats is due to a decline in the amount of enzyme protein present, presumably due to changes in both enzyme synthetic and degradative rates.

In addition, experiments in which fasted animals were treated with insulin *in vivo* (520) indicated that, in an action which is abolished by the administration of cycloheximide, the increased LPL activity found in adipose tissue following hormone treatment is associated with enhanced enzyme secretion by the adipocyte and subsequent accumulation in the tissue. On the basis of this observation, the adipocyte secretory mechanism may also be implicated as an additional site of LPL regulation in adipose tissue (see later).

As indicated previously, agents which affect intracellular cAMP concentrations *in vivo* (eg. cholera toxin) have also been shown to affect tissue LPL activities in a persistent fashion (441).

Although these and other studies using metabolic inhibitors *in vivo* (519) have provided useful information, the major advancements in the understanding of the regulation of the LPL system have come from studies carried out *in vitro*.

In the case of adipose tissue, studies *in vitro* have used a variety of preparations including isolated fat pads, isolated adipocytes, adipose cells in culture, and cell free preparations.

Taking each type of preparation separately, the first observations of note were those of Hollenberg (521) in 1959, who showed that an increase in enzyme activity could be achieved when isolated fat pads from starved animals were incubated at 37°C in a medium containing glucose and insulin. Subsequent studies have confirmed the importance of the latter components (522,523) and have shown that catecholamines, adrenocorticotropic hormone (524), glucagon, thyroid stimulating hormone (525), and, under appropriate conditions, dibutyryl cyclic AMP, caffeine and theophylline (526) also prevented the increases previously described. Particular attention has been paid to the effects of insulin and glucocorticoids in promoting the activity of pads *in vitro* by protein synthesis-dependent mechanisms (526,527). In addition, using such incubation systems, a protein synthesis-independent activation of the enzyme which is prevented or reversed by catecholamines has also been described (528,529).

As pointed out by Robinson (530) there are complications of interpretation inherent in observations made using whole fat pads *in vitro*. Particularly, either before or after incubation *in vitro*, the tissue will contain enzyme in a number of intra- and extra-adipocyte compartments. In such circumstances, the LPL activity measured in the tissue preparation will not only represent the sum of individual activities variously distributed among different sites but will also reflect the "dynamic balance of hormonal and non-hormonal effects being exerted on the synthesis/degradation and the activation/inactivation of the enzyme".

With regard to the hormonal effects on enzyme synthesis in fat pads incubated *in vitro*, a number of studies have indicated that, by comparison with the known effects of insulin and glucocorticoids in other tissues, glucocorticoids specifically stimulate the transcription of the LPL gene(s), and that insulin has its effect through its non-specific stimulation of total mRNA translation (530).

Studies with whole fat pads have also been useful with regard to the effects of catecholamines on the LPL system. Because cAMP-dependent protein kinase action appears to have no effect on adipose LPL activity directly, the possibility that the rate of enzyme degradation may be enhanced under the influence of lipolytic stimuli has received attention and experimental support. Particularly since lysosomal action (if not proteases) appears to be involved in catecholamine-stimulated LPL degradation, it has been suggested that either the rise in intracellular cAMP concentration itself (531), or the rise in intracellular unesterified fatty acids that follow catecholamine action, may enhance the fusion of transport (export) vesicles containing the enzyme with lysosomes, thus producing the observed changes (530).

In isolated fat pad systems pulse-chase studies using radioactive amino acids have shown that the extent of this intracellular degradation of LPL is highly significant (532). Approximately 40% of the enzyme synthesized is degraded in 3 hours at 37°C, under conditions where little degradation of the total adipose tissue protein is taking place. Such a possibility for regulation in the LPL system is not without precedent in that it is now evident that several secreted proteins, in tissues other than adipose, are potentially subject to degradation shortly after their synthesis (534).

In attempts to avoid the problems inherent in the use of whole fat pads incubated *in vitro*, many studies have adopted a reductionist approach and have studied isolated adipocytes *in vitro*. Clearly, the use of isolated cells introduces other problems, both operational and interpretational, which have been considered elsewhere (eg. 468,534,535). However, such studies on the LPL system of isolated adipocytes have not only revealed the susceptibility of the system to a further variety of effectors, but has identified additional levels at which a number of effectors may be operative.

For example, adenosine and its catabolite inosine produce increases in adipocyte LPL activities (536). These actions, which have been related to those of insulin in that they involve a stimulation of phosphodiesterase activity, are clearly related to a mechanism involving cAMP (538). It is as yet unknown whether this mechanism relates solely to the action of insulin on ribosomal LPL synthesis (517), or involves a modulation of enzyme degradative rates. Adipocytes have also been the subject of study when the mechanisms of enzyme export have been considered. In addition to showing that the secretion of enzyme was sensitive to effectors that interfered with micro-tubular function (538), such studies have also indicated that insulin enhances the proportion of enzyme which is rapidly released from the cells by the action of heparin (105). Further studies have indicated that this latter would appear to reflect the operation of a protein synthesis-independent action of insulin in stimulating the translocation of intracellular enzyme to a site at the cell membrane where it may be detected immunologically (539). Thus, not only does insulin have an effect on the synthesis of LPL as indicated above, but it may also stimulate the translocation of the enzymes to an extracellular site in much the same way as the hormone has been suggested to act in stimulating the intracellular movement of glucose transport units (540–543).

In the study of the LPL systems using either whole tissue or mature tissue-derived adipocytes, the time course of study is usually confined to a few hours at most. The availability of cultured cells with the capacity to differentiate into stable adipocyte-like cells *in vitro* (145–147) has, however, provided the opportunity to study the situation over more prolonged time courses. Indeed, some studies (for example, 115) have highlighted the differences that exist between short and long-term effects in such cells. Thus, when preadipocytes and cultured cardiac cells were treated with either exogenous dibutyryl cyclic AMP, 3-iso butyl-1-methylxanthine, or cholera toxin there was a large reduction in adipocyte LPL (see above) and a smaller reduction in the heart cells up to 6 hours later. However, after 24 hours, there were activity increases in both cell types, mediated via changes in intracellular cyclic AMP concentrations, which were thought to operate through changes in messenger RNA and protein synthesis.

Despite the difficulties of interpretation because of the dual effects of some hormones on cell differentiation *per se* and LPL activity (136), the use of 3T3-L_I adipocytes in culture has allowed long-term study of the effects of insulin on LPL activity (137). Thus, in such cells and in partial contradistinction to the effects on mature adipocytes, insulin was without effect on enzyme activity during the first 4 hours of treatment. However, the hormone did stimulate the release of enzyme over a short time course (i.e. within 30 minutes) and caused an increase in cellular activity over a 2 day period. Thus, as in other systems, insulin appears to favor the relocation of enzyme in this cultured cell type and has an effect at the level of enzyme translation. These studies further suggested that the hormones also stimulated gene expression and RNA synthesis. However, such effects and time courses have not been observed in other similar studies (544), and variability related to the *in vitro* life-span of the cells used appears to be of probable importance in explaining such discrepancies (135).

The emergence of LPL during the differentiation of adipocyte precursor strains obtained from adipose depots *in vivo* has been used frequently as a so-called marker of the developing adipocyte phenotype (eg. 147,157). Likewise, such cells have provided evidence that the synthesis and transport of the enzyme to the cell surface involve separate mechanisms (151) and that both may be stimulated by otherwise neglected yet potentially important effectors (155). Importantly, a mature murine adipose tissue source has been used to produce a clonal cell line of cultured adipose cells (Ob17) which has been of considerable significance to our understanding of the adipose LPL system. Thus, in a series of publications, (141,142,469,545,546) the topology of a number of intracellular events involved in the synthesis and processing of LPL in such cells has become evident.

By depleting cells of LPL, through incubation with heparin and cycloheximide, and then following the repletion of cellular enzyme protein and activity, Ailhaud and his colleagues (545,546) have been able to follow the steps necessary to the production of functionally active enzyme. As expected, the enzyme is synthesized in the endoplasmic reticulum, but in addition, these experiments show that LPL undergoes an intracellular activation event which takes place after the enzyme exits from the endoplasmic reticulum and before it reaches the trans-golgi cisternae. The experiments also suggest that the aquisition by LPL of a catalytically active conformation is linked directly or indirectly to glycosylation. However, intracellular migration in this system, unlike that seen in mature tissue-derived adipocytes

(540), does not seem to be affected by inhibitors of glycosylation such as tunicamycin. Clearly, although the general route taken by LPL is now known, as in other systems, the detailed molecular mechanisms involved in protein/membrane targetting/translocation are incompletely understood or their general applicability assured (547).

Although much information germane to the intracellular synthesis and processing of LPL in adipose systems has come from a wide range of studies *in vitro*, very little is known of the events that are involved in the transport of the enzyme from the adipocyte to the endothelium. A heparin-mediated release of the enzyme from the cell surface *in vivo* seems an unlikely event when coupled with the necessary vectoral movement towards the endothelium. In that immobilized glycosaminoglycans do not stimulate cellular enzyme release and the concentration of the free molecules in the interstitium is lower than that needed for the stimulation of release *in vitro*, the involvement of such polyanions in anything other than endothelial cell surface sequestration has been questioned (475). However, the description of membrane continuities within and between adipocytes and endothelial cells (548), together with their proposed involvement in the movement of exogenous molecules from endothelium to adipocyte endoplasmic reticulum (549), and the cell surface location of LPL (106–108,119,120,176,539) have suggested an alternative possibility. In such a proposal, the LPL molecules that are associated with the adipocyte plasma membrane may be exported to the endothelium without leaving the plane of the membrane. Thus, their movement involves lateral diffusion in the contiguous adipocyte membranes followed by association with endothelial heparan-sulphate proteoglycan which may pass from the abluminal to luminal side of the endothelial cell either via transport vesicles (513) or through the known lateral movement of this endothelial surface component (550,551). Although the lateral diffusion coefficients of most membrane associated proteins ($10^{-10} - 10^{-12}$ cm^2/second) are 10^2 to 10^4 times slower than those measured for soluble proteins in aqueous solution (ca 10^{-8} cm^2/second), the potential rate of transfer from adipocyte to endothelium may still be achieved despite this constraint (552). However, such speculation is not as yet substantiated experimentally and the tools for measuring the true diffusion rates of proteins like LPL in membranes are, as yet, not available.

Most of the relevant information about the LPL system in muscular tissues derives from studies *in vitro*, particularly those involving perfused heart muscle and isolated cells derived from cardiac tissue. However, because of the more complicated structure of cardiac tissue, compared with for example adipose tissue, the distinction between the various cellular and extracellular pools of enzyme has relied on relatively pragmatic approaches. From studies on isolated cardiac muscle cells, it is clear that as in adipocytes, cardiac LPL has an intracellular distribution compatible with the enzyme being a cell surface or secretory product of the cardiac muscle cell (112,114). What precise mechanisms operate to control the specific gene expression in heart tissue (553), the translation of the message, and the processing and translocation of the enzyme, remain less than totally clear. In the study of the perfused heart system, the pool of extracellular enzyme readily released by heparin and which can be demonstrated immunochemically at or near the endothelial surface (301) has been of particular interest. Not only is this fraction of total cardiac muscle LPL activity variable in response to many stimuli, including a variety of inhibitors of enzyme processing and secretion (see above) but it has also been suggested that it is a substrate for cAMP dependent protein kinase (554). This latter observation is in direct opposition to the lack of effect this protein kinase has on adipose tissue derived enzyme (530,555). Whether the modulation of soluble cardiac enzyme by cAMP-dependent protein kinase catalysed phosphorylation has any parallel *in vivo*, and whether there is a true distinction between adipose and cardiac enzyme in this regard, must be open to further experimental investigation. It is perhaps of interest to place the foregoing in proximity with the observation that although intact LPL is released from the cardiac endothelium by heparin, even in the absence of any other additions, this enzyme is degraded proteolytically in the perfusion medium (556). Whether the intact enzyme or the degradation product is the substrate for cAMP-dependent protein kinase remains to be seen.

Although the balance of LPL synthesis and degradation has not been addressed directly for heart muscle cells, it is clear that such cells are able to take up and degrade exogenous enzyme (511). Furthermore, although it has been suggested that insulin stimulates myocardial LPL activity by an apparent effect on protein synthesis, the action of this agent could also be related to the inhibitory effect the hormone has on cardiac lysosomal protein degradation (557). To continue in a speculative vein, it might be finally observed that by contrast to the situation in adipose tissue, although lateral motion of material in cardiac membranes is proven (558), there is at present no evidence to suggest a continuity between the sarcoplasmic reticulum and the plasma membrane of myocytes, or between the external leaflet of the endothelial cell and that of myocytes. Such questions relating to the molecular mechanisms operative in the processing and translocation of the enzyme in cardiac tissue are still outstanding. Undoubtedly, the use of isolated cardiac cells in culture will be of considerable value in addressing such problems in the future, just as they have been of help in answering related problems in the past (eg. 115). Unfortunately, the use of cultured heart cells does not circumvent the problem of the multiple lipase species present in cardiac tissue [which are variously sensitive to heparin-induced release (472)] in that all three cardiac lipases [i.e. lipoprotein (alkaline) lipase, neutral lipase and lysosomal (acid lipase)] are present in such cells (559).

It is clear that progress towards an understanding of the reciprocal nature of control that would seem to be necessary to explain the changes in adipose and muscle enzyme activities can only be made by the concerted use of experimental systems already available and by the creation of new ones.

One cell type which has recently become of interest as a potential model system for the study of the control of the LPL system is the macrophage. As a postscript to this Chapter then, it is appropriate to review briefly the characteristics of the enzyme in this cell type.

Although the macrophage is able to take up very low density lipoproteins and their partially triglyceride-depleted remnants, it is also possible for extracellular fatty acids generated by the action of macrophage-secreted LPL to be assimilated by the cells (560). It is of particular interest that the macrophage is the only cell type studied so far which secretes LPL continuously in a manner which is only slightly enhanced by the presence of heparin (130). Whether such a distinction between this and other cell types is related to the migratory capacity of the macrophage is unknown. In macrophages, this secretion of enzyme is cycloheximide sensitive (130), and both the intracellular and extracellular activities are reduced when intracellular cAMP concentrations are raised under conditions where protein synthesis rates remain unchanged. As with the other cell types discussed in detail above, (adipocytes and cardiac muscle cells) the macrophage also has cell surface-associated enzyme. This activity is distinct from that which is secreted, and it is the demonstrable lipolytic activity at this site which is able to promote the direct uptake of lipolytic products into the cells. This latter is also unique to the macrophages because in the LPL system of other cells, the site of cell surface lipolysis is remote (in cell-type terms) from the cellular site of LPL synthesis and export.

The short-term control of enzyme synthesis in this cell type may have parallels with other systems, but it is definitely characteristic of the secretory macrophage rather than its monocyte progenitor.

Finally, although much may be deduced from the many systems described here, there is much still to be learned of the physiological and molecular control of LPL. Clearly, a cognizance of the comparative view will provide one of the avenues for future progress.

References

1. Cryer, A. 1983. *In*: Biochemical Interactions at the Endothelium. A. Cryer, editor. Elsevier Science Publishers, Amsterdam, New York, Oxford. 245–274.
2. Casley-Smith, J. R. 1980. *In*: Vascular Endothelium and Basement Membranes, Advances in Microcirculation Vol. 9. B. M. Aptura, editor. S. Kager, Basel. 1–44.
3. Chapman, M. J. 1980. *J. Lipid Res.* 21:789–853.
4. Eisenberg, S. 1979. *Prog. Biochem. Pharmacol.* 15:139–165.
5. Eisenberg, S. 1975. *Adv. Lipid Res.* 13:1–89.
6. Havel, R. J., G. L. Goldstein and M. S. Brown. 1980. *In*: Metabolic Control of disease. P. K. Bondy and L. E. Rosenberg, editors. W. B. Saunders Corp., Philadelphia. 393–494.
7. Morrisett, J. D., R. L. Jackson and R. I. Levy. 1977. *Biochim. Biophys. Acta* 472:93–133.
8. Schaefer, E. J. and R. I. Levy. 1979. *Prog. Biochem. Pharmacol.* 15:200–215.
9. Mahley, R. W. 1982. *Med. Clin. North Am.* 66:375–402.
10 Mahley, R. W. and T. L. Innerarity. 1983. *Biochim. Biophys. Acta* 737:197–222.

11. Schaefer, E. J., S. Eisenberg and R. I. Levy. 1978. *J. Lipid Res.* 19:667–687.
12. Quinn, D., K. Shirai and R. L. Jackson. 1982. *Prog. Lipid Res.* 22:35–78.
13. Mahley, R. W., T. L. Innerarity, S. C. Rall and K. H. Weisgraber. 1984. *J. Lipid Res.* 25:1277–1294.
14. Dolphin, P. J. 1985. *Can. J. Biochem. Cell Biol.* 63:850–869.
15. Harlan, W. R., P. S. Winosett and A. J. Wasserman. 1967. *J. Clin. Invest.* 46:239–247.
16. Nilsson-Ehle, P. 1972. *Clin. Chim. Acta* 42:383–389.
17. Persson, B. 1973. *Acta. Med. Scand.* 193:457–462.
18. Nilsson-Ehle, P. 1974. *Clin. Chim. Acta* 54:283–291.
19. Pykalisto, O. J., P. H. Smith and J. D. Brunzell. 1975. *Proc. Soc. Ex. Biol. Med.* 148:297–303.
20. Twu, J. J., A. S. Garfinkel and M. C. Schotz. 1976. *Atherosclerosis* 24:119–128.
21. Taskinen, M. R. and E. A. Nikkila. 1979. *Atherosclerosis* 32:289–299.
22. Iverius, P. -H. and J. D. Brunzell. 1985. *Am. J. Physiol.* 249:E107–E114.
23. Dahms, W. T., P. Nilsson-Ehle, A. S. Garfinkel, R. L. Atkinson, G. A. Bray and M. C. Schotz. 1982. *Int. J. Obesity* 5:81–84.
24. Savard, R., Y. Deshaies, J. -P. Despres, M. Marcotte, L. Bukowiecki, C. Allard and C. Bouchard. 1984. *Can. J. Physiol. Pharmacol.* 62:1448–1452.
25. Janasson, L., G. K. Hansson, G. Bondjers, G. Bengtsson and T. Olivecrona. 1984. *Atherosclerosis* 51:313–326.
26. Sadur, C. N. and R. H. Eckel. 1982. *J. Clin. Invest.* 69:1119–1125.
27. Wang, C. -S., A. Kuksis, and F. Manganaro. 1982. *Lipids* 17:278–284.
28. Kotze, J. P. and J. H. Spiers. 1976. *S. Afr. Med. J.* 50:1760–1764.
29. Goldberg, I. J., J. R. Paterniti and W. V. Brown. 1983. *Biochim. Biophys. Acta* 752:172–177.
30. Cryer, A. and H. M. Jones. 1979. *Comp. Biochem. Physiol.* 63B:501–505.
31. Reichl, D. 1972. *Biochem. J.* 128:79–87.
32. Rogers, M. P. and D. S. Robinson. 1974. *J. Lipid Res.* 15:263–272.
33. Hamosh, M. and P. Hamosh. 1975. *Biochim. Biophys. Acta* 380:132–140.
34. Cryer, A., S. E. Riley, E. R. Williams and D. S. Robinson. 1976. *Clin. Sci. Molec. Med.* 50:213–221.
35. Hamosh, M., T. R. Clary, S. S. Chernick and R. O. Scow. 1970. *Biochim. Biophys. Acta* 210:473–482.
36. Carneheim, C., J. Nedergaard and B. Cannon. 1984. *Am. J. Physiol.* 246:E327–E333.
37. Enser, M. 1972. *Biochem. J.* 129:447–453.
38. Masuno, H., T. Tsujita, H. Nakanishi, A. Yoshida, R. Fukunishi and H. Okuda. *J. Lipid Res.* 25:419–427.
39. Paterniti, J. R., W. V. Brown, H. N. Guisberg and K. Artzt. 1983. *Science* 221:167–169.
40. Skowronski, G. A., S. B. Gertner, N. S. Paisley and S. I. Sherr, 1983. *Enzyme* 30:48–53.
41. Cryer, A. and A. M. Sawyerr. 1978. *Comp. Biochem. Physiol.* 61B: 151–159.
42. Barakat, H. A., E. B. Tapscott and C. Smith. 1977. *Lipids* 21:550–555.
43. Cryer, A., J. Kirtland, H. M. Jones and M. I. Gurr. 1978. *Biochem. J.* 170:169–172.
44. Robinson, D. S. 1963. *J. Lipid Res.* 4:21–23.
45. Rothwell, J. E. and M. C. Elphick. 1982. *J. Develop. Physiol.* 4:153–159.
46. F. R. Heller. 1983. *Biochim. Biophys. Acta* 752:357–360.
47. Wallinder, L. A., G. Bengtsson and T. Olivecrona. 1982. *Biochim. Biophys. Acta* 711:107–113.
48. Dark, J., G. N. Wade and I. Zucker. 1984. *Physiol. Behav.* 32:75–78.
49. Enser, M. 1973. *Biochem. J.* 136:381–385.
50. Bensadoun, A., C. Ehnholm, D. Steinberg and N. V. Brown. 1974. *J. Biol. Chem.* 249:2220–2227.
51. Ehnholm, C., P. V. J. Kinnunen, J. K. Huttenen, E. A. Nikkila, and M. Ohta. 1975. *Biochem. J.* 149:649–655.
52. Mersmann, H. J. and L. -J Koong. 1984. *J. Nutr.* 114:862–868.

53. Plaas, H. A. K., R. Harwood and A. Cryer. 1978. *Biochem. Soc. Trans.* 6:596–598.
54. Wisner, D. A. Jr., K. Shirai and R. L. Jackson. 1980. *Artery* 6:419–436.
55. Chilliard, Y. and J. Robelin. 1985. *Reprod. Nutr. Develop.* 25:287–293.
56. Tume, R. K. 1983. *Aust. J. Biol. Sci.* 36:41–48.
57. Chilliard, Y., M. Dorleans and P. Morand-Fehr. 1977. *Ann. Biol. Anim. Biochim. Biophys.* 17:1021–1034.
58. Chilliard, Y., D. Sauvant, J. Herrieu, M. Dorleans and P. Morand-Fehr. 1977. *Ann. Biol. Anim. Biochim. Biophys.* 17:1021–1034.
59. Pfaff, F. E. Jr., J. D. Benson and R. E. Austic. 1977. *Comp. Biochem. Physiol.* 58B:345–348.
60. Kompiang, I. P., A. Bensadoun, and M. -W. W. Young. 1976. *J. Lipid Res.* 17:498–505.
61. Griffin, H. 1982. *Biochem. J.* 206:647–654.
62. Cheung, A. H., A. Bensadoun and C. -F Cheng. 1979. *Anal. Biochem.* 94:346–357.
63. Husbands, D. 1972. *Br. J. Pout. Sci.* 13:85–90.
64. Gershenwald, J. E., A. Bensadoun and A. Saluja. 1985. *Biochim. Biophys. Acta* 836:286–295.
65. Kelley, J. L., C. S. Wang, H. B. Bass and R. H. Thayer. 1982. *Artery* 10:379–394.
66. Evans, A. J. 1972. *Int. J. Biochem.* 3:199–206.
67. Hogg, S. I. and A. Cryer. 1983. *Comp. Biochem. Physiol.* 74B:593–596.
68. Skinner, E. R. and A. M. Youssef. 1982. *Biochem. J.* 203:727–734.
69. Chang, F. 1977. *Comp. Biochem. Physiol.* 57B:209–214.
70. Jensen, R. G. and R. E. Pitas. 1976. *J. Dairy Sci.* 59:1203–1214.
71. Chilliard, Y. 1982. *Le Lait* 62:1–31.
72. Hernell, O. and T. Olivecrona. 1974. *J. Lipid Res.* 15:367–374.
73. Mehta, N. R., J. B. Jones and Hamosh, M. 1982. *J. Pediat. Gastroenterol. Nutr.* 1:317–326.
74. Hamosh, M. and R. O. Scow. 1971. *Biochim. Biophys. Acta* 231:283–289.
75. Abe, K. and K. Yoshimura. 1972. *J. Physiol. Soc. Japan.* 34:81–82.
76. Brady, M. and J. A. Higgins. 1967. *Biochim. Biophys. Acta* 137:140–146.
77. Hamosh, M., H. Yeager, Y. Shechter and P. Hamosh. 1976. *Biochim. Biophys. Acta* 431:519–525.
78. Skowronski, G. A., S. Varghese, S. B. Getner and S. I. Sherr. 1983. *Pharmacol. Res. Commun.* 15:661–673.
79. Okabe, T., H. Yorifuju, T. Murase and F. Takaku. 1984. *Biochem. Biophys. Res. Commun.* 125:273–278.
80. Henson, L. C. and H. C. Schotz. 1975. *Biochim. Biophys. Acta* 409:360–366.
81. Dicorleto, P. E. and D. B. Zilversmit. 1975. *Proc. Soc. Exp. Biol. Med.* 148:1101–1105.
82. Vijayakumar, S. T., S. Leelamma and P. A. Kurup. 1975. *Atherosclerosis* 21:1–14.
83. DeGasquet, P. and E. Pequignot. 1972. *Biochem. J.* 127:445–448.
84. Elphick, M. C. and D. Hull. 1977. *J. Physiol.* 273:475–487.
85. Mallov, S. and A. A. Alousi. 1965. *Proc. Soc. Exp. Biol. Med.* 119:301–306.
86. Gray, J. M. and M. R. C. Greenwood. 1983. *Am. J. Physiol.* 245:E132–E137.
87. Benson, J. D., A. Bensadoun and D. Cohen. 1975. *Proc. Soc. Exp. Biol. Med.* 148:347–350.
88. Shemesh, M., A. Bensadoun and W. Hansel. 1976. *Proc. Soc. Exp. Biol. Med.* 151:667–669.
89. Cryer, A. and H. M. Jones. 1978. *Biochem. J.* 174:447–451.
90. Hemon, P., D. Ricquier and G. Mory. 1975. *Hormon. Metab. Res.* 7:481–484.
91. Guerrier, D. and H. Pellet. 1979. *FEBS Lett.* 106:115–120.
92. Radomski, M. W. and T. Orme, 1971. *Am. J. Physiol.* 220:1852–1856.
93. Ricquier, D., G. Mory and P. Hemon. 1979. *Can. J. Biochem.* 57:1262–1266.
94. Horowitz, B. A. 1984. *Metabolism* 33:354–357.
95. Llobera, M., A. Montes and E. Herrera. 1979. *Biochem. Biophys. Res. Commun.* 91:272–277.

96. Grinberg, D., I. Ramirez, S. Vilaro, M. Reina, M. Llobera and E. Herrera. 1985. *Biochim. Biophys. Acta* 833:217–222.
97. Brecher, P. and H. T. Kuan. 1979. *J. Lipid Res.* 20:464–471.
98. Chajek, T., O. Stein and Y. Stein. 1977. *Atherosclerosis* 26:549–561.
99. Eckel, R. H. and R. J. Robbins. 1984. *Proc. Natl. Acad. Sci.* (USA) 81:7604–7607.
100. Bensadoun, A. and T. L. Koh. 1977. *J. Lipid Res.* 18:768–773.
101. Rodbell, M. 1964. *J. Biol. Chem.* 239:733–755.
102. Davies, P. and D. S. Robinson. 1973. *Biochem. J.* 136:437–439.
103. Cunningham, V. J. and D. S. Robinson. 1969. *Biochem. J.* 112:203–209.
104. Spencer, I. M., A. Hutchinson and D. S. Robinson. 1978. *Biochim. Biophys. Acta* 530:375–384.
105. Cryer, A., P. Davies, E. R. Williams and D. S. Robinson. 1975. *Biochem. J.* 146:481–488.
106. Kern, P.A., S. Marshall and R. H. Eckel. 1985. *J. Clin. Invest* 75:199–208.
107. Arnaud, J. O. and J. Boyer. 1977. *Biochim. Biophys. Acta* 486:462–469.
108. Arnaud, J. O., O. Nobili and J. Boyer. 1979. *Biochim. Biophys. Acta* 572:193–200.
109. Verine, A., P. Salers and J. Boyer. 1982. *Am. J. Physiol* 243:E175–E181.
110. Chohan, P. and A. Cryer. 1977. *Biochem. Soc. Trans.* 5:1340–1343.
111. Bagby, G., M. -S Liu, and J. A. Spitzer. 1977. *Life Sci.* 21:467–474.
112. Chohan, P. and A. Cryer, 1978. *Biochem. J.* 174:663–666.
113. Chohan, P. and A. Cryer. 1979. *Biochem. J.* 181:83–93.
114. Rajaram, O. V., M. G. Clark and P. J. Barter. 1980. *Biochem. J.* 186:431–438.
115. Vahouny, G. V., A. Tamboli, M. Vander Maten, J. -S. Twu and M. C. Schotz. 1980. *Biochim. Biophys. Acta* 620:63–69.
116. Friedman, G., T. Chajek-Shaul, O. Stein and Y. Stein. 1983. *Biochim. Biophys. Acta* 752:106–117.
117. Bravion, P. M., A. H. Cheung and A. Bensadoun. 1978. *Biochim. Biophys. Acta* 531:96–108.
118. Brannon, P. M. and H. Bensadoun. 1980. *Biochim. Biophys. Acta* 618:173–182.
119. Clegg, R. A. 1979. *Biochem. Soc. Trans* 7:1053–1054.
120. Clegg, R. A. 1981. *Biochim. Biophys. Acta* 664:397–408.
121. Clegg, R. A. 1981. *Biochim. Biophys. Acta* 663:598–612.
122. Tajima, S., R. Hayashi, S. Tsuchiya, Y. Migake and A. Yamamoto. 1985. *Biochem. Biophys. Res. Commun.* 126:526–531.
123. Balin, Z. 1984. *Bull. Cancer* (Paris). 71:412–418.
124. Stray, N., H. Letnes and J. P. Blomhoff. 1985. *Scand. J. Gastroenterol.* (Suppl) 107:67–72.
125. Yoshii, H., K. Watanabe, Y. Yanaghia and T. Shida. 1984. *Nippon Ika. Daigaku Zasshi* 51:774–775.
126. Ostlund-Lindqvist, A. -M., S. Gustafson, P. Lindquist, J. L. Witztum and J. A. Little. 1983. 3:433–440.
127. Melmed, R. N., G. Friedman, T. Chajek-Shaul, O. Stein and Y. Stein. 1983. *Biochim. Biophys. Acta* 762:58–66.
128. Wang-Iverson, P., A. Ungar, J. Bliumis, P. R. Bukberg, J. C. Gibson and W. V. Brown. 1982. *Biochem. Biophys. Res. Commun.* 104:923–928.
129. Chait, A., P. -H. Iverius and J. D. Brunzell. 1982. *J. Clin. Invest.* 69:490–493.
130. Mahoney, E. M., J. C. Khoo, and D. Steinberg. 1982. *Proc. Natl. Acad. Sci.* (USA). 79:1639–1642.
131. Khoo, J. C., E. M. Mahoney and J. L. Witztum. 1981. *J. Biol. Chem.* 256:7105–7108.
132. Bates, S. R., P. L. Murphy, Z. Feng, T. Kanazawa and G. S. Getz. 1984. *Arteriosclerosis* 4:103–114.
133. Green, H. and M. Meuth. 1974. *Cell* 3:127–133.
134. Green, H. and O. Kehinde. 1975. *Cell* 5:19–27.
135. Eckel, R. H., W. Y. Fujimoto and J. D. Brunzell. 1981. *Int. J. Obesity* 5:571–580.

136. Spooner, P. M., S. S. Chernick, M. Garrison and R. O. Scow. 1979. *J. Biol. Chem.* 254:1305–1311.
137. Spooner, P. M., S. S. Chernick, M. Garrison and R. O. Scow. 1979. *J. Biol. Chem.* 254:10021–10029.
138. Mahoney, J. R., B. A. Beutler, N. Letrang, W. Vine, Y. Ikeda and P. Krishram. 1985. *J. Immunol.* 134:1673–1675.
139. Kawakami, M., P. H. Pekala, M. D. Lane and A. Cerami. 1982. *Proc. Natl. Acad. Sci.* (USA). 79:912–916.
140. Negrel, R., P. Grimaldi and G. Ailhaud. 1978. *Proc. Natl. Acad. Sci.* (USA) 75:6054–6058.
141. Vannier, C., H. Jansen, R. Negrel and G. Ailhaud. 1982. *J. Biol. Chem.* 257:12387–12393.
142. Vannier, C., E. -Z Amri, J. Etienne, R. Negrel and G. Ailhaud. 1985. *J. Biol. Chem.* 260:4424–4431.
143. Forest, C., D. Czerucka, P. Grimaldi, C. Vannier, R. Negrel and G. Ailhaud. 1983. *In*: The Adipocyte and Obesity: Cellular and Molecular Mechanisms. A. Angel, C. H. Hollenberg and D. A. K. Roncari, Editors. Raven Press, New York. 53–64.
144. Hiragun, A., M. Sato and H. Mitsui. 1980. *In Vitro* 16:685–693.
145. Hiragun, A. 1985. *In*: New Perspectives in Adipose Tissue, Structure Function and Development. A. Cryer and R. L. R. Van, Editors. Butterworths, London. 333–352.
146. Cryer, A. 1982. *In*: Biochemical Development of the Fetus and Neonate. C. T. Jones, Editor. Elsevier Biomedical Press. 731–757.
147. Cryer, A. 1985. *In*: New Perspectives in Adipose Tissue: Structure, Function and Development. A. Cryer and R. L. R. Van, Editors, Butterworths. London. 383–405.
148. Bjorntorp, P., M. Karlsson, P. Pettersson and G. Sypniewska. 1980. *J. Lipid Res.* 21:714–723.
149. Van, R. L. R., C. E. Bayliss and D. A. K. Roncari. 1976. *J. Clin. Invest.* 58:699–704.
150. Rothblat, G. H. and F. D. DeMartinis. 1977. *Biochem. Biophys. Res. Commun.* 78:45–50.
151. Glick, J. M. and G. H. Rothblat. 1980. *Biochim. Biophys. Acta* 618:163–672.
152. Plaas, H. A. K. and A. Cryer. 1980. *J. Dev. Physiol.* 2:275–289.
153. Cryer, A. 1985. *Reprod. Nutr. Develop.* 25:159–164.
154. Cryer, A. 1985. *Reprod. Nutr. Develop.* 25:255–270.
155. Eckel, R. H., W. Y. Fujimato and J. D. Bruzell. 1979. *Diabetes* 28:1141–1142.
156. Stein, O., G. Halperin, E. Leitersdorf, T. Olivecrona and Y. Stein. 1984. *Biochim. Biophys. Acta* 795:47–59.
157. Gaben-Cogneville, A. -M., A. Quignard-Boulange, Y. Aron, L. Brigant, T. Jahcan, J. -Y. Pello and E. Swierczewski. 1984. *Biochim. Biophys. Acta* 805:252–260.
158. Glick, J. M. and S. J. Adelman. 1983. *In Vitro* 19:421–428.
159. Friedman, G., O. Stein and Y. Stein. 1978. *Biochim. Biophys. Acta* 531:222–232.
160. Chajek, T., O. Stein and Y. Stein. 1977. *Biochim. Biophys. Acta* 488:140–144.
161. Pinson, A., C. Frelin and P. Padieu. 1973. *Biochimie* 55:1261–1264.
162. Vance, J. E., J. C. Khoo and D. Steinberg. 1982. *Arteriosclerosis* 2:390–395.
163. Hulsmann, W. C., W. A. P. Breeman, H. Stam and W. J. Kort. 1981. *Biochim. Biophys. Acta* 663:373–379.
164. Fielding, P. E., V. G. Shore and C. J. Fielding. 1974. *Biochemistry* 13:4318–4323.
165. Augustin, J., H. Freeze, P. Tejada and W. V. Brown. 1978. *J. Biol. Chem.* 253:2912–2920.
166. Becht, I., O. Schrecker, G. Klose and H. Greten. 1980. *Biochim. Biophys. Acta* 620:583–591.
167. Thim, L. 1978. *Scand. J. Clin. Lab. Invest.* 38:77–81.
168. Ostlund-Lindqvist, A. -M. and J. Boberg. 1977. *FEBS Lett.* 83:231–236.
169. Ostlund-Lindqvist, A. -M. 1979. *Biochem. J.* 179:555–559.
170. Iverius, P. -H. and A. -M. Ostlund-Lindqvist. 1976. *J. Biol. Chem.* 251:7791–7795.
171. Garfinkel, A. S., E. S. Kempner, O. Ben-Zeev, J. Nikazy, S. J. James and M. C. Schotz. 1983. *J. Lipid Res.* 24:775–780.

172. Twu, J. -S., A. S. Garfinkel and M. C. Schotz. 1975. *Atherosclerosis* 22:463–472.
173. Chung, J. and A. M. Scanu. 1977. *J. Biol. Chem.* 252:4202–4209.
174. Fielding, C. J. 1976. *Biochemistry* 15:879–884.
175. Etienne, J., L. Noe, M. Rossignol, C. Arnaud, N. Vydelinghum and A. H. Kissebah. 1985. *Biochim. Biophys. Acta* 834:95–101.
176. Al-Jafari, A. A. and A. Cryer. 1986. *Biochem. J.* 236:749–756.
177. Parkin, S. M., B. K. Speake and D. S. Robinson. 1982. *Biochem. J.* 207:485–495.
178. Greten, H. and B. Walter. 1973. *FEBS Lett.* 35:36–40.
179. Etienne, J., M. Breton, A. Vanhove and J. Polonovski. 1976. *Biochim. Biophys. Acta* 429:198–204.
180. Fielding, C. J. and P. E. Fielding. 1980. *Biochim. Biophys. Acta* 620:440–446.
181. Matsumura, S., M. Matsuo and Y. Nishikura. 1976. *J. Biol. Chem.* 251:6267–6273.
182. Nieuwenhuizen, W., F. C. Remen, I. A. M. Vermeer and T. Vermond. 1976. *Biochim. Biophys. Acta* 431:288–296.
183. Bengtsson, G. and T. Olivecrona. 1977. *Biochem. J.* 167:109–119.
184. Kinnunen, P. K. J., J. K. Huffunen and C. Ehnholm. 1976. *Biochim. Biophys. Acta* 450:342–351.
185. Olivecrona, T., G. Bengtsson and J. C. Osborne. 1982. *Eur. J. Biochem.* 124:629–633.
186. Nilsson-Ehle, P., A. S. Garfinkel and M. C. Schotz. 1980. *Ann. Rev. Biochem.* 49:667–693.
187. Schotz, M. C., J. -S. Twu, M. E. Pedersen, C. -H. Chang, A. S. Garfinkel, and J. Borensztajn. 1977. *Biochim. Biophys. Acta* 489:214–224.
188. Hernell, O., T. Egelrud and T. Olivecrona. 1975. *Biochim. Biophys. Acta* 38:233–241.
189. Olivecrona, T. and G. Bengtsson. 1983. *Biochim. Biophys. Acta* 752:38–45.
190. Twu, J. -S., E. P. Nilsson-Ehle and M. C. Schotz. 1976. *Biochemistry* 15:1904–1909.
191. Morley, N. and A. Kuksis. 1972. *J. Biol. Chem.* 247:6389–6393.
192. Somerharju, P., T. Kuusi, F. Paltauf and P. K. J. Kinnunen. 1978. *FEBS Lett.* 96:170–172.
193. Morley, N. and A. Kuksis. 1977. *Biochim. Biophys. Acta* 487:332–342.
194. LaRosa, J. C., R. I. Levy, P. N. Herbert, S. E. Lux and D. S. Fredrickson. 1970. *Biochem. Biophys. Res. Commun.* 41:57–62.
195. Catapano, A. L., P. K. J. Kinnunen, W. C. Breckenridge, A. M. Gotto, R. L. Jackson, J. A. Little, L. C. Smith and J. T. Sparrow. 1979. *Biochem. Biophys. Res. Commun.* 89:951–957.
196. Kinnunen, P. K. J., R. L. Jackson, L. C. Smith, A. M. Gotto and J. T. Sparrow. 1977. *Proc. Natl. Acad. Sci.* (USA). 74:4848–4851.
197. Vernon, R. G. and R. A. Clegg. 1985. *In*: New Perspectives in Adipose Tissue, Structure, Function and Development. A. Cryer, editor. Butterworths, London. 65–86.
198. Schotz, M. C. and A. S. Garfinkel. 1972. *Biochim. Biophys. Acta* 270:472–478.
199. Garfinkel, A. S. and M. C. Schotz. 1972. *J. Lipids Res.* 13:63–68.
200. Davies, P., A. Cryer and D. S. Robinson. 1974. *FEBS. Lett.* 45:271–275.
201. Ashby, P., A. M. Tolson, and D. S. Robinson. 1978. *Biochem. J.* 171:305–311.
202. Hamosh, M. 1984. *In*: Lipases. B. Borgstrom and H. L. Brockman, editors. Elsevier Science Publishers, Amsterdam. 49–82.
203. Verger, R. 1984. ibid. 83–150.
204. Rudd, E. A. and H. L. Brockman. 1984. ibid. 151–204.
205. Kinnunen, P. K. J. 1984. ibid. 307–328.
206. Fowler, S. D. and W. J. Brown. 1984. ibid. 329–364.
207. Belfrage, P., G. Fredrickson, G. P. Stralfors and H. Tornqvist. 1984. ibid. 365–416.
208. Rapp, D. and T. Olivecrona. 1978. *Eur. J. Biochem.* 91:379–385.
209. Nilsson-Ehle, P., T. Egelrud, P. Belfrage, T. Olivecrona and B. Borgstrom. 1973. *J. Biol. Chem.* 248:6734–6737.
210. Egelrud, T. and T. Olivecrona. 1973. *Biochim. Biophys. Acta* 306:115–127.
211. Fielding, C. J. 1970. *Biochim. Biophys. Acta* 206:109–119.

212. Scow, R. O. and T. Egelrud. 1976. *Biochim. Biophys. Acta* 431:538–549.
213. Muntz, H. G., N. Matsuoka and R. L. Jackson. 1979. *Biochem. Biophys. Res. Commun.* 90:15–21.
214. Stocks, J. and D. Galton. 1980. *Lipids* 15:186–190.
215. Groot, P. H. E. and A. Van Tol. 1978. *Biochim. Biophys. Acta* 530:188–196.
216. Groot, P. H. E., M. C. Oerlemans and L. M. Scheek. 1978. *Biochim. Biophys. Acta* 530:91–98.
217. Johnson, J. D., M -R Taskinen, N. Matsuoka and R. L. Jackson. 1980. *J. Biol. Chem.* 255:3461–3465.
218. Shirai, K. and R. L. Jackson. 1982. *J. Biol. Chem.* 257:1253–1258.
219. Shirai, K., R. L. Jackson and D. M. Quinn. 1982. *J. Biol. Chem.* 257:10200–10203.
220. Baginsky, M. L. and W. V. Brown. 1977. *J. Lipid Res.* 18:423–437.
221. Brown, M. J., A. A. Belmonte and P. Melius. 1977. *Biochim. Biophys. Acta* 486:313–321.
222. Kurooka, S., M. Hashimoto, M. Tomita, A. Maki and Y. Yoshimura. 1976. *J. Biochem.* 79:533–541.
223. Goldberg, R., Y. Barenholz and S. Gatt. 1978. *Biochim. Biophys. Acta* 531:237–241.
224. Hyun, J., H. Kothari, E. Herm, J. Mortenson, C. R. Treadwell and G. Vahouny. 1969. *J. Biol. Chem.* 244:1937–1945.
225. Calame, K. B., L. Gallo, E. Cheriathundam, G. V. Vahouny and C. R. Treadwell. 1975. *Arch. Biochem. Biophys.* 168:57–65.
226. Lombardo, D., J. Fauvel and O. Guy. 1980. *Biochim. Biophys. Acta* 611:136–146.
227. Erlanson, C. 1975. *Scand. J. Gastroenterol.* 10:401–408.
228. Lynn, K. R., C. A. Chuaqui and N. A. Clevette-Radford. 1982. *Bioorg. Chem.* 11:19–23.
229. Assman, G., R. M. Krauss, D. S. Fredrickson and R. I. Levy. 1973. *J. Biol. Chem.* 248:1992–1999.
230. Ehnholm, C., W. Shaw, H. Greten and W. V. Brown. 1975. *J. Biol. Chem.* 250:6756–6761.
231. Belfrage, P. 1965. *Biochim. Biophys. Acta.* 98:660–662.
232. Newkirk, J. D. and M. Waite. 1971. *Biochim. Biophys. Acta* 225:224–233.
233. Nachbaur, J., A. Colbeau and P. M. Vignai. 1972. *Biochim. Biophys. Acta* 274:426–446.
234. Vogel, W. C. and E. L. Bierman. 1967. *J. Lipid Res.* 8:46–53.
235. Jansen, H. and Hulsmann, W. C. 1973. *Biochim. Biophys. Acta* 296:241–248.
236. Waite, M. and Sisson, P. 1974. *J. Biol. Chem.* 249:6401–6405.
237. Takano, T., W. J. Black, T. J. Peters and C. deDuve. 1974. *J. Biol. Chem.* 249:6732–6737.
238. Hajjar, D. P., C. R. Minick and S. Fowler. 1983. *J. Biol. Chem.* 258:192–198.
239. Gatt, S., Y. Barenholz, R. Goldberg, T. Dinur, G. Besley, Z. Leibovitz-Bon Gershon, J. Rosenthal, R. J. Desnick, E. A. Devine, B. Shafit-Zagardo and F. Tsuruki. 1981. *Methods in Enzymology.* 72:351–375.
240. Fredrickson, G., P. Stralfors, N. O. Nilsson and P. Belfrage. 1981. *J. Biol. Chem.* 256:6311–6320.
241. Korn, E. D. and T. W. Quigley. 1953. *J. Biol. Chem.* 226:833–839.
242. Fielding, C. J. 1973. *Biochim. Biophys. Acta* 316:66–75.
243. Hamosh, M. and R. O. Scow. 1973. *J. Clin. Invest.* 55:88–95.
244. Hamosh, M. and W. A. Burns. 1977. *Lab. Invest.* 37:603–608.
245. Vaughan, M., J. E. Berger and D. Steinberg. 1984. *J. Biol. Chem.* 239:401–409.
246. Paltouf, F., F. Esfadi and A. Holasek. 1974. *FEBS Lett.* 40:119–123.
247. Paltauf, F. and E. Wagner. 1976. *Biochim. Biophys. Acta* 431:359–362.
248. Staggers, J. E., G. J. P. Fernando-Warnakulasuriya and M. A. Wells. 1981. *J. Lipid Res.* 22:675–679.
249. Brockerhoff, H. and R. G. Jensen. 1974. Lipolytic Enzymes. Academic Press. New York. 34–90.
250. ibid. 177–192.
251. Akesson, B., S. Gronowitz and B. Herslof. 1976. *FEBS Lett.* 71:241–244.
252. Bengtsson, G., S -E. Marklund and T. Olivecrona. 1977. *Eur. J. Biochem.* 79:211–223.

253. Bengtsson, G. and T. Olivecrona. 1977. *Eur. J. Biochem.* 79:225–231.
254. Borgstrom, B. and C. Erlanson-Albertsson. 1984. *In*: Lipases. B. Borgstrom and H. L. Brockman, editors. Elsevier Science Publishers. Amsterdam. 151–183.
255. Jahn, C. E., J. C. Osborne, E. J. Schaefer and H. B. Brewer. 1981. *FEBS Lett.* 131:366–368.
256. Kubo, M., Y. Matsuzawa, S. Tajima, K. Ishikawa, A. Yamamoto and S. Tarui. 1981. *Biochem. Biophys. Res. Commun.* 100:261–266.
257. Kubo, M., Y. Matsuzawa, S. Yokoyama, S. Tajima, K. Ishikawa, A. Yamamoto and S. Tarui. 1982. *J. Biochem.* 92:865–870.
258. Krauss, R. M., H. G. Windmueller, R. I. Levy and D. S. Fredrickson. 1973. *J. Lipid Res.* 14:286–295.
259. Posner, I. 1982. *Atheroscler. Rev.* 9:123–156.
260. Bengtsson, G. and T. Olivecrona. 1983. *Biochim. Biophys. Acta* 751:254–259.
261. LaRosa, J. C., R. I. Levy, H. G. Windmueller and D. S. Fredrickson. 1972. *J. Lipid Res.* 13:356–363.
262. Scow, R. O. and T. Olivecrona. 1977. *Biochim. Biophys. Acta* 487:472–486.
263. Bengtsson, G. and T. Olivecrona. 1980. *Eur. J. Biochem.* 106:557–562.
264. Smith, L. C. and H. J. Pownall. 1984. *In*: Lipases, B. Borgstrom and H. L. Brockman, editors. Elsevier Science Publishers, Amsterdam. 263–305.
265. Vaino, P., J. A. Virtanen and P. K. J. Kinnunen. 1982. *Biochim. Biophys. Acta* 711:386–390.
266. Maylie, M. F., M. Charles and P. Desnuelle. 1972. *Biochim. Biophys. Acta* 276:162–175.
267. Chapus, C. and M. Stemeriva. 1976. *Biochemistry* 15:4988–4991.
268. Lombardo, D. 1982. *Biochim. Biophys. Acta* 700:67–74.
269. Hayase, K. and A. L. Tappel. 1970. *J. Biol. Chem.* 245:169–175.
270. Garner, C. W. 1980. *J. Biol. Chem.* 255:5064–5068.
271. Bengtsson, G. and T. Olivecrona. 1979. *Biochim. Biophys. Acta* 575:471–474.
272. Fredrickson, G. P., Stralfors, N. O. Nilsson and P. Belfrage. 1981. *Methods. Enzymol.* 71:636–646.
273. Gidez, L. I. 1968. *J. Lipid Res.* 9:794–798.
274. Jensen, G. and A. Bensadoun. 1981. *Anal. Biochem.* 113:246–252.
275. Kuusi, T. E., Nikkila, I. Virtanen and P. K. J. Kinnunen. 1979. *Biochem. J.* 181:245–246.
276. Warner, T. G., L. M. Dambach, J. H. Shin and J. S. O'Brien. 1981. *J. Biol. Chem.* 276:2952–2957.
277. Riley, S. E. and D. S. Robinson. 1974. *Biochim. Biophys. Acta* 369:371–386.
278. Olivecrona, T. and G. Bengtsson. 1984. *In*: Lipases. B. Borgstrom and H. L. Brockman, editors. Elsevier Science Publishers. Amsterdam. 205–261.
279. Robinson, D. S. 1963. *Adv. Lipid Res.* 1:133–182.
280. Riley, S. E. and D. S. Robinson. 1974. *Biochim. Biophys. Acta* 369:371–386.
281. Woollett, L. A., D. C. Beitz, R. L. Hood, and S. Aprahamian. 1984. *Analyt. Biochem.* 143:25–29.
282. Shimizu, S., K. Inoue, Y. Tani, and H. Yamada. 1979. *Analyt. Biochem.* 98:341–345.
283. Kishimoto, Y. and N. S. Radin. 1959. *J. Lipid Res.* 1:72–78.
284. Greten, H., R. I. Levy and D. S. Fredrickson. 1968. *Biochim. Biophys. Acta* 164:185–194.
285. Schotz, M. C., A. S. Garfinkel, R. J. Huebotter, and J. E. Stewart. 1970. *J. Lipid Res.* 11:68–69.
286. Nilsson-Ehle, P., H. Tornquist, and P. Belfrage. 1972. *Clin. Chim. Acta* 42:383–390.
287. Nilsson-Ehle, P. 1984. *Clin. Chim. Acta* 141:293–298.
288. Ehnolm, C., E. A. Nikkila and P. Nilsson-Ehle. 1984. *Clin. Chem.* 30:1568–1570.
289. Nozaki, S., M. Kubo, Y. Matsuzawa and S. Tarui. 1984. *Clin. Chem* 30:748–751.
290. Blache, P. J. 1983. *Clin. Chem.* 29:154–158.
291. Taskinen, M. R., E. A. Nikkila, J. K. Huttunen, and Hilden, R. 1980. *Clin. Chim. Acta* 104:107–117.

292. Huttunen, J. K., C. Enholm, P. K. J. Kinnunen and E. A. Nikkila. 1975. *Clin. Chim. Acta* 63:335–347.
293. Cryer, A. and H. M. Jones. 1981. *Int. J. Biochem.* 13:109–111.
294. Fredrickson, D. S., J. L. Goldstein and M. S. Brown. 1978. *In*: The Metabolic Basis of Inherited Disease. 4th ed. J. B. Stanbury, J. B. Wyngaarden and D. S. Fredrickson, editors. McGraw-Hill, New York. 604–655.
295. Breckenridge, W. C., J. A. Little, G. Steiner, A. Chow and M. Poapst. 1978. *New Engl. J. Med.* 298:1265–1273.
296. Yamamura, T., H. Sudo, K. Ishikawa and A. Yamamoto. 1979. *Atherosclerosis* 34:53–66.
297. Catapano, A. L., G. L. Mills, P. Roma, M. LaRosa and A. Capurso. 1983. *Clin. Chim. Acta* 130:317–328.
298. Olivecrona, T., S. S. Chernick, G. Bengtsson-Olivecrona, J. R. Paterniti, W. V. Brown and R. O. Scow. 1985. *J. Biol. Chem.* 260:2552–2557.
299. Behr, S. R., J. R. Patsch, T. Forte and A. Bensadoun. 1981. *J. Lipid Res.* 22:443–451.
300. Suri, B. S., M. E. Targ and D. S. Robinson. 1979. *Biochem. J.* 178:455–466.
301. Pedersen, M. E., M. Cohen and M. C. Schotz. 1983. *J. Lipid Res.* 24:512–521.
302. Soler-Argilaga, C., A. Danon, E. Goh, H. G. Wilcox and M. Heimberg. 1975. *Biochem. Biophys. Res. Commun.* 66:1237–1242.
303. Bjorntorp, P., G. Enzi, R. Ohlson, B. Persson, P. Sponbergs and U. Smith. 1975. *Horm. Metab. Res.* 7:230–237.
304. Ramirez, I. 1981. *Am. J. Physiol.* 240:E533–E538.
305. Nestel, P. J., W. Austin, and C. Foxman. 1969. *J. Lipid Res.* 10:383–387.
306. Hartman, A. D. 1977. *Am. J. Physiol.* 232:E316–E323.
307. Garfinkel, A. S., N. Baker and M. C. Schotz. (1967). *J. Lipid Res.* 8:274–280.
308. Maggio, C. A. and M. R. C. Greenwood. 1982. *Physiol. Behavior* 29:1147–1152.
309. Markscheid, L. and E. Shafrir. 1965. *J. Lipid Res.* 6:247–257.
310. Scow, R. O., S. S. Chernick and T. R. Fleck. 1977. *Biochim. Biophys. Acta* 487:297–306.
311. Scow, R. O., E. J. Blanchette-Mackie and L. C. Smith. 1976. *Circ. Res* 39:149–162.
312. Cryer, A. 1981. *Int. J. Biochem.* 13:525–541.
313. Reardon, M. F., H. Sakai, and G. Steirner. 1982. *Artheriosclerosis* 2(5):396–402.
314. Brunzell, J. D., W. R. Hazzard, D. Porte and E. L. Bierman. 1973. *J. Clin. Invest.* 52:1578–1585.
315. Wolfe, R. R., M. J. Durkot, and M. H. Wolfe. 1981. *Am. J. Physiol.* 241:E385–E395.
316. Wolfe, R. R. and M. J. Durkot. 1985. *J. Lipid Res.* 26:210–217.
317. Cryer, A., S. E. Riley, E. R. Williams and D. S. Robinson. 1976. *Clin. Sci. Mol. Med.* 50:213–221.
318. Linder, C., S. S. Chernick, T. R. Fleck and R. O. Scow. 1976. *Am. J. Physiol.* 231:860–864.
319. McBride, O. W. and E. D. Korn. 1963. *J. Lipid Res.* 4:17–20.
320. Felts, J. M. 1964. *Health Physics* 10:973–979.
321. Gal, S., D. J. P. Bassett, M. Hamosh and P. Hamosh. 1982. *Biochim. Biophys. Acta* 713:222–229.
322. Nathan, C. F., H. W. Murray and Z. A. Cohn. 1980. *New Engl. J. Med.* 303:622–623.
323. Mahley, R. W., K. H. Weisgrabber and T. L. Innerarity. 1979. *Atherosclerosis Rev.* 5:1–34.
324. Zilversmit, D. B. 1973. *Circ. Res.* 33:633–638.
325. Becker, G. H., B. Meyer, and H. Necheles. 1950. *Gastroenterology* 14:80–92.
326. Herzstein, J., C. -I. Wang and D. Adlersburg. 1953. *Arch. Intern. Med.* 92:265–272.
327. Hrachovec, J. and M. Rockstein. 1959. *Gerontologia* 3:305–326.
328. Carlson, L. A., S. O. Froberg, and E. R. Nye. 1968. *Gerontologia* 14:65–79.
329. Reaven, G. M. 1978. *Gerontology* 33:368–371.
330. Brodows, R. G. and R. G. Campbell. 1972. *N. Engl. J. Med.* 287:969–970.
331. Chen, Y. -D. I. and G. M. Reaven. 1981. *J. Gerontol.* 36:3–6.

332. Summerfield, J. A., D. Applebaum-Bowden and W. R. Hazzard. 1984. *Proc. Soc. Ex. Biol. Med.* 175-158-163.
333. Vijayakumar, S. T., S. Leelamma and P. A. Kurup. 1975. *Atherosclerosis* 21:1–14.
334. Rokos, J., P. Hahn, O. Koldovsky and P. Prochazka. 1963. *Physiol. Bohemoslov.* 12:213–219.
335. Fernando-Warnakulazuriya, G. J. P, J. E. Staggers, S. C. Frost and M. A. Wells. 1981. *J. Lipid Res.* 22:668–672.
336. Ferre, P., P. Satabin, L. El. Manoubi, S. Callikan and J. Girard. 1981. *Biochem. J.* 200:429–433.
337. Ravamo, L. 1984. *Pediatr. Res.* 18:642–647.
338. Cryer, A. and H. M. Jones. 1979. *Biochem. J.* 178:711–724.
339. Fernando-Warnakulasuriya, G. J. P., M. L. Eckerson, W. A. Clark and M. A. Wells. 1983. *J. Lipid Res.* 24:1626–1638.
340. Cryer, A. and H. M. Jones. 1978. *Clin. Sci. Mol. Med.* 55:121–123.
341. Planch, E., A. Boulange, P. De Gasquet and N. T. Tonnu. 1980. *Am. J. Physiol.* 238:E511–E517.
342. Chajek, T., O. Stein and Y. Stein. 1977. *Atherosclerosis* 26:549–561.
343. Schriebler, T. H. and H. H. Wolff. 1966. Z. Zellforsch. 69:22–44.
344. Glatz, J. F. C. and J. H. Veerkamp. 1982. *Biochim. Biophys. Acta* 711:327–335.
345. Hollenberg, C. H. 1966. *J. Clin. Invest.* 45:205–216.
346. Roncari, D. A. K. and R. L. R. Van. 1978. *Clin. Invest. Med.* 1:71–79.
347. O'Hea, E. K. and G. A. Leveille. 1969. *J. Nutr.* 99:338–344.
348. Ingle, D. E., D. E. Bauman and U. S. Garrigus. 1972. *J. Nutr.* 102:609–616.
349. Hanson, R. W. and J. F. Ballard. 1967. *Biochem. J.* 105:529–536.
350. Jansen, G. R., M. E. Zanetti and C. F. Hutchison. 1966. *Biochem. J.* 99:333–340.
351. Leveille, G. A. 1976. *Proc. Soc. Exp. Biol. Med.* 125:85–88.
352. Leveille, G. A., E. K. O'Shea and K. Chakrabarty. 1968. *Proc. Soc. Exp. Biol. Med.* 128:398–401.
353. Goodridge, A. G. and E. G. Ball. 1976. *Am. J. Physiol.* 213:245–249.
354. Shrago, E., T. Spennetta and E. Gordon. 1969. *J. Biol. Chem.* 244:2761–2766.
355. Das, J. B., I. Joshi and A. I. Philippart. 1982. *Biochem. J.* 206:663–666.
356. Cryer, A. and H. M. Jones. 1978. *Biochem. J.* 172:319–325.
357. Pequignot-Planche, E., P. De Gasquet, A. Boulange and N. T. Tonnu. 1977. *Biochem. J.* 162:461–463.
358. Blasquez, E., T. Sugase, M. Blasquez and P. P. Foa. 1974. *J. Lab. Clin. Med.* 83:957–967.
359. Blasquez, E., L. A. Lipshaw, M. Blasquez and P. P. Foa. 1975. *Pediatr. Res.* 9:17–25.
360. Cryer, A. and H. M. Jones. 1980. *Biochem. J.* 186:805–815.
361. Ailhaud, G. 1982. *Mol. Cell. Biochem.* 49:17–31.
362. Hietanen, E. and M. R. C. Greenwood. 1977. *J. Lipid Res.* 18:480–490.
363. Hood, R. L. 1982. *Fed. Proc.* 41:2555–2561.
364. Cryer, A., B. R. Gray and J. S. Woodhead. 1984. *J. Develop. Physiol.* 6:159–176.
365. Merkel, R. A., K. S. Sidhu, R. S. Emery, M. E. Spooner, D. R. Romsos and A. F. Parr. 1976. *In*: Biology of fat in meat animals. Madison University, Wisconsin, North Central Reg. Res. Publ., No. 234, 234–269.
366. Steffen, D. G., L. J. Brown and H. H. Mersmann. 1978. *Comp. Biochem. Physiol.* 59:195–198.
367. Cannon, B. and J. Nedergaard. 1982. *In*: Biochemical Development of the fetus and neonate. Elsevier Biomedical Press, Amsterdam. 697–730.
368. Nedergaard, J. and O. Lindberg. 1982. *Int. Rev. Cytol.* 74:187–286.
369. Schenk, H., T. Heim, T. Mende, F. Varga and E. Goetze. 1975. *Eur. J. Biochem.* 58:15–22.
370. Trayhurn, P. 1981. *Biochim. Biophys. Acta* 664:549–560.
371. Pillay, D. and E. Bailey. 1982. *Biochim. Biophys. Acta* 713:663–669.
372. Henning, S. J. 1981. *Am. J. Physiol.* 241:G199–G214.

373. Hamosh, M., M. R. Simon, H. Canter and P. Hamosh. 1978. *Pediatr. Res.*, 12:1131–1136.
374. Hietanen, E. and J. Hartiala. 1979. *Biol. Neonate.* 36:85–91.
375. Matsuo, M., N. Nakamura, S. Yamasaki, S. Mimasu and T. Matsuo. 1980. *Kobe. J. Med. Sci.* 26:229–236.
376. Farrell, P. M. and M. Hamosh. 1978. *Clin. Perinatal.* 5:197–229.
377. Weinhold, P. A., M. M. Quade, T. B. Brozowski and D. A. Feldman. 1980. *Biochim. Biophys. Acta* 617:76–84.
378. Argiles, J. and E. Herrara. 1981. *Biol. Neonate* 39:37–44.
379. Mostello, D. J., M. Hamosh and P. Hamosh. 1981. *Biol. Neonate* 40:121–128.
380. Possmayer, F. 1982. *In*: Biochemical development of the fetus and neonate. Elsevier Biomedical Press, Amsterdam. pp. 337–391.
381. Cuzner, M. L. and A. L. Davidson. 1968. *Biochem. J.* 106:29–34.
382. Sudjic, M. M. and R. Booth. 1976. *Biochem. J.* 154:559–560.
383. Rovamo, L. 1984. *Pediatr. Res.* 18:642–647.
384. Andrew, G., C. Chan and D. Schiff. 1976. *J. Pediatr.* 88:273–278.
385. Dhanireddy, R., M. Hamosh, K. N. Sivasubramanian, P. Chowdhry, J. Scanlon, and P. Hamosh. 1981. *J. Pediatr.* 98:617–622.
386. Shennan, A. T., M. H. Bryan and A. Angel. 1977. *J. Pediatr.* 91:134–137.
387. Hamosh, M. and P. Hamosh. 1983. *Molec. Aspects Med.* 6:199–289.
388. Gustafson, A., I. Kjellner, R. Olegard and L. H. Victorin. 1972. *Acta. Pediatr. Scand.* 61:149–158.
389. Olegard, R., A. Gustafson, I. Kjellner and L. H. Victorin. 1975. *Acta Pediatr. Scand.* 64:745–751.
390. De Gasquet, P., S. Griglio, E. Pequignot-Planche and Malewiak, M. I. 1977. *J. Nutr.* 107:199–212.
391. De Gasquet, P. and E. Pequignot. 1973. *Horm. Metabl. Res.* 5:440–m443.
392. Goubern, M. and R. Portet. 1980. *Horm. Metab. Res.* 12:73–77.
393. Paik, S. H. and E. S. Yearick. 1978. *J. Nutr.* 108:1798–1805.
394. Lawson, N., A. D. Polland, R. J. Jennings, M. I. Gurr and D. N. Brindley. 1981. *Biochem. J.* 200:285–294.
395. Nilsson-Ehle, P., S. Carlstrom and P. Belfrage. 1975. *Scand. J. Clin. Lab. Invest.* 35:373–378.
396. Persson, B. 1974. *Clin. Sci. Mol. Med.* 47:631–634.
397. Pav, J. and J. Wenkeova. 1960. *Nature Lond.* 185:926–928.
398. Chan, C. P. and J. S. Stern. 1982. *Am. J. Physiol.* 242:E445–E450.
399. Linder, C., S. S. Chernick, T. R. Fleck and R. O. Scow. 1976. *Am. J. Physiol.* 231:860–864.
400. Atkin, J. and A. A. Meng. 1972. *Diabetes* 21:149–156.
401. O'Looney, P., M. Vander Maten and G. V. Vahouny. 1983. *J. Biol. Chem.* 258:12994–13001.
402. Bagdade, J., D. Porte and E. L. Bierman. 1968. *Diabetes* 17:127–132.
403. Bar-on, H., E. Levy, Y. Oschry, E. Ziv and E. Shafrir. 1984. *Biochim. Biophys. Acta* 793:115–118.
404. Sadur, C. N. and R. H. Eckel. 1982. *J. Clin. Invest.* 69:1119–1124.
405. De Gasquet, P., E. Pequignot-Planche, N. T. Tonnu and F. A. Diaby. 1975. *Horm. Metab. Res.* 7:152–157.
406. Hulsmann, W. C. and M. -L Dubelaar. 1986. *Biochim. Biophys. Acta* 875:69–75.
407. Krausz, Y., H. Bar-on and E. Shafrir. 1981. *Biochim. Biophys. Acta* 663:69–82.
408. Bagdade, J. E., E. Yee, J. Albers and O. J. Pykalisto. 1976. *Metabolism* 25:533–542.
409. Pedersen, M. E., L. E. Wolf and M. C. Schotz. 1981. *Biochim. Biophys. Acta* 666:191–197.
410. Stern, M. P., O. G. Kolterman, J. F. Fries, H. O. McDevitt and G. M. Reavan. 1973. *Arch. Intern. Med.* 132:97–101.

411. Hamosh, M. and P. Hamosh. 1975. *J. Clin. Invest.* 55:1132–1135.
412. Kim, H. J. and R. K. Kalkhoff. 1975. *J. Clin. Invest.* 56:888–896.
413. Wilson, D. E., C. M. Flowers, S. I. Carlile and K. S. Udall. 1976. *Atherosclerosis* 24:491–499.
414. Gray, J. M. and M. R. C. Greenwood. 1984. *Proc. Soc. Exp. Biol. Med.* 175:374–379.
415. Ramirez, I. 1981. *Am. J. Physiol.* 240:E533–E538.
416. Wynn, V., J. W. H. Doar, G. L. Mills and T. Stokes. 1969. *Lancet* 2:756–760.
417. Zorilla, E., M. Hulse, A. Hernandex and H. Gershberg. 1968. *J. Clin. Endocrinol. Metab.* 28:1793–1796.
418. Shepherd, A. and M. P. Cleary. 1984. *Am. J. Physiol.* 246:E123–E128.
419. Steingrimsdottir, L., J. Brasel and M. R. C. Greenwood. 1980. *Am. J. Physiol.* 239:E162–E167.
420. Alousi, A. A. and S. Mallov. 1964. *Am. J. Physiol.* 206:603–609.
421. Hansson, P., G. Nordin and P. Nilsson-Ehle. 1983. *Biochim. Biophys. Acta* 753:364–371.
422. Skottova, N. L., Wallinder and G. Bengtsson. 1983. *Biochim. Biophys. Acta* 750:533–538.
423. Lithell, H., J. Boberg, K. Hellsing, S. Ljunghal, G. Lundqvist. 1981. *Eur. J. Clin. Invest.* 11:3–10.
424. Vandermarsson, S., P. Hedner and P. Nilsson-Ehle. 1982. *Eur. J. Clin. Invest.* 12:423–428.
425. Hansson, P., T. Holmin and P. Nilsson-Ehle. 1981. *Biochem. Biophys. Res. Commun.* 103:1254–1257.
426. La Fonatan, M. and M. Berlan. 1985. *In*: New Perspectives in Adipose Tissue: Structure Function and Development. A. Cryer & R. L. R. Van, eds., Butterworths, London. 145–182.
427. Garcia-Sainz, J. A. and J. N. Fain. 1982. *Trends Pharmacol. Sci.* 3:201–203.
428. Nikkila, E. A., P. Torsti and O. Penttila. 1965. *Life Sci.* 4:27–35.
429. Jansen, H., Hulsmann, W. C., A. Van Zuylen-Van Wiggen, C. B. Struijk and V. M. T. Houtsmuller. 1975. *Biochem. Biophys. Res. Commun.* 64:747–751.
430. Hulsmann, W. C., M. M. Geelhoed-Mieras, H. Jansen and U. M. T. Houtsmuller. 1979. *Biochim. Biophys. Acta* 572:183–187.
431. Stam, H., K. Schoondewoerd, W. A. P. Breeman and W. C. Hulsmann. 1984. *Horm. Metab. Res.* 16:293–297.
432. Stam, H. and W. C. Hulsmann. 1984. *Biochim. Biophys. Acta* 794:72–82.
433. Borensztajn, J., P. Keig and A. H. Rubenstein. 1973. *Biochem. Biophys. Res. Commun.* 53:603–608.
434. Kotlar, T. J. and J. Borensztajn. 1977. *Am. J. Physiol.* 233:E316–E319.
435. Simpson, J. 1979. *Biochem. J.* 182:253–255.
436. Jansen, H., H. Stam, C. Kalkman and W. C. Hulsmann. 1980. *Biochem. Biophys. Res. Commun.* 92:411–416.
437. Asayama, A., S. Amemiya, S. Kusano and K. Kato. 1984. *Metab. Clin. Exp.* 33:129–131.
438. Zinder, O., M. Hamosh, T. R. C. Fleck and R. O. Scow. 1974. *Am. J. Physiol.* 226:744–748.
439. Steingrimsdottir, L., J. A. Brasel and M. R. C. Greenwood. 1980. *Metabolism* 29:837–844.
440. Bagby, G. J. and Spitzer, J. A. 1981. *Proc. Soc. Exp. Biol. Med.* 168:395–398.
441. Knobler, H., T. Chajek-Shaul, O. Stein, J. Etienne and Y. Stein. 1984. *Biochim. Biophys. Acta* 795:363–371.
442. Odonkor, J. M. and M. P. Rogers. 1984. *Biochem. Pharmacol.* 33:1337–1341.
443. Dousset, N., R. Feliste, M. Carton and L. Douste-Blazy. 1984. *Biochim. Biophys. Acta* 794:444–453.
444. Phares, C. K. and R. M. Carroll. 1984. *J. Helmithol.* 58:25–30.
445. Hozex, P. J., N. Le Trang, A. H. Fairlamb and A. Cerami. 1984. *Parasite Immunol.* (Oxf) 6:203–210.

446. Beutler, B., J. Mahoney, N. Le Trang, P. Pekala and A. Cerami. 1985. *J. Exp. Med.* 161:984–995.
447. Bragdon, J. H. and R. S. Gordon. 1958. *J. Clin. Invest.* 37:574–578.
448. Jones, N. and R. J. Havel. 1967. *Am. J. Physiol.* 213:824–828.
449. Borensztajn, J., M. S. Rone, S. P. Babirak, J. A. McGarr and L. B. Oscai. 1975. *Am. J. Physiol.* 229:394–397.
450. Lithell, H., J. Boberg, K. Hellsing, G. Lundqvist and B. Vessby. 1978. *Arteriosclerosis* 30:89–94.
451. Pedersen, M. E. and M. C. Schotz. 1980. *J. Nutr.* 110:481–487.
452. Fried, S. K., J. O. Hill, M. Nickel and M. Di Girolamo. 1983. *J. Nutr.* 113:1861–1869.
453. Tepperman, H. M. and J. Tepperman. 1958. *Diabetes* 7:478–485.
454. Harris, K. L. and J. M. Felts. 1973. *Biochim. Biophys. Acta* 316:288–295.
455. Nestel, P. J. and P. J. Barter. 1973. *Am. J. Clin. Nutr.* 26:241–245.
456. Weisenburg-Delorme, C. L. and K. L. Harris. 1975. *J. Nutr.* 105:447–451.
457. Jacobs, I., H. Lithell and J. Karlsson. 1982. *Acta Physiol. Scand.* 115:85–90.
458. Lithell, H., R. Schele, B. Vessby and I. Jacobs. 1984. *J. Appl. Physiol.* 57:698–702.
459. Taskinen, M. R., E. A. Nikkila, S. Rehunen and A. Gordin. 1980. *Artery* 6:471–483.
460. Cybulska, B., W. B. Szostok, M. Bialkowska and K. Swiatkowska. 1973. *Mater. Med. Pol.* 5:247–249.
461. Sasinowski, F. and R. Oswald. 1981. *Lipids* 16:380–383.
462. Jansen, H., W. C. Hulsmann, A. van Zuylen-van Wiggen, C. B. Struijk and U. M. T. Houtsmuller. 1975. *Biochem. Biophys. Res. Commun.* 64:747–753.
463. Hulsmann, W. C., M. M. Geelhoed-Mieras, H. Jansen and U. M. T. Houtsmuller. 1979. *Biochim. Biophys. Acta* 572:183–189.
464. Eckel, R. H., W. Y. Fujimoto and J. D. Brunzell. 1979. *Diabetes* 28:1141–1142.
465. Bourdeaux, A. -M., Y. Giudicelli, Rebourcet, M. -C., Nordmann, J. and Nordmann, R. 1980. *Biochem. Biophys. Res. Commun.* 95:212–219.
466. Howard, B. V. 1977. *J. Lipid Res.* 18:561–571.
467. Vanhove, A., C. Wolf, M. Breton and M. -C. Glangeaud. 1978. *Biochem. J.* 172:239–245.
468. Al-Jafari, A. A., S. R. Lee, R. K. Tume and A. Cryer. 1986. *Cell. Biochem. Funct.* 4:169–179.
469. Vannier, C., J. Etienne and G. Ailhaud. 1986. *Biochim. Biophys. Acta* 875:344–354.
470. Hirsch, A. H. and O. M. Rosen. 1984. *J. Lipid Res.* 25:665–677.
472. Gartner, S. L. and G. V. Vahouny. 1966. *Am. J. Physiol.* 211:1063–1068.
472. Stam, H. and H. C. Hulsmann. 1984. *Biochim. Biophys. Acta* 794:72–82.
473. Ben-Zeev, O., H. Schwalb and M. C. Schotz. 1981. *J. Biol. Chem.* 256:10550–10554.
474. Jansen, H., H. Stam, C. Kalkman and W. C. Hulsmann. 1980. *Biochem. Biophys. Res Commun.* 92:411–416.
475. Cryer, A., F. S. Wusteman and J. J. Casey. 1984. *Cell. Biochem. Funct.* 2:53–56.
476. Calatroni, A., P. V. Donnelly and N. Di Farrante. 1969. *J. Clin. Invest.* 48:332–343.
477. Engeberg, H. 1977. *Fed. Proc.* 36:70–72.
478. Horner, A. A. 1976. *FEBS Lett.* 46:166–170.
479. Noel, S. -P. 1984. *Can. J. Biochem. Cell. Biol.* 62:89–93.
480. Bagby, G. J. 1983. *Biochim. Biophys. Acta* 753:47–52.
481. Wallinder, L., G. Bengtsson and T. Olivecrona. 1979. *Biochim. Biophys. Acta* 575:166–173.
482. Wallinder, L., J. Peterson, T. Olivecrona and G. Bengtsson-Olivecrona. 1984. *Biochim. Biophys. Acta* 795:513–524.
483. Peterson, J., T. Olivecrona and G. Bengtsson-Olivecrona. 1985. *Biochim. Biophys. Acta* 837:262–270.
484. Chajek-Shaul, T., G. Friedman, O'Stein, J. Etienne and Y. Stein. 1985. *Biochim. Biophys. Acta* 837:271–278.
485. Cryer, A. 1983. *In*: Biochemical Interactions at the Endothelium. (A. Cryer, ed.) Elsevier Science Publishers, Amsterdam. pp. 1–4.

486. Awbrey, B. J., J. C. Hoak and W. G. Owen. 1979. *J. Biol. Chem.* 254:4092–4100.
487. Shimada, K. and T. Ozawa. 1985. *J. Clin. Invest.* 75:1308–1316.
488. Bauer, P. I., R. Machovich, K. G. Buki, E. Csonka, S. A. Koch and I. Horvath. 1984. *Biochem. J.* 218:119–124.
489. Fielding, C. J., I. Vlodavsky, P. E. Fielding and D. Gospodarowicz. 1979. *J. Biol. Chem.* 254:8861–8868.
490. Fielding, C. J. and P. E. Fielding. 1983. *In*: Biochemical Interactions at the Endothelium (A. Cryer, ed.) Elsevier Science Publishers, Amsterdam. pp. 275–299.
491. Desai, K. S., A. I. Gotlieb and G. Steiner. 1986. *Can. J. Physiol. Pharmacol.* 63:809–815.
492. Barzu, T., P. Molho, G. Tobelem, M. Petitou and J. Caen. 1985. *Biochim. Biophys. Acta* 845:196–203.
493. Stout, R. W. 1983. *In*: Biochemical Interactions at the Endothelium. (A. Cryer, ed.) Elsevier Science Publishers, Amsterdam. pp. 301–312.
494. Wusteman, F. S. 1983. *In*: Biochemical Interactions at the Endothelium (A. Cryer, ed.) Elsevier Science Publishers, Amsterdam. pp. 79–109.
495. Olivecrona, T. and G. Bengtsson. 1983. *In*: The Adipocyte and Obesity: Cellular and Molecular Mechanisms. (A. Angel, C. H. Hollenberg and D. A. K. Roncari, eds.) Raven Press, New York. pp. 117–126.
496. Shimada, K., P. J. Gill, J. E. Sibert, W. H. Douglas and B. L. Fanburg. 1981. *J. Clin. Invest.* 68:995–1002.
497. Cheng, C. -F., G. M. Costa, A. Bensadoun and R. D. Rosenberg. 1981. *J. Biol. Chem.* 256:12893–12898.
498. Williams, M. P., H. B. Streeter, F. S. Wusteman and A. Cryer. 1983. *Biochim. Biophys. Acta* 756:83–91.
499. Olivecrona, T., G. Bengtsson-Olivecrona, J. C. Osborne and E. S. Kempner. 1985. *J. Biol. Chem.* 260:6888–6891.
500. Clarke, A. R., M. Luscombe and J. J. Holbrook. 1983. *Biochim. Biophys. Acta* 747:130–137.
501. Kjellen, L., I. Pettersson, and M. Hook. 1981. *Proc. Natl. Acad. Sci. U.S.A.* 78:10407–10413.
502. Matoh, S., I. Funakoshi, N. Ui and I. Yamashina. 1980. *Arch. Biochem. Biophys.* 202:137–143.
503. Wolinsky, H. 1980. *Circ. Res.* 47:301–311.
504. Bengtsson, G. and T. Olivecrona. 1981. *FEBS Lett.* 128:9–12.
505. Fielding, C. J. and Higgins, J. M. 1974. *Biochemistry* 13:4324–4329.
506. Kotlar, T. J. and J. Borensztajn. 1979. *Biochem. J.* 183:171–174.
507. Matsuoka, N., K. Shirai and R. L. Jackson. 1980. *Biochim. Biophys. Acta* 620:308–316.
508. Shimada, K., J. J. Lanzillo, W. H. J. Douglas and B. L. Fanburg. 1982. *Biochim. Biophys. Acta* 710:117–121.
509. Kazunari, W., H. Miki, H. Etoh, F. Okunda., T. Kumada and R. Kusukawa. 1983. *Japn. Circ. J.* 47:837–842.
510. Chajek-Shaul, T., G. Friedman, O. Stein, T. Olivecrona and Y. Stein. 1982. *Biochim. Biophys. Acta* 712:200–210.
511. Friedman, G., T. Chajek-Shaul, T. Olivecrona, O. Stein and Y. Stein. *Biochim. Biophys. Acta* 711:114–122.
512. Gibbs, M. E. and G. E. Lienhard. 1984. *J. Cell Physiol.* 121:569–575.
513. Williams, S. K., D. A. Greener and N. J. Solenski. 1984. *J. Cell Physiol.* 120:157–162.
514. Wing, D. R., C. J. Fielding, and D. S. Robinson. 1967. *Biochem. J.* 104:45C–46C.
515. Schotz, M. C. and A. S. Garfinkel. 1965. *Biochim. Biophys. Acta* 106:202–205.
516. Borensztajn, J., M. S. Rone and T. Sandros. 1975. *Biochim. Biophys. Acta* 398:394–400.
517. Vydelingum, N., R. L. Drake, J. Etienne and A. Kissebah. 1983. *Am. J. Physiol.* 245:E121–E131.
518. Jansen, H., A. S. Garfinkel, J. S. Twu, J. Nikazy and M. C. Schotz. 1978. *Biochim. Biophys. Acta* 531:109–114.

519. Chajek, T., O. Stein and Y. Stein. 1975. *Biochim. Biophys. Acta* 380:127–131.
520. Garfinkel, A. S., P. Nilsson-Ehle and M. C. Schotz. 1976. *Biochim. Biophys. Acta* 424:264–273.
521. Hollenberg, C. H. 1959. *Am. J. Physiol.* 197:667–670.
522. Salaman, M. R. and D. S. Robinson. 1966. *Biochem. J.* 99:640–647.
523. Wing, D. R., C. J. Fielding and D. S. Robinson. 1966. *Biochem. J.* 99:648–656.
524. Robinson, D. S. and D. R. Wing. 1970. *In*: Adipose tissue regulation and metabolic functions. B. Jeanrenaud and D. Hepp, eds. George Thieme Verlag, Stuttgart, pp. 41–51.
525. Nestel, P. J. and W. Austin. 1969. *Life Sci.* (II) 8:157–164.
526. Ashby, P., D. P. Bennett, I. M. Spencer and D. S. Robinson. 1978. *Biochem. J.* 176:865–872.
527. Ashby, P. and D. S. Robinson. 1980. *Biochem. J.* 188:185–192.
528. Cryer, A., B. Foster, D. R. Wing and D. S. Robinson. 1973. *Biochem. J.* 132:833–836.
529. Parkin, S. M., K. Walker, P. Ashby and D. S. Robinson. 1980. *Biochem. J.* 188:193–199.
530. Robinson, D. S., S. M. Parkin, B. K. Speake and J. A. Little. 1983. *In*: The Adipocyte and Obesity: Cellular and Molecular Mechanisms. (A. Angel, C. H. Hollenberg, and D. A. K. Roncari, eds.) Raven Press, New York. pp. 127–136.
531. Mooney, R. A. and M. D. Lane. 1981. *J. Biol. Chem.* 256:11724–11733.
532. Speake, B. K., S. M. Parkin and D. S. Robinson. 1985. *Biochim. Biophys. Acta* 840:419–422.
533. Bienkowski, R. S. 1983. *Biochem. J.* 214:1–10.
534. Pretlow, T., E. E. Weir and J. Zettergren. 1975. *Int. Rev. Exp. Pathol.* 14:91–204.
535. Hefley, T., J. Cushing and J. S. Brand. 1981. *Am. J. Physiol.* 240:C234–C238.
536. Bourdeaux, A. -M., M. -C. Rebourcet, J. Nordmann, R. Nordmann and Y. Giudicelli. 1982. *Biochem. Biophys. Res. Commun.* 107:59–67.
537. Bourdeaux, A. -M., R. Nordmann and Y. Giudicelli. 1984. *FEBS Letts.* 178:132–136.
538. Cryer, A., A. McDonald, E. R. Williams and D. S. Robinson. 1975. *Biochem. J.* 152:717–720.
539. Al-Jafari, A. A. and A. Cryer. 1986. *Biochem. J.* 238:239–246.
540. Cushman, S. W. and L. J. Wardzala. 1980. *J. Biol. Chem.* 255:4758–4762.
541. Czech, M. P. 1984. *Recent Prog. Horm. Res.* 40:347–373.
542. Kono, T. 1983. *Recent. Prog. Horm. Res.* 39:519–557.
543. Toyoda, N., F. W. Robinson, M. M. Smith, J. E. Flanagan and T. Kono. 1986. *J. Biol. Chem.* 261:2117–2122.
544. Eckel, R. H., W. Y. Fujimoto and J. D. Brunzell. 1978. *Biochem. Biophys. Res. Commun.* 84:1069–1075.
545. Vannier, C. and G. Ailhaud. 1986. *Biochim. Biophys. Acta* 875:324–333.
546. Ammi, E. -Z., C. Vannier, J. Etienne and G. Ailhaud. 1986. *Biochim. Biophys. Acta* 875:334–343.
547. Walter, P., R. Gilmore and G. Blobel. 1984. *Cell* 38:5–8.
548. Blanchette-Mackie, E. J. and R. O. Scow. 1981. *J. Ultrastruct. Res.* 77:277–294.
549. Blanchette-Mackie, E. J. and R. O. Scow. 1981. *J. Ultrastruct. Res.* 77:295–318.
550. Anderson, M. J. and D. M. Farnbrough. 1982. *J. Cell Biol.* 96:120a.
551. Bayne, E. K., M. J. Anderson and D. M. Fambrough. 1982. *J. Cell Biol.* 95:117a.
552. McCloskey, M. and M. -M. Poo. 1984. *Int. Rev. Cytol.* 87:19–81.
553. Ben-Zeev, O., A. J. Lusis, R. C. le Boeuf, J. Nikazy and M. C. Schotz. 1983. *J. Biol. Chem.* 258:13632–13636.
554. Oscai, L. B., A. Coruso and W. K. Palmer. 1986. *Biochem. Biophys. Res. Commun.* 135:196–199.
555. Steinberg, D. and J. C. Khoo. 1977. *Fed. Proc.* 36:1986–1990.
556. Friedman, G., T. Chajek-Shaul, J. Etienne, O. Stein and Y. Stein. 1986. *Biochim. Biophys. Acta* 875:397–399.
557. Long, W. M., B. H. L. Chua, B. L. Munger and H. E. Morgan. 1984. *Fed. Proc.* 43:1295–1300.

558. Wetzel, M. G. and R. O. Scow. 1984. *Am. J. Physiol.* 246:C467–C485.
559. Ramirez, I., A. J. Kryski, O. Ben-Zeev, M. C. Schotz and D. L. Severson. 1985. *Biochem. J.* 232:229–236.
560. Steinberg, D. 1983. *Arteriosclerosis* 3:283–301.

INDEX